Gynecological Cancer Management

Identification, diagnosis and treatment

This book is dedicated to:

Our wives, Kathleen Clarke-Pearson and Maureen Soper and our children Don, Emily, Mary and Mike Clarke-Pearson; and Emily, Will and Alex Soper for their constant support and love as we have pursued our careers.

Our mentors, Roy T. Parker, MD, William T. Creasman, MD, Charles B. Hammond, MD, Allen Addison, MD, William N. Spellacy, MD, James R. Scott, MD, and Gary H. Johnson, MD, for the standards of excellence they set for us, for the wealth of knowledge that they shared, and for their continued friendship and guidance.

Gynecological Cancer Management

Identification, diagnosis and treatment

EDITED BY

Daniel L. Clarke-Pearson, MD, FACOG, FACS

Robert A. Ross Distinguished Professor and Chair
Department of Obstetrics and Gynecology
University of North Carolina
Chapel Hill
NC, USA

John T. Soper, MD, FACOG

Charles Hendricks Distinguished Professor
Division of Gynecologic Oncology
Department of Obstetrics and Gynecology
University of North Carolina
Chapel Hill
NC, USA

(W)WILEY-BLACKWELL

A John Wiley & Sons, Ltd., Publication

Library of Congress Cataloging-in-Publication Data

﹍﹍ant gynecological cancer : evaluation and management / [edited by] Daniel Clarke-Pearson, John

 ; cm.
Includes bibliographical references and index.
ISBN 978-1-4051-9079-4 (hardcover : alk. paper)
1. Generative organs, Female–Cancer. 2. Gynecologic pathology. 3. Precancerous conditions.
I. Clarke-Pearson, Daniel L. II. Soper, John (John T.)
[DNLM: 1. Genital Neoplasms, Female–diagnosis. 2. Genital Neoplasms, Female–therapy. 3. Genitalia, Female–pathology. 4. Precancerous Conditions. WP 145 P925 2009]
RC280.G5P738 2009
616.99'465–dc22   2009031375

A catalogue record for this book is available from the British Library.

Set in 9/12pt Meridien by Aptara® Inc., New Delhi, India
Printed and bound in Singapore by Fabulous Printers Pte Ltd

1   2010

Contents

Colour plates can be found facing page 116

List of Contributors

Daniel L. Clarke-Pearson, MD, FACOG, FACS
Robert A. Ross Distinguished Professor and Chair
Department of Obstetrics and Gynecology
University of North Carolina School of Medicine
Chapel Hill, NC, USA

John T. Soper, MD, FACOG
Charles Hendricks Distinguished Professor
Division of Gynecologic Oncology
Department of Obstetrics and Gynecology
University of North Carolina School of Medicine
Chapel Hill, NC, USA

Lisa N. Abaid, MD, MPH
Gynecologic Oncology Associates
Newport Beach, CA, USA

Victoria Lin Bae-Jump, MD, PhD
Assistant Professor
Division of Gynecologic Oncology
Department of Obstetrics and Gynecology
University of North Carolina School of Medicine
Chapel Hill, NC, USA

Ursula Balthazar, MD
Fellow
Clinical Instructor
Division of Reproductive Endocrinology and Infertility
Department of Obstetrics and Gynecology
University of North Carolina School of Medicine
Chapel Hill, NC, USA

John F. Boggess, MD
Associate Professor
Division of Gynecologic Oncology
Department of Obstetrics and Gynecology
University of North Carolina School of Medicine
Chapel Hill, NC, USA

Leigh A. Cantrell, MD, MSPH
Fellow
Clinical Instructor
Division of Gynecologic Oncology
Department of Obstetrics and Gynecology

University of North Carolina School of Medicine
Chapel Hill, NC, USA

Wesley C. Fowler, Jr. MD, FACOG, FACS
Palumbo Distinguished Professor of Gynecologic Oncology
Director, Division of Gynecologic Oncology
Department of Obstetrics and Gynecology
University of North Carolina School of Medicine
Chapel Hill, NC, USA

Paola A. Gehrig, MD, FACOG
Associate Professor
Division of Gynecologic Oncology
Department of Obstetrics and Gynecology
University of North Carolina School of Medicine
Chapel Hill, NC, USA

Rabbie K. Hanna, MD
Fellow
Clinical Instructor
Division of Gynecologic Oncology
Department of Obstetrics and Gynecology
University of North Carolina at Chapel Hill, NC, USA

Chad Livasy, MD
Associate Professor
Department of Pathology and Laboratory Medicine
University of North Carolina School of Medicine
Chapel Hill, NC, USA

Alberto A. Mendivil, MD
Fellow
Clinical Instructor
Division of Gynecologic Oncology
Department of Obstetrics and Gynecology
University of North Carolina School of Medicine
Chapel Hill, NC, USA

Jennifer L. Ragazzo, MD
Assistant Professor
Division of Women's Primary Healthcare
Department of Obstetrics and Gynecology
University of North Carolina School of Medicine
Chapel Hill, NC, USA

Emma Rossi, MD
Fellow
Clinical Instructor
Division of Gynecologic Oncology
Department of Obstetrics and Gynecology
University of North Carolina School of Medicine
Chapel Hill, NC, USA

Aaron Shafer, MD
Fellow
Clinical Instructor
Division of Gynecologic Oncology
Department of Obstetrics and Gynecology
University of North Carolina School of Medicine
Chapel Hill, NC, USA

Linda Van Le, MD, FACOG, FACS
Professor
Division of Gynecologic Oncology
Department of Obstetrics and Gynecology
University of North Carolina School of Medicine
Chapel Hill, NC, USA

Denniz Zolnoun, MD, FACOG
Associate Professor
Division of Advanced Laparoscopy and Pelvic Pain
Department of Obstetrics and Gynecology
University of North Carolina School of Medicine
Chapel Hill, NC, USA

Preface

Over the past three decades, the specialty of obstetrics and gynecology has matured into a broad and diverse group of skills and disciplines. Advances in the basic science of reproduction, human physiology, genetics, oncology, surgical technology, and pharmacology have broadened our understanding of the field and at the same time provided the opportunity to provide improved health to women under our care.

The breadth of the specialty has resulted in specific areas of subspecialization recognized by the American Board of Obstetrics and Gynecology (ABOG): maternal-fetal medicine, reproductive endocrinology and infertility, female reconstructive surgery and pelvic floor medicine, and gynecologic oncology. All of these subspecialties require a minimum of 3 additional years of training beyond the traditional 4 years of training in obstetrics and gynecology. And there are specific written and oral examinations in these subspecialties that are required before ABOG will issue a "Certificate of Special Competence."

Given the subspecialists' additional skill and knowledge in their area of subspecialty training, the general obstetrician and gynecologist must decide when it is appropriate for a patient to remain under his or her care, and when it is most appropriate to refer to a subspecialist for consultation or continuing care.

In the area of gynecologic oncology, it has become apparent that there are diagnoses and conditions where the obstetrician and gynecologist has a level of uncertainty (or lack of confidence in his or her ability or knowledge base to adequately manage the patient) and therefore refers the patient to a gynecologic oncologist. For example, should every adnexal mass discovered by physical examination or ultrasound be referred to a gynecologic on-cologist because it "might" be an ovarian cancer? Clearly this triage strategy is inappropriate. We feel that the general gynecologist should manage the "benign" ovarian tumors, while referral of "probable" ovarian cancer to a gynecologist is appropriate for best patient care. So, what are the criteria that a gynecologist can use to differentiate masses that are "possibly" ovarian cancer from those that are "probably" ovarian cancer?

As educators of residents in obstetrics and gynecology, we have come to believe that many of the women we see in referral should be cared for by obstetricians and gynecologists. While we agree that referral of women with known or suspected gynecologic cancers is appropriate, we also feel that there are a number of conditions that do not require referral or consultation.

It is not our intent to explore the reasons for these referrals. The goal of this book is to review the current management of a number of gynecologic conditions that we gynecologic oncologists often see in consultation yet believe should be managed by the general gynecologist.

This text is not intended to be an extensive resource or reference encyclopedia of selected gynecologic conditions. There are several comprehensive texts of gynecology that serve as excellent reference sources. Rather, we have chosen to present each topic with a concise overview or background followed by case-based scenarios that discuss the specific management of these common problems. We hope this will be a practical guide to the management of many gynecologic conditions that the general gynecologist can and should manage.

In many instances, the pathologist serves as an important consultant. While at UNC we enjoy the consultation of pathologists who specialize in gynecologic pathology, we recognize that general gynecologists in the community must rely on their pathologists who practice the breadth of surgical pathology. The communication between the pathologist and the gynecologist is critical in decision-making. We have therefore added sections entitled "Pathology Notes," which are intended to share with the reader issues that we feel are important to establish the correct diagnosis (and therefore result in the proper treatment). Again, we do not intend this to serve as a comprehensive pathology text, but rather to highlight the important issues in the pathologic evaluation of these specific conditions. Hopefully, they will result in better understanding between the gynecologist and the pathologist.

In the end, we hope this text will provide the general gynecologist with the current clinical information necessary to manage most conditions that are not true gynecologic malignancies and at the same time identify the situations where consultation or referral to a gynecologic oncologist would be in the patient's best interest.

Daniel Clarke-Pearson
John Soper
October 2009

Acknowledgements

We wish to acknowledge our Wiley-Blackwell publisher, Martin Sugden, PhD, who helped us develop the vision of the unique content and focus for this book and for his support in launching this endeavour. We appreciate the diligent work of the Wiley-Blackwell editorial staff, especially Cathryn Gates, Rebecca Huxley and Baljinder Kaur who provided the editorial expertise to bring this book to fruition.

To our co-authors who worked diligently to complete their manuscripts on the prescribed time-line, we extend our thanks! And a special thanks to Chad Livasy, MD, Alice Chuang, MD, and Glen Yamagada, MD for providing the excellent images which further enhance the clinical scenarios.

CHAPTER 1

Vulvar Dystrophies

Denniz Zolnoun, MD
Department of Obstetrics and Gynecology,
University of North Carolina School of Medicine, Chapel Hill, NC, USA

Pathology Notes: Chad Livasy, MD
Associate Professor, Department of Pathology and Laboratory Medicine, University of North Carolina School of Medicine, Chapel Hill, NC, USA

Background

Vulvo-vaginal symptoms are among the most common reasons that women seek health care; upward of 6 million physician office visits are made by women of all age ranges for vulvo-vaginal symptoms.[1] Despite such staggering statistics, most clinicians are not adequately prepared to diagnose and treat chronic vulvo-vaginal symptoms. Overlapping clinical appearance, symptoms, and pathophysiology, compounded by nonspecific histology on biopsy, are the main causes for confusion.

This chapter will focus on the following six nonmalignant vulvo-vaginal conditions that clinically may raise concern about premalignant processes:
- Lichen sclerosis
- Contact dermatitis
- Lichen simplex chronicus
- Lichen planus
- Plasma cell vulvitis
- Desquamative inflammatory vaginitis

These conditions share overlapping symptoms of itching and burning to variable degrees. Collectively, these conditions are challenging to care for due to lack of consensus on diagnosis and treatment, intractable and fluctuating clinical course, overlapping morphology and histology, and significant individual variation in treatment response. Additionally, many of these conditions often coexist, posing yet another layer of complexity in deciphering the cause of a patient's chief complaint. Given the intertwined pathophysiology, it is no wonder that the care of these patients seems more a proverbial shot in the dark than a stepwise methodical process.

The diagnostic definition of these six conditions is based on a constellation of symptoms, morphology, and histopathology. As noted in Table 1.1, the primary complaint of the first three conditions is itching, while the primary complaints of the last three are burning, rawness, and pain with intercourse. Thus, using a symptom-based approach, the discussion of these disorders is divided into two parts: conditions with primary complaints of itching (lichen sclerosis, contact dermatitis, and lichen simplex chronicus), and those with primary complaints of burning/rawness sensation (lichen planus, plasma cell vulvitis, and desquamative inflammatory vaginitis). Vulvar intraepithelial dysplasia (VIN), which is often associated with unilateral and focal itching, will be discussed in Chapter 2.

Gynecological Cancer Management: Identification, Diagnosis and Treatment, Edited by Daniel L. Clarke-Pearson and John T. Soper. Published 2010 by Blackwell Publishing, ISBN: 978-1-4051-9079-4.

Table 1.1 Overview of vulvar dermatoses

	Symptoms	Morphology & exam	Histopathology	Comment
Presenting Chief Complaint: Itching and Secondary Burning				
Lichen sclerosis (LS)	Itching; secondary symptoms of dysparunia, dysuria, and burning develop from trauma and agglutination.	Thin, atrophic, wrinkled skin. Agglutination with loss of architectures. In addition may have superimposed features described under contact dermatitis and LSC.	Epidermal atrophy with loss of rete ridges. Upper dermis shows band-like infiltrate and homogenization of collagen. Squamous hyperplasia often present from chronic itching.	Biopsy helpful; histology similar to lichen planus. Clinical and histologic superimposed contact dermatitis and LSC may be present
Contact dermatitis	Itching, burning and "dryness" sensation. Can be acute (allergic) vs. chronic (irritant). Washing with cold water suits symptoms.	Red, classic "diaper rash," with variable excoriation in acute presentation. With chronicity appearance similar to LSC.	Dermal chronic infiltrate, spongiosis, acanthosis, parakeratosis. Similar to atopic/allergic dermatitis.	Biopsy nonspecific, common with acute itching and/or allergy to topical agents. Etiology deciphered from history.
Lichen simplex chronicus (LSC)	Prolonged bouts of itching and scratching. Itching intensifies a night with scratching during sleep. Warm water/sitz bath provokes itch–scratch cycle.	Thick, pale orange-peel appearing labia majora and minora. Progressively ashy scaly vulva with exposure to air during exam. Otherwise similar to contact dermatitis with change in pigment	Lichenification: thickening in epidermus (acanthosis) AND stratum corneum (hyperkeratosis); additional findings similar to contact dermatitis.	Biopsy nonspecific, common with chronic itching regardless of etiology. Etiology deciphered from history in the absence of premalignant (VIN) or nonmalignant (LS) conditions.
Presenting Chief Complaint: Burning & Rawness				
Lichen planus (LP)	Burning pain, rawness, postcoital bleeding.	Red, well-demarcated lesions in vulva, vagina, and gingiva. On keratinized skin, flat-toped papules with lacy white dome; lesion-specific punctuate allodynia.	Lichenoid pattern: band-like lymphocytic infiltrate in the upper dermis with basal cell damage, cell death, or vacuolar alteration.	Biopsy helpful; histology similar to lichen sclerosis.
Plasma cell vulvitis	Burning sunburn-type pain and dryness, variable dysparunia.	Normal vagina. Irregular heart's line with glossy moist well-dermacated red inner labial fold. Greater mechanical than punctate allodynia.	Lichenoid vasculopathic pattern with band-like infiltrate of mainly plasma cells in the superficial dermis and extravested RBCs.	Biopsy nonspecific; clinically similar to LP confined to vulvar mucosa.

Table 1.1 (*Continued*)

	Symptoms	Morphology & exam	Histopathology	Comment
Desquamative inflammatory vaginitis (VIN)	Discharge, vulvar burning, irritation, and dysparunia.	Normal vulva (mucosa and skin), dripping thin yellowish discharge at introitus; petechial redness on vaginal walls. Greater mechanical than punctate allodynia.	Two patterns: lichenoid inflammatory infiltrate or mixed infiltrate with lymphocytes, plasma cells, eosinophils.	Biopsy non.specific; clinically similar to LP confined to vagina with excessive discharge.

Lichen sclerosis, contact dermatitis, and lichen simplex chronicus

Lichen sclerosis

Generally, lichen sclerosis (LS), also known as lichen sclerosis et atrophicus, affects women in two extremes of reproductive life: pre-puberty and menopause.[2] While the prevalence of LS is unknown in the general population, it is estimated to be as high as 1% and constitutes the most common anogenital dermatitis.[3] While most cases of LS appear de novo, LS lesions may develop at a site of injury and traumatized skin (Kobner pheonomenon).[3] The most common symptom of LS is intractable itching with secondary burning and rawness from self-inflicted trauma (scratching and rubbing). In addition, it is common for chronic sufferers to develop superimposed contact dermatitis.[3-5] Characteristic findings on physical examination are hypopigmentation and thin wrinkled skin with atrophy of subcutaneous tissue.[4] In addition, there is loss of vulvar topography caused by agglutination of the clitoral hood, with the clitorial glans "buried" under the fused tissue, and flattening of the labia minora. Age distribution and posttraumatic development of LS suggests a hormonal etiology, but to date no association between estrogen metabolism and LS has been identified. Nevertheless, estrogen therapy for associated atrophy is a common practice.

LS is one of the few dermatoses with specific histopathology.[6] Lichenoid inflammation (a band-like upper dermal lymphocytic infiltrate) and dermal homogenization (loss of collagen) together are classic findings in LS. Although the presence of lichenoid inflammation and epidermal basal layer damage is not itself pathoneumonic of LS, this finding in association with dermal homogenization is used by dermatopathologists to render a diagnosis of LS.[6]

Complications associated with lichen sclerosis

Due to the severe itching associated with lichen sclerosis and the subsequent itch–scratch cycle, patients may develop superimposed contact dermatitis either caused by allergic reaction to a variety of topical agents or by irritation from rubbing. Intractable itching and scratching (the itch–scratch cycle) in turn gives rise to the characteristic skin changes seen with lichen simplex chronicus, namely a thick, leathery, excoriated skin. Comorbid lichen plans and malignancy has also been described in long-standing lichen sclerosis (see Clinical Scenario 1).

Contact dermatitis

Vulvar contact dermatitis is the most commonly overlooked vulvar condition, with a reported incidence of 20% to 30% in specialty vulvar clinics.[7] Although it is usually not the primary cause of vulvar symptoms, it is often a compounding factor in patients complaining of persistent vulvar pruritus (eg, primary lichen simplex chronicus), irritation (eg, plasma cell vulvitis), or burning (eg, generalized vulvodynia). This is not surprising considering the host of behavioral factors (eg, overzealous hygienic practices and self-medication) and clinical factors (eg, chronic use of high-potency steroids and polypharmacy) that are both associated with intractable vulvo-vaginal symptoms.[7,8]

Similar to lichen sclerosis, the primary complaint of contact dermatitis is itching.[7,9] An associated stinging sensation is common with allergic contact dermatitis, while an associated raw or chafing sensation is suggestive of irritant contact dermatitis (eg, diaper rash). The physical exam findings of contact dermatitis demonstrate varying degrees of redness interposed with normal skin. Although scaly skin is common with contact dermatitis in other areas of the body, it is not usually seen on the vulva.[10] The moist and warm environment of the vulvar region does not readily reveal scaly dermatosis; however, with progressive airing one begins to see a scaly dusky hue over the labia, which is suggestive of atopic dry skin.

A cotton swab test is a useful tool for the differential diagnoses of vulvovaginal conditions such as contact dermatitis. The cotton swab test is conducted by applying the tip of the cotton swab perpendicular to the vulvar skin and asking the patient to rate the sensation as "a cotton swab sensation" versus "a pinprick sensation." If the application of the cotton swab is perceived as a pinprick, then the test is abnormal (punctuate allodynia), which is indicative of an intrinsic inflammatory process of the skin, such as lichen planus. Patients with contact dermatitis, however, have a normal cotton swab test but demonstrate hypersensitivity to gentle stroking (mechanical allodynia).

Vulvar contact dermatitis can be broadly sub-classified into two categories: irritant and allergic.[7] Both variants of contact dermatitis have similar clinical appearances and often coexist. However, it is the nuances of the clinical presentation that favor one subtype over the other. The hallmark of allergic contact dermatitis in the acute phase is severe pruritus, vesiculation, and most importantly, a tendency to spread beyond the initial site of contact. Biopsy is only of value in ruling out malignant processes (squamous cell carcinoma)[5] or premalignant processes (VIN lesions). More often than

not, the biopsy results from cases of contact dermatitis are clinically vague, with descriptions such as "chronic inflammation with neurophilic infiltrate," "spongiosis," "acanthosis," and "parakeratosis." These descriptors are simply histopathologic correlates of what is observed by the clinician. For example, the clinical correlates of acanthosis are an orange peel-appearing, thick skin, while the correlates of parakaratosis are scaliness and an ashy appearance following exposure to air.

Lichen simplex chronicus

Lichen simplex chronicus (LSC) is divided into two clinical subtypes: primary and secondary.[11] Primary LSC refers to a condition that arises de novo on "normal" skin. As suggested by its alternate name, neurodermatitis,[11] primary LCS is commonly associated with anxiety disorders. In contrast, secondary LCS develops because of a preexisting dermatologic disorder such as lichen sclerosis. Although the exact prevalence of LSC is unknown, it is estimated to affect up to 0.5% of the general population in western countries.[11] In response to chronic excoriation associated with LCS, the vulvar skin thickens. It can be likened to a callous, similar to what is observed in the extremities. Histologic correlates of this thickening are described in terms of dermal (acanthosis) and epidermal (hyperkeratosis) thickening; otherwise, histologic findings in LSC are nonspecific (Table 1.1).[11] In the presence of moisture, the skin assumes a wrinkly, white appearance, similar to how fingertips will wrinkle and whiten in a long hot bath. Thus, the term lichenification is used to describe the pale, orange-peel appearing, thick skin of the vulva that is seen in LSC. Other associated findings are decreased sensation on the affected skin and a change in skin pigmentation (hypopigmentation or hyperpigmentation).

Summary

Chronic diffuse itching is rarely caused by infectious conditions[12] (eg, yeast infection) or premalignant processes such as VIN, which tend to cause focal, unilateral symptoms (Chapter 2). Many overlapping dermatoses are often present in a given patient. The key in deciphering the cause of a patient's

Table 1.2 General vulvar care

Minimizing Daytime Friction
- Liberal use of oil-based creams such as Gene's Vitamin E Cream.[a] For patients with excessivesensitivity, use Crisco shortening or shay butter.[b] Reapply throughout the day.
- Use cold water after using the bathroom to rinse the area. Ask patients to carry a water bottle for this purpose. Cold water (unlike warm water) stops itching.
- Instruct patients to not wipe but pad dry their perineum after washing with cold water.

Aborting Bouts of Intense Itching Sensation
- Apply deep pressure when faced with an itching sensation rather than rubbing of any kind.
- Reapply copious amounts of creams (as above).
- Place a bag of frozen peas wrapped in a thin towel over the labial folds and perineum.

Aborting Nighttime Scratching During Sleep
- Use a sedating agent (titrate slowly to maximal tolerance):
    Doxepin 10–50 mg 1–2 h before bedtime
    Diphendryamine 25–50 mg 30 min before bedtime
    Hydroxyzine 10–50 mg 2 h before bedtime
- Keep nails short and wear white cotton gloves at night.

[a] Can be purchased from Sam's Club or http://www.genesvitamine.com
[b] Compounding pharmacy; for assessment of qualifications please refer to http://www.pcab.info/

symptoms is to use a symptoms-based approach in alleviating symptoms, aborting the itch–scratch cycle, and ultimately promoting the skin's health (Table 1.2). Targeted biopsy can then be used to rule out premalignant processes and to guide additional therapy. The case studies at the end of this chapter will provide a guide to differential diagnosis, relief of symptoms, and treatment approach for patients with LS and contact dermatitis.

Lichen planus, plasma cell vulvitis, and desquamative inflammatory vaginitis

Whereas lichen sclerosis, contact dermatitis, and lichen simplex chronicus are characterized by a chief complaint of itching, lichen planus, plasma cell vulvitis, and desquamative inflammatory vaginitis are primarily associated with symptoms of burning, pain with intercourse, and discharge (Table 1.1).

Lichen planus
Classical lichen planus (LP) is characterized by shiny, flat-topped, firm papules (bumps) on the extremities, trunk, and mucosa. The most common form of this mucocutaneous dermatosis that is seen in gynecology is known as vulvo-vaginal-gingival syndrome. Vulvo-vaginal-gingival syndrome typically presents as a single or multiple well-demarcated, intensely red lesions with a reticular appearance.* In cases with extensive vaginal involvement, synechiae and varying degrees of vaginal obliteration are common. While oral lesions can vary from painless white lacy streaks to desquamative gingivitis, vulvo-vaginal lesions tend to consistently show lichenoid inflammation.

While lesions of LP on the mucosal surface are tender, lesions on the extremities (eg, wrist or ankles) are typically nontender. LP is a relatively rare condition (1–2% of the U.S. population); nevertheless the prevalence of LP is reported to be as high as 8% in the referral setting.[13, 14] Histolopathology in LP is characterized by lichenoid inflammation with basal layer damage (Table 1.1). As described earlier, lichenoid inflammation is also seen with lichen sclerosis. What sets LP apart from LS,

---

* Photo discussion of LP and other dermatologic lesions in differential diagnosis can be found at http://dermnetnz.org/scaly/lichen-planus

however, is the histologic absence of dermal homogenization (loss of collagen and sclerosis). Interestingly, the histopathology and morphology of LS and LP may converge over time. For example, it is common for patients with long-standing lichen sclerosis to develop clinical and histologic features of erosive LP. Similar to other inflammatory vulvo-vaginal conditions, the etiology of LP remains elusive. Similar to many such ulcerative lesions, LP is highly responsive to steroids and therapy with immunomodulators. Mucosal responsiveness to treatment varies depending on anatomic location. While oral mucosal lesions are highly responsive to treatment with steroids, vulvo-vaginal lesions tend to be more resistant and in fact more painful.[14]

Plasma dell vulvitis

Plasma cell vulvitis, or Zoon balanitits (the common term for the condition in men), is a benign but chronic and erosive inflammatory condition of the genital skin. While this condition is most often reported in uncircumcised men, its manifestation and prevalence in women is not well described. In either gender, however, plasma cell balanitis and vulvitis are often difficult diagnoses to make histologically and need to be correlated with clinical presentation. Histologic and clinical similarity between plasma cell vulvitis and LP has raised debate as to whether this is a distinct entity or a disorder within the spectrum of LP.[15]

The most common compliant is persistent rawness and sunburn sensation, painful intercourse, and pruritus. The diagnosis is rendered after excluding infectious conditions, specifically fungal infection. It is not uncommon for patients to have been treated with a variety of antifungal and/or antibacterial therapy before receiving the definitive diagnosis. Extensive and well-demarcated moist erythema in plasma cell vulvitis is confined to the vulvar mucosa, especially in the inner labial folds. Speculum examination is otherwise normal. Excessive discharge, loss of architecture, and agglutination are not characteristically observed. The clinical diagnosis can be confirmed by a biopsy showing a band-like infiltrate of plasma cells in the surperficial dermis. The most effective treatment in men is circumcision when possible; otherwise, use of topical corticosteroids and immunomodulators such as tacrolimus is the mainstay of therapy. Because the pathogenesis of this condition remains unclear, variable response to treatment is common in clinical practice. Thus, trial and error using a variety of medications alone or in combination is a mainstay of practice.

Desquamative inflammatory vaginitis

Desquamative inflammatory vaginitis (DIV) is a specific inflammatory condition of the vagina and the subject of much controversy. The etiology and the population prevalence of DIV are unknown. While some authorities view DIV as an independent entity, others view it along the continuum of inflammatory conditions of the vulvo-vaginal region. Clinically, the diagnosis of DIV is rendered in patients who complain of increased vaginal discharge and pain with intercourse when no identifiable cause of vaginitis can be identified. Because postmenopausal atrophic vaginitis may have similar presentations, empiric therapy with topical estrogen should be considered as first-line therapy. Failure to respond after 3 to 6 months of estrogen therapy supports the diagnosis of inflammatory vaginitis such as DIV when all known etiologies been eliminated. Unlike LP and plasma cell vulvitis, however, the vulvar region in a DIV case is normal in appearance. DIV is characterized primarily by a sterile discharge that is a watery and yellow, and by painful intercourse. Examination of the vulva is often normal, although discharge of variable consistency may be present. Speculum examination may reveal synechiae, vaginal stenosis, and most commonly, erythema. Stroking the vaginal walls with a cotton swab is commonly associated with an intense burning sensation. Generally, histology shows nonspecific inflammation. Because DIV patients present with nonspecific symptoms of burning and pain, and because cursory examinations reveal limited clinical findings, it is important to conduct a detailed assessment of the vaginal wall and to specifically look for erythema and mechanical allodynia (burning sensation on stroking of the vaginal wall with a q-tip).

Summary

It is apparent from the above description of these six vulvo-vaginal conditions that there is much overlapping morphology and pathophysiology. Diagnosis of any these conditions can be confusing and is further complicated by the fact that there are three embryologically distinct skin types (juxtaposed on the labia) unlike any other area of body. Consider, for example, how dermatitis is a scaly disease in other parts of the body, yet the scales are typically absent in the vulvar region and even a sophisticated observer is likely to see only shiny, glazed skin.

Clearly, the treatment approach in clinical practice is symptoms-based in that it is more guided by ameliorating the symptoms than untangling key driving factors. For example, as will be demonstrated in the upcoming case discussions, overlapping histopathologic and clinical presentation are common in seemingly diverse pathophysiologic processes such as lichen simplex chronicus, contact dermatitis, and lichen sclerosis. Dermatologic responses to irritant and/or chronic inflammation, regardless of the triggering event, have a similar appearance. Hypopigmentation and/or hyperpigmentation, atrophy, excoriation, and leather-like thickening of the skin are the end result of a number of interrelated or superimposed pathophysiologic processes. A prototypical patient with itching from lichen sclerosis may develop irritant dermatitis (chafing) from frictional forces. Chronic use of corticosteroids may in turn exacerbate the associated atrophy. Atrophy and the loss of protective layers then intensifies the symptoms of contact dermatitis. Lastly, use of topical anesthetics in an attempt to bring about relief may backfire and lead to an allergic response, resulting in a new onset of itching and burning suggestive of allergic contact dermatitis. Thus, unlike many medical conditions in which treatment follows a stepwise approach, it is not surprising that the care of these patients is complex, often involving diverse treatment approaches tailored to the individual's needs.

The following section presents representative case studies of each of these six vulvo-vaginal conditions. The cases are structured in order to demonstrate the overlap between conditions and to detail the means by which clinicians can determine the primary diagnosis and treatment approach.

Clinical Scenario 1

A 55-year-old woman presents with lichen sclerosis that was first diagnosed 15 years earlier. She reports a worsening of her symptoms over the past 3 years since menopause. She readily admits a chronic itch–scratch cycle, especially after taking a warm bath or shower. Recently, she has noticed postcoital bleeding. She has been using a high-potency steroid (clobetasol propionate cream 0.05%). While the steroid initially helped, with progressive use she experienced worsening symptoms after 6 months of daily treatment. She then tried tacrolimus (Protopic) and pimecrolimus (Elidel) without any improvement in symptoms.

How should this patient be evaluated?

When presented with steroid-resistant dermatoses and exacerbation after a long hiatus, superimposed malignancy should be excluded, because it is identified in 4% to 6% of patients with lichen sclerosus.[11] In chronic sufferers, comorbidity with other dermatoses is the rule rather than the exception. In addition to malignancy, superimposed infection and cellulitis from chronic itching should be ruled out. Lastly, it is common for lichen sclerosis and lichen planus to coexist, and their histopathology would reflect this overlap. For this reason, several biopsies representative of the different abnormal areas observed on the individual patient's vulva should be obtained.

Consistent with acute exacerbation, there is redness extending to the thighs (Plate 1.1). The labial skin is otherwise thick and pale, with superficial excoriation from itching. Bilateral fissuring is present in the lower labia majora (Plate 1.1), where none had been evident in the preceding visit. Two representative biopsies werey obtained, which showed two different histologies: lichen simplex chronicus and lichenoid dermatitis favoring lichen planus. The following excerpt is directly taken from the patient's pathology report:

The lesions near lateral thigh are similar to previous biopsies. Epidermal hyperplasia is more marked than previous biopsy [consistent with clinical and histologic diagnosis of LSC, and clinical exacerbation]. The features in LSC are all secondary to rub or scratch and are not specific to the etiology (Plate 1.2A).

The medial labial lesions have different features with sparse to moderate lichenoid inflammatory infiltrate in addition to hyperkeratosis [consistent with LSC] and epidermal hyperplasia [another feature of LSC]. [Previous biopsies] do not exhibit any evidence of lichenoid inflammation favoring lichen planus (Plate 1.2B).

How should you treat this complex case?

The pathologist has rendered the diagnoses of lichen sclerosis, lichen planus, and lichen simplex chronicus. It is recognized that these conditions can coexist (sometimes referred to as "the three lichens"[16]), and a targeted biopsy based on the patient's localization and topography is most useful in finding the cause of new-onset symptoms or symptom exacerbation.

Reviewing and re-reviewing skin care is a must in patients with chronic vulvar dermatoses. It is common for patients to try a number of over-the-counter or "girlfriend-endorsed" remedies in an attempt to find relief. Overzealous hygiene from fear of infection is common in this population of patients. In this particular case, the patient was asked to stop using all of her medications, including any self-medication. The patient should be instructed as to the importance and rational for NOT using soap in the vulvar region; the vulva needs its natural oil to maintain its barrier mechanisms against constant contact, moisture, and irritants.[10] The patient should be further advised to avoid lukewarm water. While the sitz bath is a common practice in obstetrics, exposure to heat may precipitate intense itching and should be avoided in patients with an itch–scratch cycle.

Lastly, copious use of vitamin E cream or other nonirritating thick petroleum-based compounds should be recommended since these medications make a barrier between the vulvar surface and clothing. In cases like this, patients in our practice are also instructed to apply a "Press'n Seal" barrier similar to plastic wrap, to the crotch of their underwear, in order to keep the maximum amount of cream on the vulva. Again, the overarching objective in these measures is to avoid contact to the irritated skin while aggressively controlling bouts of the itch–scratch cycle.

In this situation we also prescribed Doxepine, titrated up by 10 mg every 3 to 5 days to a total of 50 mg nightly, in order to decrease the likelihood of nighttime scratching. In addition, we prescribed our "plan B topical regimen"[†] as a last resort. Our Plan B topical regimen consists of a combination of topical 5% lidocaine and 0.05% estradiol compounded in hydrophilic petrolatum. While the exact mechanism by which this cream brings about relief is unknown, a higher dose of topical estrogen in combination with a topical anesthetic decreases the skin's propensity toward itching and promotes estrogen-mediated "thickening" of the skin. Due to severity of this case, a nighttime sedative, reestablishment of dermatologic health, and the plan B regimen were instituted concurrently. But typically we reserve our plan B regimen for patients who have failed to respond to our standard skin care (Table 1.1) while being off of any topical agents. The plan B regimen is typically used for a short duration (8–12 weeks), in order to abort the itch–scratch cycle and restore vulvar skin health in patients with long-standing dermatoses and polypharmacy. Caution should be exercised in that application of this compound on the mucosal surface is associated with systemic absorption to varying degrees. At the end of the 8 to 12 weeks of therapy with this regimen and concurrent skin

---

[†] Lidocaine 5% and estradiol 0.5 mg/g in hydrophilic petrolatum, 60-g tube formulated by Triangle Compounding Pharmacy, Cary, NC. Note: It is best to use high-volume pharmacies that are registered by the board. For further information on compounding pharmacies visit http://www.pcab.info/ and http://www.pcab.org/

care, we prescribe a progestational agent in menopausal patients with an intact uterus, and switch patients back to their mainstay therapy for lichenoid conditions. In our experience, most patients can be maintained using a multitier therapy using intermittent topical anti-inflammatory medications (eg, every month), topical estrogen, and attention to skin care.

Clinical Scenario 2

A 36-year-old who reports being in good health until a year ago presents with a chief complaint of a "burning sensation" in the vulvar region. On initial evaluation, she had been empirically treated with topical antifungal creams. With persistent symptoms, she had been offered various topical treatments including topical steroids. After a week of using topical steroids, she noticed a burning sensation that became progressively worse. When she called her physician's office, she was reassured that her symptoms would improve with ongoing steroid use. She finally discontinued the treatment after 3 to 4 weeks. Since then, she experienced worsening of her symptoms to the point where she is no longer able to wear fitted pants. She also has developed an itching sensation in addition to burning. She denies having an itch–scratch cycle and has no exacerbation of her symptoms with intercourse. The generalized vulvar discomfort and rawness, nevertheless, has affected her interest in intimacy.

Based on the historical information, what is the differential diagnosis?

Based on her history and her presentation, the top two differential diagnoses in most clinicians' minds would be an infectious etiology (eg, yeast or bacterial vaginosis) or an idiopathic pain disorder (eg, vulvar vestibulitis syndrome). When faced with persistent vulvo-vaginal symptoms, empiric treatment with a host of antibacterial and antifungal[17] creams is not only ineffective but in most cases counterproductive and even harmful. While the discussion and management

of idiopathic pain disorders is beyond the scope of this chapter, this diagnosis is considered when no dermatologic and pathologic explanation can be identified.[16, 18] In this case, the best course of action would be to obtain a vaginal and vulvar culture prior to empiric treatment.[12]

Non-judicious use of over-the-counter medications, steroids, and prescription medications may trigger an allergic reaction. Regardless of her initial diagnosis, because the likely trigger of her symptoms was steroid use, she was likely to have superimposed allergic dermatitis.

On physical examination, the labia majora are diffusely red without visible scaling (Plate 1.3), but the vulvar surface is progressively dry and dusky with air exposure. There is tenderness to a cotton swab test, a glossy appearance, and small fissures in the folds of both the labia majora and minora. Although minimal punctuate allodynia (pinprick sensation with a cotton swab) is observed during the examination, significant mechanical allodynia (hypersensitivity on gentle stroking of vulvar surface) is observed. The vestibular mucosa is pale and atrophic with mild tenderness (Fig. 1.1). What is the most likely diagnosis?

The examination confirms the likely diagnosis of allergic dermatitis as noted by the expansion of a rash beyond the affected region of the labia. In addition to allergic dermatitis, she is likely to have a component of irritant dermatitis due to dryness, superimposed irritation, and friction from clothing on the irritated skin. The cause of her initial presentation cannot be evaluated at this time because of her superimposed dermatologic condition. Thus, the initial goal of the treatment should be to address her symptoms and restore her dermatologic health.

What additional diagnostic and treatment approaches should be considered?

Cultures from labial folds for yeast were obtained and returned negative. The treatment approach was aimed at (1) aborting the cycle of irritation and rawness, (2) minimizing the sensation of itching, and (3) promoting general vulvar health. The patient was instructed to discontinue the use

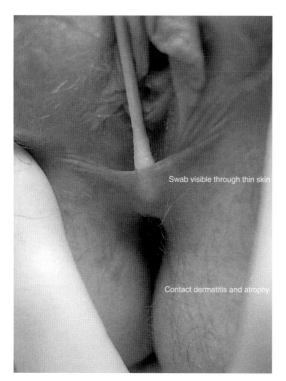

Swab visible through thin skin

Contact dermatitis and atrophy

Figure 1.1 Pale atrophic thinning of the skin in context of contact dermatitis.

of topical agents and was started on vitamin E cream and general vulvar skin care (Table 1.2). After 4 to 6 weeks of topical vulvar skin care and nightly application of Estrace cream, her dermatologic symptoms resolved.

On repeat examination 3 months to the date of her initial visit, she had no abnormal dermatologic findings. Her labia exhibited no tenderness to a point palpation with a cotton swab (punctuate allodynia). Although her labia were normal, they were sensitive to a gentle stroke of a cotton swab (mechanical allodynia), as it caused a sensation of rawness and burning.

What could be causing these symptoms?

She was diagnosed with generalized vulvodyina and started on slowly accelerating doses of amitriptyline (10 mg at bedtime, increasing by

10-mg increments every 3–5 days to a total daily dose of 75–100 mg). She reported an 80% improvement in symptoms with 75 mg of nightly amitriptyline. A detailed discussion on the management of idiopathic vulvo-vaginal pain disorders (eg, vulvar vestibulitis syndrome) can be found in Consensus Statement 2005.[18]

Clinical Scenario 3

A 37-year-old woman presents with a chief complaint of intractable pain with intercourse that started 5 years ago. Up until then, she had no history of pain with intercourse. Over the years, her symptoms have progressively worsened to a point where she now reports daily unprovoked pain. Her last attempt at intercourse was 2 years earlier, during which she experienced bleeding. She also has noted a progressive increase in vaginal discharge, especially during menses, which tends to linger on as ongoing spotting. She denies an itch–scratch cycle but does report an "itchy-burning sensation" of her vulva.

Previously, she had undergone a laparoscopy where a diagnosis of endometriosis was rendered. She was given a trial of Lupron, which co-incided with the exacerbation of her symptoms, including a progressive increase in dryness and burning. Otherwise, she has not sought care for this condition for the past 2 years.

What is her differential diagnosis based on history?

In the absence of an acute infectious process, as in this case, the likely differential diagnosis is a chronic inflammatory vulvo-vaginal process. The age of this patient, however, warrants a careful assessment of the vulvo-vaginal region. A simple magnifying glass will provide sufficient power to rule out any raised, atypical lesions suggestive of VIN. Also, it is unlikely that her condition could be explained by endometriosis alone. Histologic findings suggestive of endometriosis during laparoscopy may be an incidental finding and not the cause of dysparunia. Administration of Lupron for treatment of endometriosis not suprisingly exacerbated her condition by causing a hypoestrogenic state with worsening atrophy and dryness sensation.

Exam findings included tender, well-circumscribed mucocutanous lesions of the vulva (Plate 1.4). While the vaginal lesions were not distinct enough to be seen with a speculum exam, the posterior cervix was agglutinated to the posterior vaginal wall, which could be "softened" and separated with gradual genital digital pressure application.

What physical exam findings confirm your diagnosis?

It is imperative that the physical exam include a full dermatologic assessment. In the author's experience, patients rarely voluntarily disclose symptoms related to the oral cavity or other "unrelated" parts of the body. On exam and subsequent questioning, this patient reported a long-standing problem of recurrent oral burning and a previous diagnosis of oral lichen planus (Plate 1.5). Due to financial reasons, she has not had an additional workup and evaluation for her erosive oral lesion. Incidentally, on further query, it was found that the fluctuation in oral lesions closely mirrored that of the vulvo-vaginal regions. A prototypical fluctuation consisted of a worsening of burning in the mouth followed by an immediate increase in oral cavity redness. Even though the appearance of the vulvar lesions took an average of 3 weeks to develop, they rapidly became painful and more resistant to healing. Unlike oral lesion, the vulvar lesion showed non-specific inflammation. However, cliniopathologic diagnosis of lichen planus was rendered based on history and exam findings. While it is true that many women with vulvar lesions seem to also suffer from oral lesions, the converse is not true in the author's experience. And in this case, history and biopsy findings would have been sufficient in making the diagnosis once other known etiologies had been ruled out (eg, infectious, atrophy).

What is the appropriate treatment?

A three-pronged treatment approach should be used in order to (1) promote healing of the current ulcer, (2) reduce pain and suffering, and (3) induce long-term remission. In general, when faced with extensive systemic lesions or resistant/intractable local lesions, oral steroids and steroid-sparing adjunct treatments such as methotrexate should be used in combination. Thus, consultation with a dermatologist with experience in the treatment of ulcerative mucocutaneous lesions should be initiated in the first visit. Treatment with topical anti-inflammatory agents and local anesthetics can then be used to treat the inflammation and pain associated with active lesions. In this case, a pulse oral steroid regimen was used starting with a 40-mg dose, tapered very slowly over 4 months to 2.5 mg/day. In addition, in order to decrease the probability of flares, she was started on weekly intramuscular methotrexate.

While her oral lesions rapidly responded to steroids (within 2 weeks), her vulvo-vaginal lesions were more resistant (4–6 weeks), necessitating a concurrent use of vaginal hydrocortisone suppositories. In our experience, a prolonged titration regimen (up to 3–4 months) is required with vulvar lesions. This patient was co-managed by our colleagues in dermatology. Please note the discussion below about the role of topical agents in treating inflammation localized to the vulva (plasma cell vulvitis) and vagina (DIV).

In our experience, commercially available topical anesthetic agents (especially Benzocaine) are allergenic and are not well tolerated. Thus, we often use a compounding pharmacy in order to develop individualized treatment. While a detailed discussion of compounding medications, including the pros and cons, are beyond the scope of this chapter, most specialized compounding pharmacies with a focus on women's health can serve as a valuable resource for busy clinicians (http://www.pcab.info/). Our typical regimen for the management of pain with active ulcers is as follows: 5% lidocaine and 10% benzocaine compounded in hydrophilic petrolatum. For oral lesions or excessively moist vulvar lesions, we change the formulation to an Orogel base, which is more paste-like and adheres better to a moist surface.

Clinical Scenario 4

A 52-year-old presents with a chief complaint of vulvo-vaginal pain, specifically a burning and raw sensation, which began around the time of menopause at age 48. After a year of monthly treatment with a variety of antifungal and antibacterial medications for presumed yeast and bacterial vaginosis, she was treated with boric acid for an intractable vulvo-vaginal yeast infection. Application of boric acid precipitated severe burning and a diffuse rash, for which she was treated with daily steroids. After 3 months of steroid therapy, her symptoms improved, but her burning persisted and progressively became worse. At this point, the diagnosis of generalized vulvodynia was made by the third clinician who had examined her, and she was started on amitriptyline about 6 months prior to this clinic visit. She reports that she is "over the acute flare caused by medication" and her symptoms are back to the baseline of "sunburn-type rawness and burning in her inner labial lips," pain with intercourse, and a general sensation of dryness. Her previous two biopsies indicated "chronic nonspecific inflammation and epithelial atrophy" and "no malignant or premalignant lesions were identified." Thus she was told that her biopsies were "normal" and was left with the perception that nothing was wrong with her.

What is her differential diagnosis based on history?

Based on her history, iatrogenic allergic dermatitis caused by boric acid is the likely cause of her initial flare. Because it is extremely unlikely that infectious processes are the cause of her persistent symptoms, this case emphasizes the importance of confirming the diagnosis of infectious processes prior to embarking on em-

piric treatment. Whereas the itch–scratch cycle is an unlikely cause of her symptoms, the presence of atrophy and chronic inflammation favors dermatopathology. The least likely cause of her symptoms based on her history and workup to date is an idiopathic pain disorder such as generalized vulvodynia.

On physical exam, no abnormality on the labia major and external surface of labia minora was noted. With the patient's guidance the "irritation" was localized to the inner lips of the labia minora. On close inspection, glossy "wet" redness was noted in the inner folds of the labia minora with irregular and asymmetric margins of "heart's line" (Plate 1.6). Both tactile and mechanical allodynia were present on sensory examination. Gental stroking with a cotton swab (mechanical allodynia), however, reproduced over 80% of her chief complaint of "rawness and sunburn type irritation."

Given these findings, what is your presumed diagnosis and what other evaluation is appropriate?

This case clearly illustrates the diagnostic conundrum that gynecologists encounter. Faced with clinical signs of inflammation, our immediate instinct is to perform a biopsy from representative areas in order to appropriately rule out premalignant and malignant processes. In evaluation of vulvar dermatoses, biopsies serves not only to eliminate the possibility of premalignant processes, but the "histologic features" of the biopsies are useful in arriving at a clinicopathologic diagnosis.[11] Unfortunately, most of us (as gynecologists) are not trained in dermatopathology and in fact have limited knowledge of how to go about arriving at a clinicopathologic interpretation of the histology and the presenting signs and symptoms. In this case, biopsy showed band-like plasma cell infiltrate in the upper dermis, and in conjunction with findings of moist erythema confined to the inner labial fold, the diagnosis of plasma cell vulvitis was rendered.

Close collaboration and guidance from our colleagues in dermatopathology (pathologists with specialized training in dermatoses) are imperative in arriving at a diagnosis and tailoring an individualized treatment plan. In this case, the biopsies were mailed to our institution and read by dermatopathologists. Based on the histologic feature and clinical presentation, this patient was diagnosis with Zoon balinitis or plasma cell vulvitis.

What is your treatment approach?

As in earlier cases, the general approach for treatment is to (1) eliminate irritation and restore dermatologic health (Table 1.2), (2) reduce pain and suffering, and (3) induce remission. The cardinal rule of therapy is to find the right combinations of dose, frequency, and intervals that give maximal benefit with limited side effects. To this end, some general guidelines are noteworthy. First, higher frequency and potency of anti-inflammatory agents are most effective in inducing remission but should only be used for a brief period of 3 to 4 weeks. Second, titration should be done slowly, expanding each step over a period of 2 weeks in order to assess the consequence of tapering. Third, the order of tapering should be that of decreasing frequency first, followed by decreasing the potency. Further decrease in the frequency (eg, from once a day to once every other day) should be the last step before final titration. This less-frequent, lower-potency dosage should be maintained for 4 weeks before final titration. Not surprisingly, it is not uncommon for the optimal therapy or combination of therapies to be arrived at after a year of trial and error.

In line with the above-mentioned principle, nonsteroid immunomodulators are first-line therapies, with topical steroids and oral medications reserved for intractable cases. Similarly, topical steroid therapy should start with less potent formulation first (eg, hydrocortisone), with a more potent formulation (eg, clobetasole) reserved for intractable cases.

In this case, the patient was started on tacrolimus and instructed on a regimen of topical skin care (Table 1.2). For pain management, she was started on topical lidocaine ointment (5%). Lastly, she was asked to contact us if she experienced burning with any of the topical treatments (eg, allergic dermatitis). After 4 weeks of therapy, her symptoms were markedly improved. Subsequently, over the ensuing 6 to 8 months, her treatment was titrated down to biweekly application of topical tacrolimus (0.03%). Vaginal estrogen tablets (Vagifem) and vitamin E cream were concurrently used throughout this period in order to correct atrophy and minimize superimposed dermatitis.

Pathology notes

Vulvar dystrophy

Vulvar punch biopsies may be interpreted by pathologists with various backgrounds, including dermatopathologists, general pathologists, and gynecologic pathologists. For inflammatory dermatoses involving the vulva, the first task of the pathologist is to integrate clinical history, physical exam findings, and histopathology to make as specific a diagnosis as possible to guide therapy. It is therefore important for the clinician to communicate physical exam findings, including description of affected nongenital sites, and clinical history to the pathologist. The second task for pathologists interpreting vulvar dystrophy biopsies is to exclude vulvar neoplasia and infectious conditions, sometimes with the help of special stains. The terminology used in articles and textbooks to describe vulvar inflammatory dermatoses is inconsistently applied. Classification of vulvar dermatoses using the same specific terminology applied to conditions affecting nongenital skin is advised. Descriptive diagnoses are not encouraged and are likely to be of little utility in determining the clinical management of the patient. Use of consistent terminology helps ensure that the clinician is more likely to understand the terminology and will be able to

Pathology notes (*continued*)

use the pathology report information to optimize patient therapy. A brief discussion of important pathologic aspects for the most common vulvar inflammatory dermatoses follows.

The most common inflammatory disorder involving the vulva is eczematous dermatitis, which is characterized histologically by the presence of intercellular edema, "spongiosis" within the epidermis, and a variably intense dermal chronic inflammatory infiltrate. There are several clinical variants of eczematous dermatitis based on clinical features of the condition; these variants usually cannot be subtyped on histology alone. Once the pathologist has made the diagnosis of eczematous dermatitis and excluded other dermatoses, it is then up to the clinician to then search for the specific etiology. Eczematous dermatitis is the histopathologic counterpart to contact dermatitis in most patients, with the differential diagnosis including both irritant contact dermatitis and allergic contact dermatitis. Common causes of irritant contact dermatitis include soaps, perfumes, cleansers, topical over-the-counter medications, urine, sweat, and friction. Irritant contact dermatitis results from direct damage to the skin by exogenous agents. Allergic contact dermatitis is rarer and may be more difficult to confirm without skin patch testing. Histopathologic features in skin biopsies favoring allergic contact dermatitis include the presence of increased eosinophils around superficial venules and occasionally within the spongiotic epidermal layer, and intraepidermal microgranulomas consisting of Langerhans cells. Allergic contact dermatitis represents a type IV hypersensitivity reaction to a specific allergen. Fungal infections may occasionally show histopathologic features similar to eczematous dermatitis and should be excluded by the pathologist, especially given the different treatment implications. The absence of fungal organisms in the biopsy can be confirmed with special stains such as the periodic acid–Schiff (PAS) stain.

Lichen simplex chronicus (LSC) is a reactive condition often seen in association with eczematous dermatitis. LSC is characterized histologically as showing epidermal acanthosis, hyperkeratosis, and hypergranulosis. LSC represents a cutaneous reaction to repeated physical trauma such as chronic scratching. LSC is not a distinct entity that explains the patient's condition. The pathologist is expected to make an attempt to identify the underlying cause of LSC if possible. If there are no histopathologic features that identify an underlying etiology, the pathology report can so state. Eczematous dermatitis is the most common specific inflammatory condition to be seen in association with LSC. The differential diagnosis for LSC includes VIN simplex-type.

The diagnosis of well-established lichen sclerosus (LS) is typically straightforward due in large part to the characteristic homogenized dermal sclerosis seen on light microscopy. It should be noted that early lesions of LS may be difficult to diagnose and can show overlapping histologic features with lichen planus (LP). The presence of even subtle dermal sclerosis favors the diagnosis of LS over LP. Some cases of LS may be associated with superimposed LSC and have an unusual appearance on physical exam. The presence or absence of atypia should be noted in biopsies from elderly women showing LS. LS does appear to be associated with some risk for developing vulvar squamous cell carcinoma and VIN simplex-type in elderly women.

A whole host of other inflammatory disorders may involve the vulva, including infections, psoriasis, lichen planus, Behçet disease, Crohn disease, plasma cell vulvitis, and various acantholytic disorders. Biopsy evaluation by a pathologist with experience in evaluating inflammatory skin conditions is optimal to help ensure all diagnostic possibilities have been considered in a biopsy, especially for unusual or problematic cases.

References

1. Eckert LO. Clinical practice. Acute vulvovaginitis. *N Engl J Med*. 2006;355:1244–1252.

2. Edwards QT, Saunders-Goldson S. Lichen sclerosus of the vulva in women: assessment, diagnosis, and management for the nurse practitioner. *J Am Acad Nurse Pract*. 2003;15:115–119.

3. Funaro D. Lichen sclerosus: a review and practical approach. *Dermatol Ther*. 2004;17:28–37.

4. Scurry J, Whitehead J, Healey M. Histology of lichen sclerosus varies according to site and proximity to carcinoma. *Am J Dermatopathol*. 2001;23:413–418.

5. Scurry JP, Vanin K. Vulvar squamous cell carcinoma and lichen sclerosus. *Australas J Dermatol*. 1997;38(suppl 1):S20–S25.

6. Lynch PJ, Moyal-Barracco M, Bogliatto F, Micheletti L, Scurry J. 2006 ISSVD classification of vulvar dermatoses: pathologic subsets and their clinical correlates. *J Reprod Med*. 2007;52:3–9.

7. Margesson LJ. Contact dermatitis of the vulva. *Dermatol Ther*. 2004;17:20–27.

8. Moyal-Barracco M, Edwards L. Diagnosis and therapy of anogenital lichen planus. *Dermatol Ther*. 2004;17:3846.

9. O'Hare PM, Sherertz EF. Vulvodynia: a dermatologist's perspective with emphasis on an irritant contact dermatitis component. *J Womens Health Gend Based Med*. 2000;9:565–569.

10. Farge MaM, Howard. The vulvar epithelium differs from the skin: implications for cutaneous testing to address topical vulvar exposures. *Contact Dermatitis*. 2004;51:201–209.

11. Lynch PJ. Lichen simplex chronicus (atopic/neurodermatitis) of the anogenital region. *Dermatol Ther*. 2004;17:8–19.

12. Edwards L. The diagnosis and treatment of infectious vaginitis. *Dermatol Ther*. 2004;17:102–110.

13. Yoshido M. Effective treatment of erosive lichen planus with thalidomide and topical tacrolimus. *International J Dermatol*. 2006;45:1244–1245.

14. Kennedy CM, Galask RP. Erosive vulvar lichen planus: retrospective review of characteristics and outcomes in 113 patients seen in a vulvar specialty clinic. *J Reprod Med*. 2007;52:43–47.

15. Scurry J, Wilkinson EJ. Review of terminology of precursors of vulvar squamous cell carcinoma. *J Low Genit Tract Dis*. 2006;10:161–169.

16. Foster DC. Vulvar disease. *Obstet Gynecol* 2002;100:145–163.

17. Nyirjesy P, Seeney SM, Grody MH, Jordan CA, Buckley HR. Chronic fungal vaginitis: the value of cultures. *Am J Obstet Gynecol*. 1995;173:820–823.

18. Haefner HK, Collins ME, Davis GD, *et al.* The vulvodynia guideline. *J Low Genit Tract Dis*. 2005;9:40–51.

CHAPTER 2

Vulvar Intraepithelial Neoplasia and Cancer

Leigh A. Cantrell, MD, MSPH
Department of Obstetrics and Gynecology, University of North Carolina School of Medicine, Chapel Hill, NC, USA

Linda Van Le, MD, FACOG
Department of Obstetrics and Gynecology, University of North Carolina School of Medicine, Chapel Hill, NC, USA

Pathology Notes: Chad Livasy, MD
Associate Professor, Department of Pathology and Laboratory Medicine, University of North Carolina School of Medicine, Chapel Hill, NC, USA

Background

Vulvar intraepithethial neoplasia (VIN) is the current accepted term for squamous intraepithelial neoplasia of the vulva. Between 1973 and 2000, the reported incidence rose by 411%, from 0.6 cases per 100,000 women to 2.9 cases per 100,000 women.[1] This may be causally linked to changes in sexual practices, as more than 90% of high-grade VIN cases are associated with human papilloma virus (HPV). The incidence of VIN has almost tripled in women younger than 35 years old.[2,3] Although rates of VIN are increasing, the incidence of invasive vulvar cancer has remained stable at approximately 4,000 cases diagnosed annually in the United States.[3] This may reflect an increase in reported incidence of VIN due an increased awareness and diagnosis of vulvar dysplasias or an improvement in treatment and follow-up.

The term "vulvar intraepithethial neoplasia" was adopted by the International Society for Study of Vulvar Disease in 1986, and subsequently by the WHO/International Society of Gynecologic Pathologists in 1994. VIN was initially divided into categories of severity or level of epidermal involvement by cellular changes, nuclear atypia, and mitotic activity similar to cervical intraepithelial neoplasia (CIN). In 1986, the International Society for the Study of Vulvar Disease (ISSVD) classified VIN in three categories (VIN I, II, and III). Abnormal epithelial development is present in the lowest third of the epithelium for a diagnosis of VIN I; in the lower two-thirds of the epithelium for VIN II; and in greater than two-thirds of the epithelium for VIN III. This system was revised in 2004, as it became apparent that the 1986 nomenclature did not reflect natural disease progression. VIN I was not found to be a precursor for invasive cancer, nor was the diagnosis readily reproducible among pathologists, and it was therefore dropped in the 2004 system. It is thought that VIN I findings are HPV-related or reactive.[4]

The current classification system describes two types of VIN. The most common type is the "*usual type*", also called warty, basaloid, bowenoid, or mixed. This type is found in younger women (30s and 40s) who are often smokers (60–80%).

Gynecological Cancer Management: Identification, Diagnosis and Treatment, Edited by Daniel L. Clarke-Pearson and John T. Soper. Published 2010 by Blackwell Publishing, ISBN: 978-1-4051-9079-4.

Other risk factors include neoplasia of the lower genital tract, immunosuppression (transplant patients, HIV disease, etc), and prior condylomas. Usual VIN is often associated with herpes simplex virus, lichen sclerosus, lichen planus, and Paget's disease. The *usual type* of VIN has been shown to progress to invasive squamous cell carcinoma in approximately 6.5% of patients, with 3.2% having occult disease.[4, 5]

A distinct, second type of VIN is the *differentiated* or *simplex type*. Simplex VIN accounts for 2% to 10% of vulvar intraepithelial neoplasia cases. Twenty-five percent of patients have a history of smoking, and multicentric lesions are less often found. It is more common in older women. The mean age of patients diagnosed with simplex VIN lesions is 67 years, and they are almost always found in the postmenopausal woman (two to three decades later than the classic VIN lesion). This variant is a more common precursor of invasive squamous cell carcinoma of the vulva and is often found adjacent to invasive squamous cell carcinoma of the vulva. Van Seters and associates reviewed the natural history of differentiated VIN and found that in 9% of untreated patients, and 3% of treated patients, the disease will progress to invasive vulvar cancer.[5]

Simplex VIN may be associated with lichen sclerosus and lichen simplex chronicus, but generally not with HPV. Eighty-three percent of simplex VIN is found adjacent to vulvar lichen sclerosis or squamous hyperplasia lesions. Fifty percent of patients with vulvar carcinoma have lichen sclerosus.[3]

Many pathology reports still use the terms VIN I, II, and III to describe vulvar lesions. The term carcinoma in situ is also used interchangeably with VIN III. We will utilize the terms VIN I, II, III in this chapter (Table 2.1).

Table 2.1 Classification system for vulvar intraepithelial neoplasia

ISSVD[a], 2004 modified terminology	Prior terminology
Flat condyloma/HPV effect	VIN I
VIN, usual type, warty type	VIN II, III
Basaloid type, mixed (warty/basaloid)	
VIN, differentiated	Differentiated VIN

[a]International Society for the Study of Vulvar Diseases.

Pathology notes

The grading schema for vulvar intraepithelial neoplasia (VIN) parallels that of cervical intraepithelial neoplasia (CIN): VIN I (mild squamous dysplasia), VIN II (moderate squamous dysplasia), and VIN III (severe squamous dysplasia). Unlike the cervix, where CIN I is very common, the diagnosis of VIN I is quite uncommon. In fact, non-neoplastic reactive atypia secondary to dermatitis conditions should first be considered and excluded by the pathologist before making the diagnosis of VIN I. The hallmark histologic features of classic (HPV-associated) VIN consist of a progressive loss of maturation within the epidermis (from VIN I to VIN III) associated with increased nuclear/cytoplasmic ratios, increased mitotic figures, coarse chromatin, and scattered apoptotic bodies. A surface reaction of hyperkeratosis or parakeratosis is often present. In classic VIN, koilocytic atypia may or may not be found. Some authors have also used the terms warty VIN or basaloid VIN to further describe morphologic variants of classic VIN. Similar to the cervix, strong staining for p16 and increased Ki-67 index have been described in classic VIN, and on rare occasion these markers may be helpful in distinguishing classic forms of VIN from their mimics. However, immunohistochemical stains are generally not required for the diagnosis of most cases of classic VIN.

There is convincing evidence that cancer of the vulva arises not only from classic (HPV-associated) VIN, but also from a more histologically subtle form of VIN termed simplex or differentiated VIN.[6] Simplex VIN is estimated to

Pathology Notes (*continued*)

account for approximately 2% to 5% of VIN cases and is not associated with HPV infection. Simplex VIN is typically identified in postmenopausal women and may be seen in association with vulvar dystrophy such as lichen sclerosus or lichen simplex chronicus. This form of VIN deserves special mention because it can be easily overlooked by the pathologist and misinterpreted as a benign reactive condition such as vulvar dystrophy. Unlike classic VIN, which shows a progressive loss of maturation from VIN I to VIN III, the epidermis in VIN simplex shows evidence of maturation with preservation of low nuclear/cytoplasmic ratios within keratinocytes. VIN simplex typically shows thickening of the epidermis by a proliferation of atypical keratinocytes with large vesicular nuclei, prominent nucleoli, and brightly eosinophilic cytoplasm (Fig. 2.1A). The rete ridges may show elongated and branched architecture. Biomarkers p53 and Ki-67 are helpful in evaluating suspicious lesions, as both show suprabasilar extension of nuclear positivity compared to adjacent normal epidermis (Fig. 2.1B).[7] Pathologists should be particularly aware of the possibility of VIN simplex when evaluating biopsies of new vulvar lesions in postmenopausal women with a history of vulvar carcinoma. Simplex VIN is by definition a carcinoma in situ and appears to have a greater potential for progression to invasive squamous cell carcinoma than classic VIN. Conservative excision of lesions is recommended with clinical follow-up.

Perhaps the most challenging component of pathologic evaluation of vulvar neoplasia is assessing for the presence or absence of early stromal invasion in cases showing extensive VIN III. This difficulty is due to multiple factors, including tangential sectioning of biopsy specimens, extension of VIN into cutaneous adnexal structures, subtle forms of stromal invasion, and extremely well-differentiated forms of squamous cell carcinoma. As a result of these factors, it may be difficult on some small biopsies to give a definitive diagnosis of invasion or report specific tumor

A

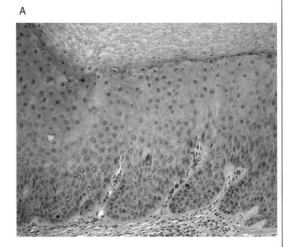

B

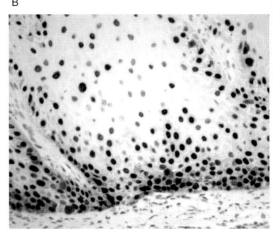

Figure 2.1 VIN simplex. **A.** VIN simplex showing epidermal acanthosis with elongated rete ridges, cytologic atypia including nucleoli, hypereosinophilic cytoplasm, and overlying parakeratosis and hyperpkeratosis. **B.** Immunohistochemistry for p53 shows suprabasilar nuclear immunoreactivity, supportive of the diagnosis of VIN simplex.

measurements such as depth of invasion. In most cases, however, the presence or absence of invasion can be definitively assessed. When invasive carcinoma is found in a specimen, every attempt should be made by the pathologist to measure

Pathology notes (*continued*)

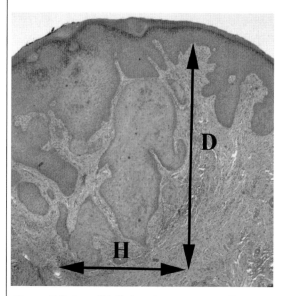

Figure 2.2 Superficially invasive squamous cell carcinoma of the vulva. The depth of invasion (*D arrow*) is measured from the adjacent most superficial dermal papillae to the deepest point of invasion. The greatest horizontal extent of tumor (*H arrow*) should also be reported in the pathology report.

both the depth of invasion and greatest horizontal extent of tumor, and comment on the presence/absence of lymphovascular space invasion by tumor. The important cutoffs for superficially invasive squamous cell carcinoma of the vulva are 1.0 mm in depth and 2.0 cm in greatest diameter. The depth of invasion for vulvar cancers is defined as the measurement from the epithelial stromal junction of the adjacent most superficial dermal papillae to the deepest point of invasion (Fig. 2.2). This depth should be measured by the pathologist with an ocular micrometer.

It should be noted that the diagnosis of verrucous carcinoma will typically require a large, deep biopsy or excisional biopsy, as this rare very-well-differentiated tumor requires detailed examination of the epithelial–stromal interface to be recognized. Small superficial biopsies of these tumors will often return with a pathologic diagnosis of a nonspecific benign condition or possibly condyloma.

Paget's disease of the vulva

Paget's disease is another premalignant condition of the vulva. It accounts for less than 1% of vulvar neoplasia. Paget's disease of the breast was initially described by Sir James Paget in 1874. Since that time, it has been described in numerous other tissues, including the vulva, and is classified as mammary or extramammary Paget's disease. Most patients with vulvar Paget's disease are postmenopausal (average age, 59–67 years) and Caucasian. The main presenting symptoms are pruritis, burning, and irritation. Paget's disease is of apocrine origin and the anogenital region is the most common site of extramammary Paget's disease.

Paget's disease appears as erythematous, eczematous, indurated lesions. Histologically, the presence of intracellular acid or neutral mucopolysaccharide demonstrated by special stains is diagnostic of Paget's disease. Sometimes lesions are ulcerated and bleed on contact. Most frequently the labia majora are affected and the extent of disease is directly correlated with the duration of disease.

Paget's disease must be surgically excised because there is a 4% to 15% chance of underlying vulvar adenocarcinoma. These patients are also at risk for synchronous primaries of other organs (20–30%) and should be screened for lesions of the breast, rectum, bladder, urethra, cervix, or ovary.[8–12] Positive margins are common in the resection of this disease. Unfortunately, Paget's disease of the vulva often recurs, regardless of margin status.[13]

Pathology notes

Paget's disease

Paget's disease of the vulva is characterized by infiltration of the epidermis by neoplastic glandular cells. Most cases of vulvar Paget's disease are thought to have a primary cutaneous origin from malignant transformation of adnexal apocrine or eccrine cells or possibly pluripotential stem cells in the epidermis. Secondary Paget's disease may be seen in association with adenocarcinomas arising in nearby organs such as the Bartholin glands, rectum, or genitourinary tract. Histologic mimics of Paget's disease include malignant melanoma and VIN, but these diagnoses can usually be easily excluded with special stains for mucin (positive in Paget's disease), S100 (melanoma marker), and p63 (marker of squamous differentiation). Once a diagnosis of Paget's disease is confirmed, the pathologist should evaluate for the presence of dermal invasion. If dermal invasion is found to be present, the depth of invasion should be measured with an ocular micrometer and reported.

Clinical course

The majority of VIN lesions will not progress to vulvar carcinoma and some spontaneously regress. A small percentage will develop malignant changes. Patients often have recurrent vulvar dysplasia, though some recurrences may actually be persistent disease. The clinical course is variable based on disease and host factors that are incompletely understood, making this disease difficult and frustrating for treating physicians.

Studies have shown that some lesions will spontaneously regress. Jones and Rowan studied 14 women diagnosed with VIN II-III whose lesions regressed in a median of 9.5 months. The median age of these patients was 19.5 years (range, 15–27 years), and all lesions were multifocal and pigmented. All women who demonstrated regression of their lesion were asymptomatic and quite young as compared to the majority of women diagnosed with VIN II-III (median age, 19.5 vs. 35 years).[14] The terms reversible vulvar atypia and bowenoid papulosis were used in the 1970s to describe a variant of VIN II-III seen in young women with multifocal pigmented papular vulvar lesions that often regressed spontaneously. Unfortunately, there have been reports of such lesions progressing to invasive carcinoma. Given that there is no reliable way to predict which lesions will progress, it is advisable that treatment should be offered when VIN II or III is present.[15, 16]

Conversely, in van Seters review, 9% of patients (61 untreated patients and 27 patients with macroscopic disease left behind) had progression of VIN III to cancer over 1 to 8 years. Of these 8 patients, 4 had received prior radiation therapy and 1 was immunosuppressed.[5] Most think that VIN III has an overall low invasive potential of around 6%; others have shown a difference in patients treated for VIN III (3.8% progressed to invasive cancer) and those left untreated (87.5% progressed to invasive cancer). In excised lesions, occult invasion is noted in 6% to 7%.

Screening/Physical exam

There is no specific screening test for VIN. Physicians should evaluate the vulva at every annual exam. The vulva, perineum, and anus should be assessed for areas that appear raised, erythematous, excoriated, or ulcerated. Patients should be questioned regarding symptoms of pain or pruritis. The most common presenting symptom of a vulvar dysplasia is pruritis. Other symptoms include chronic itching, erythema, burning, and pain. Erythema of the vulva may have been noted by the patient. Approximately 50% of patients will be asymptomatic. Lesions may be unifocal or multifocal, and white, gray, or red. Lesions of the hair-bearing cutaneous surfaces of the vulva are usually white, while mucous membrane lesions in the inner labia are often macular and pink to red in color.[3] Hyperpigmented lesions are present in 10% to 15% of patients.[14]

Patients who are identified with symptoms or lesions should undergo an extensive vulvar examination. Evaluation of the vulva following the application of 4% acetic acid followed by inspection with a coloposcope or a handheld magnifying glass must be performed in identified patients. Because of the upper keratinized layer of epidermis, the acetic acid should be in contact with vulvar skin for several minutes, rather than the shorter contact times required for cervical or vaginal mucous membranes. The keratinized layer also most often obscures underlying vascular changes, with dysplastic lesions most often appearing as dense acetowhite lesions on the vulvar skin.

The use of toluidine blue to identify lesions has also been described. The technique applies a 1% aqueous solution of toluidine blue to the entire vulva. The area is allowed to dry for several minutes and then washed with a 1% to 2% acetic acid solution. Areas of increased nuclear activity stain blue. Many find this technique limited due to the high false-positive rate associated with areas of infection, non-neoplastic ulceration, or excoriation. The increased nuclear activity of these areas results in a high uptake of toluidine blue. False negatives are also noted in hyperkeratotic lesions, as little dye is absorbed.

Treatment

Treatment for VIN includes observation, surgical excision, and nonsurgical management. The Society of Gynecologic Oncologists published a list of accepted treatment modalities for VIN in 1996. This list included wide local excision of all gross disease with a 0.5- to 1.0-cm margin, using skinning vulvectomy with or without skin graft for more extensive disease, CO_2 laser therapy, or application of 5-fluorouracil.[17] More recently, imiquimod (Aldara) has been reported to be effective in eliminating some cases of VIN III. Observation is usually the mode of management for VIN I lesions. On the other hand, treatment is recommended for VIN II or III lesions. Selection of treatment modality should be individualized based on patient preferences, the location of disease, and the extent of the lesion.

Specifics of treatment options will be outlined in the Clinical Scenarios later in the chapter.

Prevention

The HPV-related variants of VIN would logically be prevented by targeted strategies such as vaccination. HPV type 16 DNA has been shown to exist in VIN and VAIN specimens more than 70% of the time. No preventative vaccine trials have specifically targeted prevention of VIN. VIN was postulated to be prevented as a beneficial "side effect" of ongoing vaccination for CIN and cervical cancer.[18,19] The 5-year follow-up of patients randomized to the quadrivalent HPV vaccine showed no cases of HPV-related CIN or external anogenital or vaginal disease in the treatment population.[17] Gardasil (Merck) is a prophylactic vaccine against four strains of HPV (6, 11, 16, and 18). As previously noted, the most common HPV type in VIN is HPV 16. Gardasil is currently recommended for women aged 9 to 26 who are not currently infected with HPV. For women already infected, a therapeutic vaccine would be necessary. Small trials of a therapeutic vaccine have shown promising results, but remain investigational.[20]

Unfortunately, there is no way to predict the behavior of a single lesion in your patient. Risk factors for progression include age greater than 40 and immunosuppression. The recommendations for observation alone in this subset of women are cautionary and patients must be reliable for follow-up. Recurrent VIN may occur years after treatment, especially in the immunosuppressed or radiated. Therefore treated patients should be educated that they should be screened for VIN for the long term.

Clinical Scenario 1

A 42-year-old female with a 20 pack-year history of smoking is concerned that she has a genital wart. On physical exam the patient is noted to have three lesions, two flesh-colored lesions on the left labia majora and one smaller periclitoral lesion.

What is the differential diagnosis?

While the patient's plaques could be genital condyloma, as she is concerned, these lesions could be VIN, vulvar carcinoma, or any of a variety of benign vulvar lesions. HPV-related VIN (classic or bowenoid type) has various appearances from erythematous to white, verruciform, polypoid, or papular and pigmented. Fifty-three percent to ninety percent of classic VIN lesions have HPV nucleic acids associated and therefore are associated with other HPV genital disease (genital warts, cervical dysplasia, etc).

What would you do to evaluate these lesions?

All patients who are symptomatic or have noted lesions should undergo a vulvar exam including evaluation of the vulva following the application of 4% acetic acid with gauze followed by inspection with a colposcope or a handheld magnifying glass. This technique was outlined in the background section.

Because of the possibility that these lesions represent VIN, at least one of the patient's lesions should be biopsied for a definitive diagnosis. Biopsy technique is important, as a poor-quality or tangentially cut biopsy can obscure the exact diagnosis.

How should the biopsy be performed?

Although the vulvar Pap smear has been studied as a screening modality, sensitivity is limited because of the keratinized upper layers of epidermis. Therefore, biopsy of suspicious lesions remains the gold standard for diagnosis. Vulvar biopsy is performed with a Keyes punch biopsy (4–6 mm) after injection of local anesthesia.[21] Others advocate use of an alligator-jaw instrument (often used for cervical biopsy). The danger with this method is that unless care is taken, only the superficial epithelium will be sampled.[3] Hemostasis of biopsy sites can be obtained with

Table 2.2 Surgical strategies for management of VIN

1. Excise whenever there is any question of possible invasion.
2. Excise lesions that may be easily closed primarily.
3. Laser-ablate multifocal lesions.
4. Laser-ablate lesions too large to close primarily.
5. Laser-ablate clitoral, urethral, or anal lesions.
6. In all cases a margin of at least 0.8 cm is advised.

Monsel's solution or silver nitrate, and occasionally a suture will be necessary. After undergoing biopsy, it is recommended that patients undergo pelvic rest and wait to bathe for 24 hours. No topical antibiotic ointments are necessary.

The biopsy returns as VIN III. No invasion is identified.

What treatment options would you consider for this patient?

Despite multiple trials, the most effective treatment for VIN has not been established. Surgical options, based on particular clinical circumstances, are outlined in Table 2.2. Retrospective studies suggest that surgical excision results in the best complete response rates (77%) as compared to ablational techniques such as laser therapy (21–33%) or topical immunotherapy (33%).[22] Surgical excision is often favored because the specimen may be completely studied for early invasive cancer and surgical margins may be evaluated. Superficial wide local excision with primary closure can be performed in most cases. More extensive lesions may require a split-thickness skin graft for closure.

The most important factor in surgical management, often difficult to obtain in women with multifocal disease, is negative surgical margins. When excision margins are positive, the recurrence was 2.5 times that of women with negative margins (46% vs. 17%).[22, 23] Should excision margins return positive for VIN, the patient does not need to undergo re-excision, but should be followed closely.

Local destruction using CO_2 laser is another therapeutic option. Hoffman and associates presented a case series of 18 women with VIN treated with laser vaporization. After single laser vaporization, 15 or 18 women remained free of recurrent disease, with a mean follow-up of 129.5 weeks.[24] However, studies comparing laser ablation with excisional methods demonstrated increased risk of recurrent disease in patients treated by laser vaporization alone.[25]

In non–hair-bearing areas, laser treatment should penetrate to 1 to 2 mm of depth. In hair-bearing areas, treatment must extend to 3 mm of depth to the base of the hair follicles. Given that it is impossible to measure the depth of treatment, surgeons should appreciate the deep dermal (yellow) layer. This usually is appreciated after wiping off the charred tissue. A margin of 1 cm is adequate. Complications reported with laser use include bleeding, pain, extensive scarring of the vulva, and fever. These are relatively uncommon, however, and there remains a role for this modality in the treatment of VIN. This is especially true in peri-urethral and peri-clitoral lesions, where excision may be surgically challenging and may compromise functional status.

Nonsurgical treatment

Other approaches to treating VIN include topical treatments. The Society of Gynecology Oncology list of treatment modalities included 5-FU topical therapy. Since that time other topical therapies have been studied. Imiquimod (Aldara) and 5 – FU are the most commonly utilized topical treatments.

Imidazoquinolones modulate cell-mediated immune response. The only imidazoquinolone currently available is imiquimod (Aldara; 3M Pharmaceuticals, Minneapolis). Imiquimod has been proven efficacious in the therapy of genital warts and now several studies have shown it to be effective in the treatment VIN. Van Seters and associates studied patients with VIN II-III and 81% of the patients treated with imiquimod experienced a reduction is lesion size by more than 25% at 20 weeks. Thirty-five percent of patients had a complete response at 20 weeks and were free of disease at 1 year. One patient progressed

to invasion (depth < 1 mm) at 12 months. HPV DNA was cleared in 58% of patients treated with imiquimod as compared to 8% of placebo patients. Similar results have been seen in other studies. No long-term studies have been performed to determine recurrence rates.[26] The regimen for treatment is a slow dose-escalation of 5% cream to the affected area once per week for 2 weeks, followed by 2 times per week for 2 weeks, and then 3 times per week for a total of 16 weeks. If 3 times/week dosing causes side effects, the dose can be reduced to twice weekly.

5-FU is a pyrimidine analogue that inhibits DNA synthesis and causes a chemical desquamation. While this treatment for VIN II-III has been shown to be reasonably effective, it has lost popularity due to its side effects (pain, blistering, and necrosis) and the inability of many patients to complete the prescribed course of treatment. If topical 5-FU 5% (Effudex cream) is chosen as a treatment, the commonly used regimens vary from one to three times per day application with duration from 7 days to 4 months. Given that frequent dosing will likely lead to patient self-discontinuation due to side effects, once to twice daily dosing for 3 to 6 weeks is likely most advisable.

Interferons have also been used topically and as intralesional injections. They have an antiviral and immunomodulatory effect. Interferon use has been shown to have a favorable response rate (30–40%); however, studies have been limited to small populations.[27] The regimen used by Spirtos and colleagues was a-IFN (10 ^ 6 IU/3 in 3.5% aqueous methylcellulose base) that patients applied 3 times daily until the lesions went away. In complete respondents, lesions disappeared by 4 months of treatment.

Clinical Scenario 2

A 35-year-old presents for repeat Pap smear. Six months ago she had a LGSIL pap smear, positive for high-risk HPV. She has a history of therapy for genital warts 10 years ago

Should this patient be evaluated for VIN?

This patient fits the risk profile of the younger patient with HPV-related dysplasias. Although the Pap smear and cervical colposcopy are the reason for her visit, as her physician you realize that she is at risk for developing VIN, and specifically inspect her vulva for a screening exam. No visible lesions are noted, and this is recorded in her record.

What if the patient had the above history as well as complaints of intense vulvar pruritis that had led to vulvar excoriation due to scratching?

The presence of inflammatory plaques of hyperkeratosis and diffuse erythema caused by chronic inflammation may obscure the recognition of VIN lesions. The itch–scratch cycle must be aborted prior to biopsy, because the biopsy from areas of inflammation will most often demonstrate acute and chronic inflammation with squamous hyperplasia or be diagnosed as VIN I. Topical steroids used for a short duration (2–4 weeks) will improve symptoms and vulvar inflammation, allowing an adequate evaluation for VIN. Please refer to the Chapter 1 for specific treatment recommendations. Ultimately this patient will need a vulvar biopsy to confirm the nature of her symptoms.

If the patient was pregnant and described multiple small raised purplish nodules affecting her anogenital area, what condition would you suspect and what treatment would you recommend?

Multicentric pigmented Bowen disease or bowenoid papulosis are terms used to describe these slightly raised, reddish-brown to violaceous papules. These lesions occur in young girls and older women. The mean affected age is 32 years. Approximately 10% of patients are pregnant at the time of diagnosis. These lesions have been described as self-regressing; however, the histologic findings often confirm the concomitant presence of dysplasia. We recommend biopsy and treatment as necessary, similar to other types of VIN.[14]

Clinical Scenario 3

A 43-year-old woman presents with vulvar pruritis. Vulvar exam with acetic acid application shows micropapillary changes with faint acetowhite staining of the posterior inner labia minora; biopsy returns VIN I.

What is the appropriate plan of therapy?

If the lesion noted and biopsied is the only abnormality noted, then the patient can be managed expectantly. In the new classification system VIN I was dropped and not felt to be a precursor of vulvar cancer, but rather HPV or reactive changes. The patient should undergo another exam in 6 to 12 months.

Clinical Scenario 4

A 29-year-old with prior condylomas treated several years ago presents with perineal pruritis and inspection reveals a 3 × 2-cm hypertrophic white plaque of the posterior intoitus at 5:00 and a similar 2 × 2-cm lesion at 7:00. Evaluation with 4% acetic acid reveals no other lesions. Biopsies of the noted lesions return VIN III. Cervical cytology is negative.

What treatment should the patient undergo?

The patient should undergo surgical excision or laser therapy, as invasion has been excluded.

Assuming that the patient has surgical excision and the margins are positive for VIN II-III, what should be done?

Positive margins are not ideal; however, do not mandate re-excision. As mentioned previously, the rate of recurrence in patients with positive margins is around 40%. The patient has a higher likelihood of recurrence of disease and can be offered close follow-up, versus re-excision, laser therapy, or topical agents.

Alternatively, what if the excision reveals focal invasion and negative margins?

Microinvasive squamous cell carcinoma of the vulva or stage Ia vulvar cancer is treated with local excision followed by observation. Stage Ia disease is defined as a lesion less than or equal to 2 cm in diameter on fresh specimen (specimens shrink on pathologic preparation), less than or equal to 1 mm of invasion (invasion is defined from the epithelial–stromal junction at the most superficial adjacent dermal papilla to the deepest point of invasion) with no lymphovascular space invasion.

If the excised lesion met the above criteria, then the patient can be followed with vulvar exams every 3 to 4 months for 4 years. While it is reasonable for patients to be followed by a general gynecologist, often patients wish an oncology consultation.

Clinical Scenario 5

A 40-year-old patient presents with diffuse VIN III found on multiple biopsies involving the entire labia minora and perineum (Plate 2.1).

What is the appropriate management?

For large areas of disease, the options for treatment include ablation with a CO_2 laser or a skinning vulvectomy with split-thickness skin grafting. Laser therapy might require more than one session given the extent of disease and would likely be quite painful for the patient. Surgical excision would not allow primary closure and therefore consideration of a split-thickness skin graft would need to be planned. While few general gynecologists are trained in skin grafting, joint treatment with plastic surgery can be arranged. Alternatively some gynecologic oncologists have been trained in skin grafting, and such patients could be referred to a trained specialist.

Are any nonsurgical options available to this patient?

This patient could also be treated initially with topical agents as outlined in Clinical Scenario 1. Topical agents may be curative, but would more likely reduce the lesion size and extent, allowing for a smaller surgical excision or laser treatment. Topical therapy is often poorly tolerated and therefore is rarely used with extensive lesions.

Clinical Scenario 6

A 50-year-old Caucasian female presents with localized vulvar pruritis and burning. On exam you note a 4-cm lesion with a patchy, velvet-like, reddish and whitish appearance (Plate 2.2).

What is your differential diagnosis of this lesion?

Differential diagnosis includes Paget's disease, melanoma, leukoplakia, basal cell or squamous cell carcinoma, condyloma acuminata, hidradenitis suppurativa, psoriasis, fungal infection, seborrheic or contact dermatitis, and lichen sclerosis.

A biopsy is obtained and is reported to demonstrate extramammary Paget's, disease.

What additional care does this patient require?

Surgical excision with wide margins should be undertaken. Commonly the lesions extend beyond the clinically apparent margins. Recurrences develop in 28% to 38% of patients after surgery, and more than half of these women develop recurrence within 18 months of initial treatment.

Is there any way to assure a negative margin?

Negative margins can be evaluated by obtaining frozen pathologic section at the time of excision, although Paget cells are often found well away from the clinically obvious lesion.

Is there an association with invasive vulvar cancer?

Paget's disease is associated with concurrent, invasive vulvar cancer in 4% to 15% of cases. Women with Paget's disease of the vulva should also be evaluated for Paget's synchronous neoplasms, as approximately 20% to 30% of these patients have a noncontiguous carcinoma (eg, involving breast, rectum, bladder, urethra, cervix, or ovary).[8–13]

What is the prognosis for patients with Paget's disease?

The overall prognosis is good unless there is an underlying invasive carcinoma. In patients with invasive disease, however, there is a high rate of nodal metastasis, recurrence, and death from disease. Paget's disease of the vulva is also associated with malignancies at other sites. An estimated 30% have synchronous or metasynchronous malignancies at other sites, most commonly breast, rectum, cervix, uterus, bladder, and skin. It is recommended that patients diagnosed with Paget's disease of the vulva should undergo careful breast screening and thorough recto-vaginal exam, and be made aware of the possibility of carcinoma at other sites so that appropriate screening is undertaken.[8] Patients with lesions involving the anus or urethra in particular should be evaluated with colonoscopy or cystocopy, respectively, to exclude synchronous malignancies of adjacent organs.

Clinical Scenario 7

An 80-year-old female presents for her annual exam and mentions that she is having genital itching. On the external pelvic exam, she has a unifocal raised irregular lesion on the perineum, as well as atrophic hypopigmented areas consistent with LSA. You perform a biopsy of the raised lesion which returns as VIN III.[5]

What is the most likely subtype of VIN III in this patient?

Given the patient's age and associated lichen sclerosis, the VIN III identified in this patient is likely simplex or differentiated type. Although rare, it is most common in the postmenopausal woman and is often associated with squamous cell carcinoma of the vulva.

What treatment modality is most appropriate for this patient? Should you refer this patient?

This patient should undergo surgical excision of the lesion. She has a substantial risk of having an invasive lesion, which would first be identified by excision and then further surgery performed based on the depth of invasion and size and location of the lesion. The initial excision need not be performed by a sub-specialist; however, care must be made to obtain grossly negative margins.

Clinical Scenario 8

A 55-year-old woman with a recent diagnosis of VIN II-III on vulvar biopsy returns to discuss biopsy results and treatment options.

What are the treatment options for this patient?

A number of medical and surgical treatment options exist for VIN (HPV related). However, invasive disease must be excluded initially **before initiating any therapy.** In a study of 73 women with VIN III on biopsy treated with surgical resection reported by Modesitt and associates, 22% had an underlying squamous vulvar cancer.[22] For patients whose specimen showed residual VIN III at the surgical margins, 46% recurred compared to 17% of patients with negative margins.

What is your response to the patient's query regarding the likelihood of progression to invasive squamous cell carcinoma of the vulva?

The clinical behavior of VIN varies. Seven percent to thirty-two percent of cases recur locally or persist after local excision/total vulvectomy. Some lesions will spontaneously regress after biopsy. Occult invasion is noted in 6% to 7% of excised specimens. Three percent to ten percent of patients treated for classic VIN ultimately develop invasive squamous cell carcinoma. Unfortunately, there is no way to predict the behavior of a single lesion. Risk factors for progression include age greater than 40, immunosuppression, and smoking.

What is your recommended treatment for this patient?

Given the patient's age and her concern about carcinoma, recommendation for surgical excision gives her the highest likelihood of cure and identification of invasive disease.

Clinical Scenario 9

A 27-year-old female presents for evaluation of new vulvar lesions. On examination, it appears that she has multiple vulvar condylomata. All are 2 to 3 cm in dimension. You prescibe management with a course of imiquimod (Aldara) and she returns in 8 weeks for reevaluation. At her return appointment all of her condylomatous lesions have regressed.

Is any additional evaluation recommended before initiating imiquimod therapy?

A speculum examination and thorough pelvic examination should be performed. Because this patient is presenting with multifocal lower genital tract condylomata, she should undergo screening for other sexually transmitted diseases (GC, *Chlamydia*) and should be offered HIV screening. If any of the lesions have an atypical appearance, biopsies should be performed. Cervical cytology should be performed.

What follow-up should the patient have?

This patient should be followed for vulvar dysplasia. Frequent, careful vulvar exams should be performed every 6 months. Because she has had HPV-related disease, she should be screened for cervical dysplasia according to ACOG guidelines.

What education should she have regarding her risk of vulvar dysplasia?

It is crucial that her risk for development of vulvar dysplasia be recognized and that she be made aware of this. The patient should be educated to report new vulvar lesions to her primary care physician. If dysplasia is identified, the primary physician has the responsibility to treat or refer for consultation and management.

References

1. Judson PL, Habermann EB, Baxter NN, Durham SB, Virnig BA. Trends in the incidence of invasive and in situ vulvar carcinoma. *Obstet Gynecol.* 2006;107:1018–1022.
2. Buscema J, Naghashfar Z, Sawada E, Daniel R, Woodruff JD, Shah K. The predominance of human papillomavirus type 16 in vulvar neoplasia. *Obstet Gynecol.* 1988;71:601–606.
3. Creasman WT. Preinvasive disease of the vagina and vulva and related disorders. In: DiSai PJ, Creasman WT, eds. *Clinical Gynecologic Oncology.* 7th ed. 2007:37–54.
4. Sideri M, Jones R, Wilkinson E, et al. Squamous vulvar intraepithelial neoplasia: 2004 modified terminology, ISSVD Vulvar Oncology Subcommittee. *J Reprod Med.* 2005;50:807–810.
5. van Seters M, van Beurden M, de Craen AJ. Is the assumed natural history of vulvar intraepithelial neoplasia III based on enough evidence? A systematic review of 3322 published patients. *Gynecol Oncol.* 2005;97:645–651.

6. Hart WR. Vulvar intraepithelial neoplasia: historical aspects and current status. *Int J Gynecol Pathol.* 2001:20;16–30.

7. Yang B, Hart WR. Vulvar intraepithelial neoplasia of the simplex (differentiated) type: a clincopathologic study including analysis of HPV and p53 expression. *Am J Surg Pathol.* 2000;24:429–441.

8. Tebes S, Cardosi R, Hoffman M. Paget's disease of the vulva. *Am J Obstet Gynecol.* 2002;187:281–284.

9. Parker LP, Parker JR, Bodurka-Bevers D, et al. Paget's disease of the vulva: pathology, pattern of involvement and prognosis. *Gynecol Oncol.* 2000;77:183.

10. Shepherd V, Davidson EJ, Davies-Humphreys J. Extramammary Paget's disease. *BJOG.* 2005;112:273.

11. Fanning J, Lambert HC, Hale TM, et al. Paget's disease of the vulva: prevalence of associated vulvar adenocarcinoma, invasive Paget's disease and recurrence after surgical excision. *Am J Obstet Gynecol.* 1999;180:24.

12. Feuer GA, Sheychuk M, Calanog A. Vulvar Paget's disease: the need to exclude an invasive lesion. *Gynecol Oncol.* 1990;38:81.

13. Black D, Tornos C, Soslow RA, Awtrey CS, Barakat RR, Chi DS. The outcomes of patients with positive margins after excision for intraepithelial Paget's disease of the vulva. *Gynecol Oncol.* 2007;104:547–550.

14. Jones RW, Rowan DM, Stewart AW. Vulvar intraepithelial neoplasia: aspects of the natural history and outcome in 405 women. *Obstet Gynecol.* 2005;106:1319–1326.

15. Jones RW, Rowan DM. Spontaneous regression of vulvar intraepithelial neoplasia 2-3. *Obstet Gynecol.* 2000;96:470–472.

16. Fu YS. *Pathology of the Uterine Cervix, Vagina and Vulva.* 2nd ed. 2002:168–231.

17. Society of Gynecologic Oncologists Medical Practice and Ethics Committee. *SGO Clinical Practice Guidelines: Management of Gynecologic Cancers.* Chicago: Society of Gynecologic Oncologists; October 1996.

18. Hampl M, Sarajuuri H, Wentzensen N, et al. Effect of human papillomavirus vaccines on vulvar, vaginal, and anal intraepithelial lesions and vulvar cancer. *Obstet Gynecol.* 2006;108:1361.

19. Srodon M, Stoler MH, Baber GB, Kurman RJ. The distribution of low and high-risk HPV types in vulvar and vaginal intraepithelial neoplasia (VIN and VAIN). *Am J Surg Pathol.* 2006;30:1513.

20. Davidson EJ, Faulkner RL, Sehr P, et al. Effect of TA-CIN (HPV 16 L2E6E7) booster immunisation in vulval intraepithelial neoplasia patients previously vaccinated with TA-HPV (vaccinia virus encoding HPV 16/18 E6E7). *Vaccine.* 2004;22:2722–2729.

21. Bae-Jump VL, Bauer M, Van Le L. Cytological evaluation correlates poorly with histological diagnosis of vulvar neoplasias. *J Low Genit Tract Dis.* 2007;11:8–11.

22. Modesitt SC, Waters AB, Walton L, Fowler WC, Van le L. Vulvar intraepithelial neoplasia III: occult cancer and the impact of margin status on recurrence. *Obstet Gynecol.* 1998;92:962–966.

23. Heaps JM, Fu JS, Montz FJ, et al. Surgical-pathologic variables predictive of local recurrence in squamous cell carcinoma of the vulva. *Gynecol Oncol.* 1990;38:309–314.

24. Hoffman MS, Pinelli DM, Finan M, et al. Laser vaporization for vulvar intraepithelial neoplasia III. *J Reprod Med.* 1992;37:135.

25. Leuchler RS, Townsend DE, Hacker NF, et al. Treatment of vulvar carcinoma in situ with the CO_2 laser. *Gynecol Oncol.* 1984;19:214.

26. Van Seters M, van Buerden M, ten Kate FJW, et al. Treatment of vulvar intraepithelial neoplasia with topical imiquimod. *N Engl J Med.* 2008;358:1465–1473.

27. Spirtos NM, Smith LH, Teng NN. Prospective randomized trial of topical alpha-interferon (alpha-interferon gels) for the treatment of vulvar intraepithelial neoplasia III. *Gynecol Oncol.* 1990;37:34–38.

28. Sillman FH, Sedlis A, Boyce JG. A review of lower genital intraepithelial neoplasia and the use of topical 5-fluorouracil. *Obstet Gynecol Surv.* 1985;40:190.

29. Krupp PJ. 5-fluorouracil topical treatment of in situ vulvar cancer. *Obstet Gynecol.* 1978;51:702.

CHAPTER 3

Vaginal Intraepithelial Neoplasia

Leigh A. Cantrell, MD, MSPH
Department of Obstetrics and Gynecology, University of North Carolina School of Medicine, Chapel Hill, NC, USA

Linda Van Le, MD, FACOG
Department of Obstetrics and Gynecology, University of North Carolina School of Medicine, Chapel Hill, NC, USA

Pathology Notes: Chad Livasy, MD
Associate Professor, Department of Pathology and Laboratory Medicine, University of North Carolina School of Medicine, Chapel Hill, NC, USA

Squamous vaginal intraepithelial neoplasia (VAIN) is rare, with an estimated annual incidence of 0.2 to 2 per 100,000 women. VAIN was first described in 1952 by Graham and Meigs, when they observed neoplastic vaginal changes in women who had undergone hysterectomy for carcinoma in situ (CIS) of the cervix.[1] Its invasive counterpart, primary vaginal cancer, is equally rare, and accounts for only 1% to 4% of malignant tumors of the female reproductive tract. The National Cancer Institute estimates that there will be 2160 cases of vaginal cancer and 770 deaths in the year 2009 in the United States.[2] Squamous cell carcinomas account for 90% to 95% of primary vaginal cancers. It should be recognized that most vaginal malignancies are secondary neoplasms, arising from adjacent organs via direct extension or lymphatic or hematogenous spread, with the cervix, endometrium, and colon/rectum being the most common primary sites of malignancies involving the vagina.[3]

Risk factors

VAIN usually occurs in women 40 to 60 years of age. Risk factors for developing VAIN include residual dysplasia after treatment (loop electrosurgical excision procedure or cryotherapy) or removal (hysterectomy) of the cervix for squamous intraepithelial lesions, a history of human papilloma virus (HPV) infection, prior radiation therapy, DES exposure, or previous cervical dysplasia or cancer. HPV infection seems to be the primary causative agent. Over three-fourths of women diagnosed with VAIN have a history of cervical dysplasia or cancer of the vulva or cervix, implicating the "field effect" of an HPV infection in the squamous epithelium of the entire lower genital tract. Prior pelvic radiation is also a risk factor for VAIN. This may be due to recurrence of prior cervical or vaginal cancer or secondary to radiation changes in the vaginal tissues.[4,5] Patients with a history of radiation therapy for cervical cancer preceding a diagnosis of VAIN are in general older than the typical patient with VAIN.[3] Smoking, immunocompromise

Gynecological Cancer Management: Identification, Diagnosis and Treatment, Edited by Daniel L. Clarke-Pearson and John T. Soper. Published 2010 by Blackwell Publishing, ISBN: 978-1-4051-9079-4.

(such as in women following renal transplantation or those with prior chemotherapy), and chronic irritation associated with pessary use also increase the risk of developing VAIN.

A high proportion of women diagnosed with VAIN also carry high-risk HPV types (16, 18, 31, 33, 35, 45, 51, 56, 58, and 59). Similar to CIN and VIN, VAIN lesions have been shown to have a high rate of incorporation of high-risk HPV types. Persistent infection with high-risk HPV types has been shown to be an essential, although not exclusive, factor in the pathogenesis of anogenital cancers. HPV infection leads to incorporation of two HPV genes, E6 and E7, into the host genome. E6 and E7 interfere with normal cell control mechanisms, including apoptosis and chromosomal stability.[6] Sugase and Matsukura documented the presence of HPV DNA in 71 vaginal specimens of VAIN.[7] Given the lower rate of VAIN, compared to VIN or CIN, there is overall a lower rate of HPV infection of the vaginal tissues. This may be related to the lack of an active transformation zone in vaginal mucosa and less potential for inflammation, compared to cervical and vulvar tissues. HPV types with a preference for the infection of vaginal tissues may also be less oncogenic.[8] The high-risk HPV 16 strain is most commonly identified, and is isolated in approximately 52% of VAIN lesions.[6] Ninety percent of high-grade lesions are associated with high-risk HPV (unadjusted OR = 5.01), although 64% of low-grade VAIN lesions also are associated with high-risk HPV types. High-risk HPV types are not associated with recurrence of VAIN after treatment.[6]

Smoking further increases the risk of VAIN in patients with oncogenic HPV subtypes. There was no difference in the rate of high-risk HPV infection between smokers and nonsmokers. Among patients infected with a high-risk HPV type, however, smoking increases the risk of having a high-grade VAIN (83% versus 59%, $p = 0.02$). Neither smoking nor high-risk HPV type increases the risk of recurrence.[9] Other researchers have shown that the risk of vaginal cancer increased as the number of cigarettes a patient had per day increased, and that the risk decreased once a patient stopped smoking.[10]

Prevention

A phase II trial evaluated the safety and efficacy of a candidate therapeutic vaccine against HPV in 12 women (aged 42–54) with VIN (N = 11) or VAIN (N = 1) who were also positive for high-risk HPV subtypes. Participants received a live recombinant vaccinia virus with E6 and E7 open reading frames from HPV-16 and HPV-18. All participants had high-grade lesions and results suggested a positive effect of the therapeutic vaccine on lesion size. Further study is needed in this area to validate a therapeutic role for vaccine therapy.[11]

Prophylactic vaccination with Gardasil (a quadrivalent vaccine against HPV types 6, 11, 16, and 18) has also been studied with regard to cervical dysplasia and cervical cancer. It is logical that the use of prophylactic HPV vaccination for the prevention of HPV-related disease will have an impact on the incidence of VAIN, especially since the most common isolated HPV subtype is 16. Indeed, the 5-year follow up of patients randomized to the quadrivalent HPV vaccine for prevention of cervical dysplasia and cancer has supported this logic and showed no cases of HPV-related CIN or external anogenital or vaginal disease in the treated protocol population.[12]

Diethylstilbestrol exposure

Intraepithelial dysplasia of glandular origin, or atypical vaginal adenosis, is a separate entity from VAIN. Vaginal adenosis has a well-established association with in utero diethylstilbestrol (DES) exposure. Notably, intrauterine exposure to this synthetic estrogen also predisposes women to a higher rate of VAIN due to abnormal location of the transformation zone, which extends into the vagina in 30% to 40% of DES-exposed women. Administration of DES prior to the 18th week of gestation can lead to the disruption of the normal transformation of Müllerian columnar epithelium to stratified squamous epithelium. Retention of the Müllerian epithelium leads to adenosis, which has a variety of manifestations. These include glandular cells replacing the squamous vaginal lining, glandular cells beneath an intact squamous vaginal lining, or an area of squamous metaplasia when new squamous cells attempt to replace glandular cells. Additionally, 20% of women exposed to DES have anatomic deformities of the upper vagina and cervix that can make the boundaries of the vagina and cervix difficult to ascertain.

DES exposure increases the risk for clear cell adenocarcinoma up to age 40 through unknown mechanisms. The incidence of clear cell adenocarcinoma is 1 per 1000 by age 40, with the peak incidence between ages 15 and 25. The risk of clear cell carcinoma or other malignancies in women older than 40 is still unknown, because these women are only now approaching menopause. Other abnormalities associated with DES exposure include vaginal adenosis, cockscomb cervix, cervical collar, and a transverse vaginal septum.[13, 14]

DES exposure increases the occurrence of vaginal dysplasia slightly (1.3–4.8%). The highest risk is in women whose mother received DES before 12 weeks of gestation. In general, most dysplasia occurs in the cervix rather than the vagina. However, the increased rate of VAIN dictates that DES-exposed patients should undergo close follow-up with regular cervical and vaginal cytology and colposcopy of the cervix and vagina at least yearly.[2]

VAIN diagnosis

Criteria for a cytologic diagnosis of VAIN are described according to the Bethesda system and are defined by squamous cell atypia without invasion. Classification is similar to that used for the cervix. A histologic diagnosis of VAIN is made based on the degree of cellular differentiation, maturation sequence, mitotic activity and nuclear atypia. VAIN I comprises mild dysplasia, with maintenance of the normal maturation pattern from parabasal to superficial layers with atypical cells in the lower one-third. VAIN II is moderate dysplasia, and normal cellular maturation is maintained in the upper third of the epithelium; however, in the lower two-thirds of the epithelium there is greater cell proliferation and higher mitotic activity. VAIN III constitutes severe dysplasia or CIS, in which immature cells with scanty cytoplasm and mitotic figures have a disordered arrangement throughout the epithelium. In severe dysplasia there is very little or absent squamous differentiation.[15]

Clinical presentation

Most patients with VAIN are asymptomatic and do not have a grossly visible lesion. In the uncommon scenario when gross lesions are present however, they may be raised, white, or pink. They are often multifocal in nature and it is important to examine the entire vagina. Infrequent symptoms include postcoital spotting, pruritis, burning, leucorrhea, and dyspareunia. Abnormal cytology is the most common means by which VAIN is diagnosed. VAIN usually occurs in the upper vagina or apex and is often associated with cervical or vulvar dysplasia. Care should be taken to evaluate the entire vagina, as multifocal disease is very common and treatment will only be successful if all lesions are removed.

Treatment

Given the rarity of disease, treatment of VAIN has been studied retrospectively. There are a paucity of prospective data and currently no prospective randomized trials that have established the best treatment modality. Therefore treatment options are based on what has worked in patient case series. Treatment options include surgical resection, laser ablation, and application of topical agents. If the lesion is isolated, surgical resection appears to be associated with the lowest recurrence rate among treatment options.

In treatment planning, several factors should be considered, including prior treatment failures, the patient's medical risks, desire for sexual function after treatment, and the certainty with which invasive disease has been excluded. Low-grade VAIN appears to have a regression rate of up to 78% in observational studies.[3] Conversely, VAIN III lesions have a higher rate of underlying invasive disease and disease progression; this should be taken into consideration during treatment planning.[3] Excision with subsequent pathologic evaluation rather than ablation or topical therapy is therefore preferable in most patients with unifocal high-grade VAIN lesions. However, VAIN is often a multifocal disease, which requires treatment of the entire vaginal canal. In this setting, surgical excision is less effective and also exceedingly morbid.

Radiation

In the past, radiation therapy was utilized in the treatment of VAIN. It is rarely used for this purpose today given the number of other options available and possible side effects of vaginal stricture, vaginal mucosal changes, and rectal or bladder symptoms. In a retrospective study of 13 Japanese patients treated with intracavitary brachytherapy for VAIN III after hysterectomy, all were free of disease at 127 months of follow-up. Observed side effects included rectal bleeding, hematuria, and vaginal mucosal changes in 3 of the 13 patients.[16]

Pathology notes

The histologic appearance and grading scheme for VAIN parallels that of CIN: VAIN I (mild squamous dysplasia), VAIN II (moderate squamous dysplasia), and VAIN III (severe squamous dysplasia). The grading of SIL (HSIL, LSIL) in vaginal Pap smears is also the same as cervix. Many of the patients with VAIN also have a history of CIN. The ratio of LSIL:HSIL observed in vaginal dysplasia is approximately 3:1. The natural history of VAIN is not well studied, but the peak incidence of vaginal squamous cell carcinoma is significantly later in life than for cervical squamous cell carcinoma. VAIN has been shown to be associated with HPV infection and the same risk factors as CIN. HPV infections may present as either flat condyloma or exophytic condyloma (HPV subtypes 6 and 11). One benign condition not to be confused with HPV infection is vestibular papillomatosis. This finding is typically seen in reproductive-aged patients and presents as multiple small polypoid excrescences involving the introitus. Biopsy specimens from these specimens reveal benign squamous papillomas without evidence of HPV infection.

Interpretation of vaginal biopsies and Pap smears may be complicated in postmenopausal patients with atrophic vaginitis and in patients with a prior history of radiation therapy. The combination of atrophy and inflammation may result in cytologic changes to cells that can mimic HSIL or even carcinoma. The pathologist may suggest brief treatment with hormones such as topical estrogen to diminish the atrophic changes and repeating the Pap smear in a short interval. If dysplasia is present, the atypical cells will persist following hormone treatment. For patients with a prior history of radiation therapy, it is important to communicate this important piece of information to the pathologist on the cytology request form. Radiation therapy induces several changes to cells that mimic LSIL. Radiation-induced changes can even be confused with carcinoma if the pathologist is not aware of a patient's prior history of radiation therapy. For biopsy specimens in patients with atrophic atypia or radiation atypia, immunohistochemical stains such as p16 and Ki-67 can be employed to exclude dysplasia. Currently, such ancillary tests are not available for vaginal Pap smears, but HPV testing can be very helpful in cases where atypia of uncertain significance is present.

Primary malignant vaginal tumors are usually squamous cell carcinoma (85%) and most occur in the 6th and 7th decades of life. Most vaginal squamous cell carcinomas appear histologically similar to those seen in the cervix. One particular variant of squamous cell carcinoma, papillary squamous cell carcinoma, is seen more commonly in the vagina and is characterized by a pushing margin of invasion and prominent papillary architecture. This subtype is worth mentioning because of the difficulty associated with confirming

Pathology notes (*continued*)

stromal invasion in biopsy specimens from these tumors. Superficial biopsies from these biopsies often return as VAIN III. Another rare variant of squamous cell carcinoma, verrucous carcinoma, can also be seen involving the vagina. Verrucous carcinoma is also particularly challenging to recognize in superficial biopsies due to its bland cytology and pushing margin of invasion.

Vaginal adenocarcinomas may be primary or metastatic, with most cases representing metastasis from endocervix, endometrium, ovary, or colorectum. It is the pathologist's task to work up vaginal adenocarcinoma to determine, if possible, whether the tumor represents a primary case or a metastasis. Variants observed in primary vaginal adenocarcinoma include endometrioid adenocarcinoma (may be seen in association with endometriosis), mucinous adenocarcinoma with or without intestinal differentiation, adenosquamous, serous adenocarcinoma, clear cell adenocarcinoma, and adenoid cystic carcinoma. Clear cell adenocarcinoma of the vagina is rare in women without a history of in utero DES exposure.

Clinical Scenario 1

A 50-year-old woman presents for an annual exam. She had a hysterectomy 8 years ago for persistent cervical intraepithelial neoplasia and asks if she should continue to have a vaginal Pap smear.

What is your response to the patient?

This patient is at risk for vaginal and vulvar dysplasia. A significant risk factor is a history of hysterectomy for cervical neoplasia and probable HPV infection. The patient is at risk of developing vaginal neoplasia and should be screened annually.

Conversely, most women have had a hysterectomy for other indications and should not continue to need Pap smears of the vagina. Current guidelines for vaginal pap smears state that cytology is not indicated after hysterectomy for benign disease unless the woman has a history of cervical dysplasia, DES exposure, or is immunosuppressed.

What will your examination consist of?

The cytologic exam should include sampling of the vaginal apex and sidewalls. On palpation, attention should be paid to the presence or absence of vaginal nodularity and induration. These findings should be documented.

When should a patient be referred to a specialist?

Referral of a patient with biopsy-proven VAIN should be made if a physician is not experienced in treating these patients.

What is the risk of progression to invasive vaginal carcinoma?

VAIN I has a high regression rate of approximately 78% to 88%. However, VAIN III can be associated with underlying invasive disease and demonstrates higher rates of progression to cancer (8%) and recurrence after treatment.[3]

What is the role of the primary care physician in caring for patients with VAIN?

The main role of the primary care physician is to be aware of the risk factors for development of VAIN and to evaluate patients appropriately. Once abnormal cytology is obtained, the physician should proceed with colposcopy or refer the patient for colposcopic exam by another provider.

What historical question should be asked of all patients born between 1938 and 1971?

Exposure status to DES in utero should be ascertained in all women born within this time-frame, as their risk of cervical and vaginal cancer places them into a unique screening group. The CDC website offers excellent information for patients and physicians (http://www.cdc.gov/DES).

Clinical Scenario 2

A 45-year-old presented several weeks ago for annual examination. She underwent hysterectomy for CIN 10 years ago and recent vaginal cytology returned HSIL. She returns to your office for further evaluation.

What evaluation should be performed?

Once a cytologic diagnosis of VAIN is made, colposcopic evaluation is recommended. In general, vaginal colposcopy is more difficult to perform than cervical colposcopy due to the presence of vaginal rugae and abnormal recesses at the cuff after hysterectomy. Colposcopy should be performed using the largest speculum the patient will tolerate followed by application of 4% acetic acid. (Plate 3.1). If the limits of a vaginal lesion cannot be appreciated with the colposcope and 4% acetic acid, then iodine staining (Schiller or Lugol solution) can assist in visualization.

Use of Lugol solution allows for visualization of lesions more rapidly than other methods, as lesions appear as nonstaining areas and are more apparent among the vaginal rugae. Lugol solution stains normal squamous cells dark brown as abundant intracellular glycogen will take up iodine. Nonglycogenated cells (including most dysplasic cells with large nuclei and smaller amounts of cytoplasm, non-neoplastic glandular cells, and squamous cells in atrophic mucosa) will not take up iodine and remain light yellow or white, making the lesions to distinguish from the surrounding normal tissue (Plate 16.2). In postmenopausal women, pretreatment with vaginal estrogen (Premarin cream nightly) for 3 to 4 weeks will improve the glycogen content of atrophic mucosa, improving the sensitivity of both colposcopy and Lugol staining.

If the patient is allergic to iodine, a 1% aqueous solution of toluidine blue can alternatively be utilized for visualization. The solution is applied to the vagina, allowed to dry for several minutes, and then washed with a 1% to 2% acetic acid solution. Suspected areas of VAIN will stain blue. Unfortunately a high false-positive rate is noted with this method, as areas of inflammation, non-neoplastic ulceration, or excoriation will have high uptake of blue stain. False-negative results are also noted in hyperkeratotic lesions because little dye is absorbed through the layer of hyperkeratotic epithelium. After hysterectomy, lesions in the recesses of the vaginal cuff may be difficult to visualize by any of these techniques.

All visualized acetowhite lesions, and in particular lesions with abnormal vascularity (mosaicism or punctuation), should be biopsied. Multiple small biopsies can be obtained with alligator-jaw forceps. A skin hook may be useful for manipulating the vaginal wall to allow visualization in vaginal folds or recesses caused by scarring from prior hysterectomy. VAIN is more often multifocal than CIN, and a thorough exam of the entire vagina must be undertaken when one lesion is identified. The cervix (if present) and vulva should also be evaluated to exclude concurrent lesions. A thorough digital exam should also be performed to examine for thickening, irregularity, or nodularity, and results should be included in documentation of the vaginal evaluation.[9]

In this patient colposopy identifies a 3 × 3-cm lesion in the posterior fornix which is faint white in color. Topical benzocaine is applied and a biopsy is obtained. The pathology report is consistent with mild dysplasia (VAIN I).

What are the treatment options for VAIN I? Does it need to be treated?

Low-grade VAIN appears to have a high regression rate in observational studies (78%), with

9% progression to invasive cancer and 13% persistent disease.[3] Many treatment options for VAIN have been studied, but due to the rarity of disease, most are retrospective, and therefore recommendations for the best therapy are limited. Observation or topical therapy for VAIN I would likely be sufficient; however, laser treatment or superficial excision could be considered, especially if the patient had a large or symptomatic lesion. In this case, a 3 × 3 cm lesion will be most quickly treated with a laser.

Office loop excision was described as a novel approach to treatment of VAIN in 1999 by Fanning and colleagues.[17] The initial description was in 15 patients who underwent office loop excision followed by postoperative 5FU in those with VAIN III.[17] Massad described the use of loop excision for women with unifocal or clustered multifocal VAIN lesions.[18] After local lidocaine was injected into the lesion to raise the vaginal epithelium from the underlying tissue, a 7 × 10-mm loop was used to remove the lesion with cutting current at 50 W. Defects healed secondarily. Women undergoing a loop excision of VAIN had low recurrence or progression rates, and this appears to be a safe, effective method of treatment.[18] Caution should be exercised when resecting lesions adjacent to the bladder and rectum, to avoid deep resection below the level of the endopelvic fascia, because there have been anecdotal reports of fistulas after loop excisions of vaginal lesions.

Carbon dioxide laser therapy has mixed results for treatment of VAIN, likely due to differences in depth of treatment and adequate visualization of all lesions in the vagina. At least one quarter of all patients undergoing laser therapy will need additional therapy. Overall laser therapy is well tolerated and heals well, with little sexual dysfunction. Laser therapy requires that the lesion be easily visualized and that invasion is not suspected. Colposcopic control for laser ablation of the vagina is recommended. The use of skin hooks during surgery facilitates visualization of lesions that extend into vaginal recesses. It is recommended that laser ablations are carried to a depth of 1.5 to 2 mm using continuous mode at a power density of 750 to 1000 W/mm^2. Retrospective studies have reported curative rates as high as 69%,[19] with recurrence rates of up to 38%.[20]

What treatment options are recommended if the biopsy of this lesion is VAIN II-III?

For higher grades of VAIN, surgical excision is recommended both as the primary treatment and to confirm the absence of an invasive vaginal cancer.

Surgical excision of a focal lesion at the vaginal cuff is usually done in the operating room under regional or general anesthesia. Once adequate anesthesia is achieved, the patient is placed in lithotomy position. After gentle prep of the vagina is performed, either colposcopy is performed or Lugol solution is placed to identify the area to be excised. After infiltrating the vaginal mucosa with 1% xylocaine/epinephrine, a circumferential mucosal incision with a scalpel (#15 blade) is made around the lesion. Next, the vaginal mucosa is dissected away from the endopelvic fascia with Metzenbaum or Struli scissors. Placement of a suture in the incised margin may provide better traction for dissection rather than using toothed forceps for manipulating the lesion, which might denude the mucosa by repetitive grasping. Individual bleeding sites are addressed either by placing hemostatic sutures or cauterization. Closure of the defect is left to the surgeon's discretion, but often these are able to heal spontaneously without the need for closure. Care must be taken to avoid excessive traction or electrocautery of the specimen to allow adequate pathology assessment. Possible surgical complications include hemorrhage, shortening of the vagina, or damage to bladder and/or rectum.

In a retrospective study of 105 patients who underwent partial vaginectomy for the treatment of high-grade VAIN, 12% had an underlying malignancy, 22% had negative findings on final pathology, and 88% remained without recurrence during a mean follow-up of 25 months.[21] Other retrospective series have noted short-term cure rates between 68% and 83%. A longer-term retrospective study reported a 34% recurrence rate and 66% disease-free status at 44 months after surgical resection.[22]

Clinical Scenario 3

A 38-year-old woman presents for evaluation of a low-grade squamous intraepithelial lesion (LGSIL). She has 15 to 20 colposcopically identified lesions measuring 5 to 10 mm that had the colposcopic appearance of flat condylomata, distributed from the upper fornices to the lower one-third of the vagina. She had a renal transplant 4 years ago and is maintained on cyclosporine and prednisone. She underwent a vaginal hysterectomy 10 years ago for benign disease, but the pathology report from hysterectomy was not available. Multiple biopsies returned VAIN I-II.

What treatment modalities might be considered in this patient?

Surgical options would be limited in this patient. Given chronic immunosuppression, her likelihood of spontaneous regression would be less than expected in immunocompetent patients, and she would likely be at an increased risk for progression to invasive disease. Total vaginectomy with reconstruction using spit-thickness skin grafts would be a potentially morbid procedure. Laser vaporization of the entire vagina would have a high risk of recurrence and would be quite morbid.

Topical therapies would be the first consideration for this patient. Topical 5-fluorouracil (5-FU) and imiquimod have been studied in the treatment of VAIN. Topical treatments are relatively inexpensive compared to surgical modalities. They hypothetically permeate vaginal mucosa and recesses well, which is beneficial in multifocal disease. Topical therapy is often the choice for poor surgical candidates, and may be ideal for women with larger low-grade lesions or

Table 3.1 5 Flurouricil (5-FU/Effudex) treatment regimens for treatment of VAIN (apply 1 g with vaginal applicator)

Cycle Length	Daily Application(s)
14 days (repeat for 2 or more cycles)	Once-daily application
7–14 days	Twice-daily application
8–12 weeks	2–3 times per week application

multifocal disease. Remission of VAIN lesions occurs in about 60% of patients, though up to 40% of patients may recur.[23–26]

5-fluorouracil (5-FU)

There are several treatment regimens that have been described for 5-FU treatment of VAIN. Topical 5-FU usually given as a dose of 1 to 1.5 g is applied via vaginal suppository or cream, although the FDA has not approved 5-FU for intravaginal application. A variety of treatment durations and schemas have been utilized (Table 3.1).

Researchers have noted complications of 5-FU therapy to include vaginal irritation, discharge, burning, and chronic mucosal ulceration. Approximately 8% of patients had epithelial ulcers at 6 months after treatment. They reported that the rate of vaginal ulceration was directly correlated with the length of treatment with 5-FU, especially prevalent in those with more than 10 weeks of therapy.[23] In general, because of concern for vaginal ulcer formation, use of 5-FU has fallen out of favor despite evidence indicating this to be an effective topical agent.[23–26]

Imiquimod (Aldara)

Imiquimod is an immune-modulating therapy. It induces secretion of interferon alpha, interleukin 12, and TNF alpha from local mononuclear cells. Buck and Guth studied the use of imiquimod in a small group of young patients (18–26 years) who had low-grade VAIN and no prior treatments. Imiquimod 5% cream (0.25-g sachet) was placed per vagina via an applicator once a week for 3 consecutive weeks. Eighty-six percent of patients were clear of VAIN after 1 treatment cycle, while 6 of the 37 patients required 2 cycles and one required 3 cycles. At 6 months following therapy, 92% remained clear of recurrent lesions.[25] Other investigators have placed imiquimod directly on visualized lesions at the time of colposcopic exam over several treatment appointments and noted lesion regression.[26, 27] Currently imiquimod is only approved for the treatment of genital warts.

Clinical Scenario 4

A 55-year-old with a prior hysterectomy for fibroids, who is taking black cohash for hot flashes, presents with an LSIL Pap. Vaginal colposcopy reveals no lesions, but is consistent with atrophic vaginal mucosa.

What treatment should be recommended?

Most likely this patient's abnormal Pap smear is the result of atrophic vaginal mucosa. Given the negative vaginal colposcopy, the most reasonable treatment would be to place her on vaginal estrogen for 1 to 2 months and repeat a Pap smear at that time. Either vaginal estrogen cream or estradiol suppositories could be used. Treatment with topical 5-FU or imiquimod would not be indicated at this time.

The patient is followed with serial Pap smears, and repeat Pap smears at 6 and 12 months continue to reveal LSIL despite estrogen therpy. Colposcopy remains negative.

What further evaluation should be performed?

If HPV typing was not performed earlier, it should be performed at this time. Population studies have shown a second peak of HPV prevalence in women older than 55 years of age. It appears that if women fail to eradicate high-risk HPV infection until menopause, often the virus has become integrated into host DNA, thus allowing possible progression towards dysplasia. One could also obtain "blind biopsies" of the up-

per vagina to exclude high-grade VAIN needing treatment. Regardless, the patient will need close follow-up with Pap smear and colposcopy.[28]

Clinical Scenario 5

A 55-year-old nulligravida is referred for evaluation of a vaginal Pap smear that revealed atypical glandular cells of uncertain significance (AGUS), suspect neoplasia. She underwent hysterectomy with removal of the cervix and a transverse vaginal septum 10 years ago for bleeding, with benign pathology. She was adopted, and details of family medical history are unknown.

What evaluation is needed?

Unfortunately, a history of in utero DES exposure could not be obtained for this patient. Her history of prior gross identification of upper genital tract anatomic anomalies must raise the suspicion for in utero DES exposure in a patient of this age group. Even though the patient is outside of the age group of DES-exposed women at highest risk for vaginal clear cell carcinomas, this lesion must be considered in the differential diagnosis, along with vaginal glandular dysplasia and squamous dysplasias involving vaginal adenosis. A thorough visual and digital vaginal examination should be performed because most vaginal clear cell carcinomas are detected as palpable submucosal nodules involving the vaginal canal. Complete vaginal colposcopy with acetic acid staining, augmented by Lugol solution staining, should be performed.

Colposcopy reveals multiple (> 10) 0.5 to 1-cm islands of acetowhite lesions in the upper vagina that have no atypical vascularity. These lesions do not take up Lugol solution. Biopsies reveal adenosis with squamous metaplasia and focal squamous VAIN II involving the glands.

What further evaluation or treatment would you recommend?

Involvement of vaginal adenosis by squamous dysplasia certainly could explain the cytologic abnormalities observed in this patient. However, given the multifocal nature of her adenosis and degree of cytologic abnormality, it would be prudent to perform an upper colpectomy as definitive treatment of VAIN and to exclude an invasive lesion in one of the multiple lesions that were observed by colposcopy. Colposcopy and staining with Lugol solution should be used at the time of vaginectomy to define the extent of resection needed to encompass all lesions.

References

1. Graham JB, Meigs JV. Recurrence of tumor after total hysterectomy for carcinoma in situ. *Am J Obstet Gynecol*. 1952; 64:1159.

2. NCI. http://www.cancer.gov/cancertopics/types/vaginal/. Last accessed 7/31/2008.

3. Aho M, Vesterinen E, Meyer B, et al. Natural history of vaginal intraepithelial neoplasia. *Cancer*. 1991;68:195.

4. Koss LG, Melamed MR, Daniel WW. In situ epidermoid carcinoma of the cervix and vagina following radiotherapy for cervical cancer. *Cancer*. 1961;14:353.

5. Pride GL, Buchler DA. Carcinoma of vagina 10 or more years following pelvic irradiation therapy. *Am J Obstet Gynecol*. 1977;127;513–517.

6. Wentzensen N, Vinokurova S, von Knebel Doeberitz M. Systematic review of genomic integration sites of human papillomavirus genomes in epithelial dysplasia and invasive cancer of the female lower genital tract. *Cancer Res*. 2004;64:3878–3884.

7. Sugase M, Matsukura T. Distinct manifestations of human papillomaviruses in the vagina. *Int J Cancer*. 1997;72:412.

8. Castle PE, Rodriguez AC, Porras C, et al. A comparison of cervical and vaginal human papillomavirus. *Sex Transm Dis*. 2007;34:849–855.

9. Sherman JF, Mount SL, Evans MF, Skelly J, Simmons-Arnold L, Eltabbakh GH. Smoking increases the risk of high-grade vaginal intraepithelial neoplasia in women with oncogenic human papillomavirus. *Gynecol Oncol*. 2008;72:412–415.

10. Daling JR, Sherman KJ, Hislop TG, et al. Cigarette smoking and the risk of anogenital cancer. *Am J Epidemiol*. 1992;135:180–189.

11. Baldwin PF, Van Der Burg SH, Boswell CM, et al. Vaccinia-expressed human papillomavirus 16 and 18 E6 an E7 as a therapeutic vaccination for vulval and vaginal intraepithelial neoplasia. *Clin Cancer Res*. 2003;9:5205–5213.

12. Villa LL, Costa RL, Petta CA, et al. High sustained efficacy of a prophylactic quadrivalent human papillomavirus types 6/11/16/18 L1 virus-like particle vaccine through 5 years of follow-up. *Expert Rev Vaccines*. 2007;6:141–145.

13. Waggoner SE, Mittendorf R, Biney N, et al. Influence of in utero diethylstilbestrol exposure on the prognosis and biologic behavior of vaginal clear-cell adenocarcinoma. *Gynecol Oncol*. 1994;55:238.

14. Robboy SJ, Noller KL, O'Brien P, et al. Increased incidence of cervical and vaginal dysplasia in 3,980 diethylstilbestrol-exposed young women. *JAMA*. 1984;252:2979.

15. Fu YS. *Pathology of the Uterine Cervix, Vagina and Vulva*. 2nd ed. Philadelphia: Saunders; 2002:239–251.

16. Teruya Y, Sakumoto K, Moromizato H, et al. High dose-rate intracavitary brachytherapy for carcinoma in situ of the vagina occurring after hysterectomy: a rational prescription of radiation dose. *Am J Obstet Gynecol*. 2002;187:360–364

17. Fanning J, Manahan KJ, McLean SA. Loop electrosurgical excision procedure for partial upper vaginectomy. *Am J Obstet Gynecol*. 1999;181:1382–1385.

18. Massad LS. Outcomes after diagnosis of vaginal intraepithelial neoplasia. *J Low Gen Tract Dis*. 2008;12:16–19.

19. Rome RM, England PG. Management of vaginal intraepithelial neoplasia: a series of 132 cases with long-term follow-up. *Int J Gynecol Cancer*. 2000;10:382–390.

20. Dodge JA, Eltabbakh GH, Mount SL, Walker RP, Morgan A. Clinical features and risk of recurrence among patients with vaginal intraepithelial neoplasia. *Gynecol Oncol*. 2001;83:363–369.

21. Indermaur MD, Martino MA, Fiorica JV, Roberts WS, Hoffman MS. Upper vaginectomy for the treatment of vaginal intraepithelial neoplasia. *Am J Obstet Gynecol*. 2005;193:577–580; discussion 580–581.

22. Cheng D, Ng TY, Ngan HYS, Wong LC. Wide local excision (WLE) for vaginal intraepithelial neoplasia (VAIN). *Acta Obstet Gynecol Scand*. 1999;78:648–652.

23. Krebs HB, Helmkamp BF. Chronic ulcerations following topical therapy with 5-fluorouracil for vaginal human papillomavirus-associated lesions. *Obstet Gynecol*. 1991;78:205–208.

24. Murta EF, Neves MA, Sempionato LR, Costa MC, Maluf PJ. Vaginal intraepithelial neoplasia: clinical-therapeutic analysis of 33 cases. *Arch Gynecol Obstet*. 2005:272:261–264.

25. Buck HW, Guth KJ. Treatment of vaginal intraepithelial neoplasia (primarily low grade) with imiquimod 5% cream. *J Low Genit Tract Dis*. 2003;7:290–293.

26. Diakomanolis E, Haidopoulos D, Stefanidis K. Treatment of high-grade vaginal intraepithelial neoplasia with imiquimod cream. *N Engl J Med*. 2002;347:374.

27. Haidopoulos D, Diakomanolis E, Rodolakis A, Voulgaris Z, Vlachos G, Intsaklis A. Can local application of imiquimod cream be an alternative mode of therapy for patients with high-grade intraepithelial lesions of the vagina? *Int J Gynecol Cancer*. 2005;15:898–902.

28. Syrjanen K, Kulmala SM, Shabalova I, et al. Epidemiological, clinical and viral determinants of the increased prevalence of high-risk human papillomavirus (HPV) infections in elderly women. *Eur J Gynecol Oncol*. 2008;29:114–122.

CHAPTER 4

Cervical Neoplasia

Jennifer L. Ragazzo, MD
Department of Obstetrics and Gynecology, University of North Carolina School of Medicine, Chapel Hill, NC, USA

Daniel L. Clarke-Pearson, MD, FACOG, FACS
Department of Obstetrics and Gynecology, University of North Carolina School of Medicine, Chapel Hill, NC, USA

Pathology Notes: Chad Livasy, MD
Associate Professor, Department of Pathology and Laboratory Medicine, University of North Carolina School of Medicine, Chapel Hill, NC, USA

Background

From the discovery of a screening test to the evolution of a vaccine, significant advances have been made against cervical cancer in the last 65 years. It began with Georges Papanicolau, deemed the "father of cytology" after publishing his work "Diagnosis of Uterine Cancer by the Vaginal Smear" in 1943. The Pap test was born, and never since has a more effective cancer screening test been produced. Today, with little modification in the basic methods described by Papanicolau, the "Pap smear" remains the cornerstone for the detection of premalignant and malignant changes of the cervix.

The initial proposal that cervical cancer was a sexually transmitted disease was made in 1842, by Dr. Rigoni-Stern, when he reported that prostitutes were afflicted by cervical cancer but nuns were not. While epidemiologic studies confirmed that sexual contact (early onset of sexual intercourse, multiple sexual partners, high-risk males, and herpes simplex virus infections) was a risk for cervical cancer, the true cause was not identified until the late 1970s, when zur Hausen discovered the human papilloma virus (HPV) in cervical cancer and genital warts. It is now known that certain types of HPV cause almost all cervical cancers.

As neoplastic changes precede cervical cancer, the ability to intervene and stop progression to cancer is possible. In this decade alone, there have been considerable changes in the way cervical neoplasia is diagnosed and treated. The 2001 Bethesda System is the current way of reporting cervical cytology (Table 4.1). Treatment guidelines have been created and revised, mostly based on evidence but sometimes on expert opinion. The largest consensus group, the American Society of Colposcopists and Cervical Pathologists (ASCCP), published their management recommendations in 2007.[1,2] The following is an overview of cervical neoplasia, highlighting the newest treatment guidelines as well as complicated clinical scenarios that a general obstetrician/gynecologist might face in his or her practice.

Epidemiology

A substantial decrease in the rate of cervical cancer was seen after development of the Pap smear for screening. Between 1955 and 1992, the rate of death from cervical cancer decreased by 74%. Screening for and decreasing cervical cancer incidence and mortality is an increasing challenge in developing nations, where health care and

Gynecological Cancer Management: Identification, Diagnosis and Treatment, Edited by Daniel L. Clarke-Pearson and John T. Soper. Published 2010 by Blackwell Publishing, ISBN: 978-1-4051-9079-4.

Table 4.1 2001 bethesda system for reporting epithelial cell abnormalities on cytology (abridged)

Squamous Cell
Atypical squamous cells (ASC)
    ASC of undetermined significance (ASC-US)
    ASC, cannot exclude high-grade squamous
    intraepithelial lesion (ASC-H)
Low-grade squamous intraepithelial lesion (LSIL)
    Encompassing human papillomavirus, mild dysplasia,
    and cervical intraepithelial neoplasia (CIN) 1
High-grade squamous intraepithelial lesion (HSIL)
    Encompassing moderate and severe dysplasia,
    carcinoma in situ, CIN 2, and CIN 3
Squamous cell carcinoma

Glandular Cell
Atypical glandular cells (AGC)
    Specify endocervical, endometrial, or glandular cells
    not otherwise specified
Atypical glandular cells, favor neoplastic
    Specify endocervical or not otherwise specified
Endocervical adenocarcinoma in situ (AIS)
Adenocarcinoma

Abridged from Solomon D, Davey D, Kurman R, et al. The 2001 Bethesda system: terminology for reporting results of cervical cytology. *JAMA.* 2002;287:2116.

preventative medicine are limited. Cervical cancer is the most common cause of cancer-related death in women worldwide, with over 200,000 deaths annually. Even in the United States, where cervical cancer screening is widely available, the SEER data estimate that 11,070 women will be newly diagnosed with cervical cancer and 3870 women will die from it in 2008.[3]

As HPV is the cause of 99% of all cervical cancers, the rate of HPV infection is a key factor in the development of cervical neoplasia (CIN). The prevalence of HPV in all age groups is estimated to be about 30%. By far the largest group affected is young sexually active women. In a study of 1921 women in the United States ages 14 to 59, the highest prevalence was reported in women age 20 to 24, at 44.8%.[4] In the course of a woman's lifetime, it is almost expected that she will have been exposed to HPV. Franco and associates estimate a cumulative incidence of HPV infection over 50 years to be as high as 80%.[5]

Multiple factors have been implicated in the risk for cervical cancer, but none as strongly as those that put a woman at risk for becoming infected with HPV. Sexual behavior is the principal determinant for infection with HPV. Age at first intercourse, total number of sexual contacts, and the past sexual experience of a woman's partner are all factors that increase the chance for exposure to the virus.[6] Other indicators of a greater number of sexual contacts have also been linked, including high parity, use of oral contraceptives, and a prior STD history.

Once a woman becomes infected with HPV, the risk for her to develop cervical neoplasia is associated with the presence of other factors that influence her ability to clear the virus. Cigarette smoking is associated with at least a twofold increased risk for cervical cancer. The mechanism by which cigarette smoke affects cervical cancer is not entirely clear, but thought to be a potential cause of cellular abnormalities and impaired immunity. Sexually transmitted diseases, specifically *Chlamydia* and herpes simplex virus, are also thought to modulate immunity. Any type of immunosuppression (eg, solid organ transplant recipients) promotes the persistence of HPV infection. HIV infection and chronic immunosuppressive therapy can both make a woman more susceptible to persistent HPV infection and cervical neoplasia.

Natural history of disease

Cervical cancer is one of the few cancers in which we are able to identify a precursor lesion and intervene to prevent progression of intraepithelial neoplasia to invasive cancer. It is believed that the progression of carcinoma in situ to invasive cancer occurs after a period of 10 to 15 years. Certainly the other risk factors mentioned could hasten the process. But if women are routinely screened and treated for neoplasia, cervical cancer can be prevented.

Understanding the natural history of HPV infection is essential because it relates to the development of cervical dysplasia. An HPV infection is typically cleared rapidly. The majority of infections are no longer detected by sensitive HPV testing within 6 to 9 months from the first positive HPV test. A study by Rodriguez and colleagues estimated that 67% of infections clear by 12 months. Younger patients were more likely to clear infection than women over the age of 30 years.[7]

Regression of cervical neoplasia occurs most frequently with low-grade lesions. Between 70% and 90% of CIN 1 lesions and 40% of CIN 2 lesions will resolve spontaneously.[8] These patients will also test negative for high-risk HPV within 6 to 24 months. High-grade cervical neoplasia is more likely to develop in the face of persistent HPV infection and particular HPV types. In a prospective study using HPV testing in conjunction with cervical biopsy, 33 out of 353 women reached clinical progression to CIN 3 and all had persistent infection with high-risk HPV.[9] When CIN 3 is detected, progression to invasive cancer can occur over a period that averages 10 years. It occurs over an extended period of time as cervical cells accumulate the mutations required for invasion.

The HPV virus is a double-stranded DNA virus that induces epithelial cell proliferation or papillomas. There are over 100 different types of HPV; about 40 types infect the genital tract. Each type varies by a portion of its DNA genome and is divided into two groups. The low-risk HPV types are associated with benign changes such as condyloma. The high-risk types are known as oncogenic types and are detected in CIN and cervical cancer. These oncogenic types incorporate their DNA into the genome of human cells and block the cell's ability to repair or destroy itself when it begins to accumulate mutations. All human papilloma viruses contain seven early genes (E1–E7) and two late genes (L1–L2), depending upon where they fall in the genomic sequence of the virus. E6 and E7 are known oncogenes of the high-risk types of HPV. They produce proteins that inhibit human tumor suppression genes, notably p53 and Rb. E6 protein binds and inactivates p53, a protein that is responsible for repairing damaged DNA or apoptosis (programmed cell death) in damaged human cells. E7 protein binds primarily to pRB (retinoblastoma gene), which is responsible for stopping DNA synthesis in a damaged cell. These oncoproteins deregulate cell proliferation, thus promoting tumor growth and malignant transformation.

Clinical Scenario 1

A 21-year-old college student, who has recently become sexually active, presents to Student Health seeking a prescription for oral contraceptives. She inquires if it is appropriate for her to have a Pap smear.

What are the current recommendations for cervical cancer screening?

As of 2003, recommendations for cervical cancer screening changed, allowing more time before first screening. A woman should undergo her first Pap smear 3 years after first intercourse or at age 21, whichever comes first.[10]

In addition to this change, intervals for screening have increased in low-risk women. Before age 30, it is still recommended that women undergo annual Pap smears, as this is the age where HPV infection is more likely. There are two options for women in the age group older than 30:

1 If a woman has had three consecutive normal Pap smears, she can be screened every 2 to 3 years with cytology alone.

2 If the HPV test is used in conjunction with cytology, a woman can undergo screening every 3 years if she tests negative for high-risk HPV and has a normal Pap smear. Contrary to some opinions expressed in the lay press, HPV testing is not considered the "standard of care," although it may be added to Pap smear screening as outlined above.

There is still some controversy as to when cervical cancer screening can be discontinued, as evidence is inconclusive. The U.S. Preventative Service Task Force recommends cessation of Pap smears after age 65, as long as a woman has had adequate recent screening and is at low-risk for developing cervical cancer. The American Cancer Society recommends cessation of screening at age 70. However, the American College of Obstetrics and Gynecology has not designated an age cutoff for screening, leaving it to the discretion of the physician based on the patient's age and risk factors.

With respect to women who have had a hysterectomy (including removal of the cervix), all three organizations agree that cytology can be discontinued if the following criteria are met: the hysterectomy was performed for benign reasons, the patient had routine screening prior to surgery, and the patient has no history of abnormal Pap smears. With a history of CIN 2 or 3 preceding hysterectomy, once she has had three consecutive normal Pap smears following the hysterectomy, cytology may be discontinued.

Her Pap smear returns as low-grade squamous intraepithelial lesion (LSIL).

What is the appropriate management of abnormal cytology?

When a patient has an abnormal Pap smear, in almost all circumstances she should undergo colposcopy. The exceptions to this are discussed below. The patient in this clinical scenario with an LSIL Pap smear should undergo colposcopy with colposcopic-directed biopsies. Multiple studies have shown that biopsy of lesions visualized by colposcopy is necessary to determine the grade of

the lesion and to exclude invasive carcinoma.[11] Thus management should not be based upon colposcopic impression alone. If the colposcopy is unsatisfactory because the whole transformation zone cannot be visualized or if the entire lesion cannot be seen, then an endocervical curettage (ECC) is recommended. Also, if ablation is being considered for treatment (cryotherapy or CO_2 laser) pending biopsy results, then an ECC should also be performed to rule out dysplasia that cannot be seen in the endocervical canal.

Patients with an abnormal Pap smear of LSIL or greater should be evaluated with colposcopy, with the exception of two groups. In women age 20 or less, the ASCCP guidelines recommend following a patient with ASC-US (atypical squamous cells of undetermined significance) or LSIL with annual Pap smears for up to 2 years. This age group is the most likely to clear infection from HPV and should only be evaluated with colposcopy for persistent dysplasia that persists for more than 2 years or if her Pap smear returns as ASC-H, HGSIL, or AGC. It is also reasonable to defer colposcopy for low-grade changes in pregnancy until the patient is postpartum, although colposcopy is preferred in non-adolescents.

Pathology notes

The Pap smear is the most effective cancer screening test ever developed. That being said, the following discussion will cover specific problem areas related to the Pap smear and the implications for clinical management. The take-home message for several of these problems related to the Pap smear is that HPV testing with the current FDA-approved methodology is very helpful in guiding patient management. The first issue is the sensitivity of the Pap smear. Randomized clinical trials have shown that the sensitivity of a single Pap smear to detect HSIL/carcinoma is in the range of 50% to 60%.[1] HPV testing used in conjunction with cytology improves the sensitivity to detect HSIL/carcinoma to approximately 95%.[12] It is likely that in the near future, HPV testing will become part of the general screening process in

some fashion. HPV testing is likely to be most beneficial in women over 30 years of age where the positive predictive value of the test is higher due to the overall lower prevalence of HPV infection in this age group.

Approximately 4% to 5% of all Pap smear tests return with the diagnosis of ASC-US. ASC-US is not a distinct biologic entity and encompasses both neoplastic and non-neoplastic conditions. One should expect that approximately 50% of women with the diagnosis of ASC-US are infected with high-risk HPV and approximately 10% to 20% of women with ASC-US have CIN 2 or CIN 3. HPV testing effectively segregates the 50% of women with ASC-US with true cancer risk from those patients with essentially no risk. While studies are not as clear for guiding the

Pathology notes (*continued*)

management for ASC-H, HPV testing may eventually become part the clinical algorithm for managing patients with this diagnosis as well.

Approximately 0.14% of Pap smears return with the diagnosis of atypical glandular cells of undetermined significance (AGC-US). Recognition of glandular neoplasia in the Pap smear is particularly difficult for the pathologist due to the subtle cytologic findings associated with many of these lesions. Roughly 30% to 45% of patients with an AGC-US diagnosis are subsequently found to have significant pathology. It should be noted that when dysplasia is found in patients with prior diagnosis of AGC-US on Pap smear, the abnormality is most commonly HSIL. This is due to the glandular appearance of dysplastic squamous cells in HSIL cases associated with endocervical gland involvement. In postmenopausal women, significant pathology is more often located in the endometrium including endometrial hyperplasia and carcinoma. Again, HPV testing is likely to be helpful in guiding the management of patients with a diagnosis of AGC-US on Pap smear and significant underlying cervical neoplasia including SIL, endocervial adenocarcinoma in situ, and invasive cervical carcinoma. The probability of detecting high-risk HPV for each of these lesions in patients with a diagnosis of AGC-US is approximately 95%.

It is common for many institutions to directly correlate Pap smear findings with colposcopy- directed cervical biopsy findings as a QC function. These correlations can be very helpful for problematic cases, especially when done in real time, but it should be noted that cyto/histo discrepancies are likely to be commonplace due to a number of factors, particularly those related to sampling. Although histology has traditionally been considered the gold standard, the sensitivity of colposcopy has been shown to be similar to that observed for cytology. The bottom line is that detection of high-grade SIL, regardless of methodology, requires intervention.

Issues related to pathologist interobserver reproducibility need to be briefly discussed. For Pap smear specimens, LSIL shows good interobserver reproducibility while HSIL shows lower interobserver reproducibility. For biopsy specimens, it is the just the opposite. There is significant interobserver variability distinguishing biopsies with focal LSIL changes from those without LSIL. HSIL in biopsy specimens shows good interobserver reproducibility. Immunohistochemistry for p16 has been shown to significantly improve pathologist interobserver variability in biopsy specimens and can be extremely helpful in problematic cases. HPV-related squamous dysplasias typically show up-regulation of p16 expression. Positivity for p16 expression is particularly useful in confirming the presence of HSIL in biopsy or ECC specimens when the volume of suspicious cells is low, limiting interpretation.

What is the role for HPV typing?

Currently the technology is available for the clinician to test for the presence of high-risk and low-risk HPV types. The test will detect any of the high-risk or low-risk types, but does not determine the specific type(s) present. High-risk types detected in the current panel include 16, 18, 31, 33, 35, 39, 45, 51, 52, 56, 58, 59, and 68. Low-risk types detected are 6, 11, 40, 42, 43, 44, 53, 54, 61, 72, 73, and 81. (The technology exists to test for a specific HPV type, but is currently expensive, not clinically available, and of no known clinical value.)

The combination of Pap smear with HPV testing increases the sensitivity of screening for cervical neoplasia. In a randomized trial by Mayrand and associates, the detection of CIN 2 and CIN 3 by Pap smear alone was 55% and 94.6%, respectively. However, when the Pap smear was combined with HPV testing, sensitivity to detect either CIN 2 or 3 was 100% and sensitivity of testing did not severely compromise the test's specificity.[13]

HPV typing is commonly used to triage patients with abnormal Pap smears, specifically ASC-US. As the adolescent population is most likely to test positive for HPV in the face of an ASC-US Pap smear, performing HPV typing on a Pap specimen is not helpful. However, in women age 21 or greater, HPV typing can be helpful in determining risk for high-grade neoplasia. It is unlikely that a patient will develop CIN 3 if she has an ASC-US Pap smear but is negative for high-risk HPV. For this reason, colposcopy should only be performed for patients with ASC-US who also test positive for high-risk HPV. Using HPV triage in this way will cut the number of colposcopies in half, and at the same time reduce costs.[14] If HPV testing is not available, then colposcopy for ASC-US should be performed after the patient has had two consecutive ASC-US Pap smears 6 months apart.

Another application of HPV typing is to increase screening intervals in low-risk women over age 30. When HPV typing does not identify any high-risk HPV type (and the woman has a negative Pap smear), a woman in this age group can be screened every 3 years. A positive high-risk HPV test does not indicate the need for colposcopy as long as the Pap smear is negative. With a positive high-risk HPV test and a negative Pap smear, the patient should continue to be screened annually.[15]

Should screening change if the patient has received the HPV vaccine?

The HPV vaccine, Gardasil, was approved in 2006 by the FDA for use in girls and women age 9 to 26 years old. It is a quadrivalent vaccine that protects against two oncogenic types of HPV, types 16 and 18, as well as two condyloma-causing types, types 6 and 11. Although HPV types 16 and 18 are associated with about 70% of all cervical cancers, there are still almost a dozen more high-risk HPV types. For this reason, the HPV vaccine does not replace routine cervical cancer screening. In addition, the long-term efficacy has only been shown for up to 5 years. Research is still underway to determine the length of time before immunity wanes.

The patient undergoes colposcopy with biopsy and endocervical curettage (ECC). Cervical biopsy returns as CIN 1 and the ECC is negative.

What is the management for abnormal histology?

Management of CIN is decided based on the natural history of the disease. In this clinical scenario, the patient is a young woman with a CIN 1 lesion. The chance for regression is upwards of 90%, so she may be followed with observation by repeat cytology. If she undergoes two serial Pap smears 6 months apart that are both normal, she may return to annual screening. If an abnormal Pap returns, a repeat coloposcopy is necessary. Persistent CIN1 is less likely to resolve, thus treatment might be considered in certain patients. However, there is no harm in following the patient clinically because the risk for disease progression in the face of persistent CIN 1 is very low. Bansal and associates reported a risk for progression to HGSIL after 6 months of persistent disease to be only 4%.[16] We recommend that, especially in young nulliparous patients, persistent CIN 1 should be managed with observation rather than ablative or excisional therapies that might compromise fertility and obstetrical outcomes.

As there is less chance for regression and a higher risk for disease progression, CIN 2 and CIN 3 lesions are typically managed with either an ablative or excisional procedure. It is estimated that almost half of CIN 2 lesions will regress, but since the majority will either persist or progress, treatment is indicated in most scenarios. If a patient is compliant and prefers to be followed, she should undergo cytology and colposcopy at 6-month intervals. This should be undertaken only if the entire lesion and transformation zone can be evaluated.

In a large retrospective study, where treatment of CIN 3 was withheld, 50.3% of women developed invasive cancer, versus 0.7% in women who were treated adequately.[17] Thus, all cases of CIN 3 should be treated. An ablative procedure can be chosen only in the event that endocervical sampling is negative and the entire lesion is visible. Otherwise an excisional procedure is recommended.

How does the management of CIN change based on age?

The newest ASCCP guidelines factored age in the treatment algorithms for cervical neoplasia. For women age 20 and less, observation is a key role in the management of CIN. Low-grade lesions are very likely to resolve in this age group. Haidopoulos and colleagues described a 93% regression rate of CIN1 after 2 years in women age 16 to 20 years old.[18] For this reason, if colposcopy is performed and the biopsy returns as CIN1, the recommendation is to follow the patient with yearly Pap smears for 2 years and only repeat colposcopy if cytology remains abnormal after 2 years or if it returns as greater than LSIL.

With higher-grade lesions, observation is still a possible option in this younger age group. Regression of CIN 2 in adolescent and young women has been reported between 39% and 65%.[19, 20] Thus, if colposcopy is satisfactory, it is reasonable to follow these patients closely with cytology and colposcopy at 6-month intervals. Limited data on regression of CIN 3 in adolescents is available. Thus, when CIN 3 is specified, treatment with either ablation or excision of the transformation zone is preferred.

Clinical Scenario 2

At the new obstetrical exam, a woman who is 18 weeks pregnant is found to have an abnormal Pap smear.

How should this patient be evaluated during pregnancy? Is the management different than in the non-pregnant patient?

Women of childbearing age are most at risk for cervical neoplasia. Of the 4 million women who become pregnant each year in the United States, it is estimated that between 2% and 7% will have abnormal cervical cytology on a Pap smear. Cervical cancer screening guidelines are no different for pregnant women. Likewise, an abnormal Pap smear in pregnancy should be evaluated with colposcopy under the same circumstances as in a non-pregnant patient. The only exception is that colposcopy can be postponed until postpartum for LSIL or less, although it is preferred at the time of diagnosis in a non-adolescent.

Multiple factors make colposcopy during pregnancy more difficult, including increased pelvic congestion, vaginal wall laxity, and an enlarged cervix. Just as in a non-pregnant state, an adequate colposcopy with visualization of the transformation zone is ideal. Providers may be wary to perform the necessary evaluation of cervical neoplasia during pregnancy because of the concern of bleeding and complications. However, there is good evidence that cervical biopsy is safe during pregnancy. A biopsy should be performed in any patient for whom CIN 2, CIN 3, or invasive cancer is suspected. Endocervical curettage should be avoided as the risk to pregnancy is unknown. In the face of atypical glandular cells, colposcopy with cervical biopsy can be performed, but endocervical curettage and endometrial biopsy are contraindicated.

Similar to a non-pregnant patient, CIN1 can be followed by observation with cytology at the 6-week postpartum visit. Progression of CIN 2 or CIN 3 to invasive cancer is unlikely during pregnancy. Repeat colposcopy later in pregnancy can be performed to exclude this possibility, with biopsy only if the lesion appears worse. Otherwise, treatment of high-grade dysplasia should be postponed until postpartum.[21]

Clinical Scenario 3

A 35-year-old woman who is HIV positive but otherwise healthy, has a Pap smear showing HGSIL.

How should this immunocompromised patient be treated?

Women who are immunocompromised are more likely to develop cervical dysplasia because an intact immune system is necessary to clear infection with HPV. This includes women with HIV as well as women on immunosuppression secondary to chronic disease, such as autoimmune conditions or organ transplantation. Studies have shown at least a five-fold higher incidence of cervical dysplasia in women who are on immunosuppression.[22, 23] In women with HIV, Wright and associates showed that Pap smears were as effective a screening tool compared with women who were HIV-seronegative.[24] A large prospective cohort study of 855 HIV-seropositive women compared with HIV-seronegative controls showed that in the face of normal cytology and negative HPV DNA, there was no difference in the incidence of cervical dysplasia in the two groups. This suggests that screening practices in women with HIV can be similar to the standard guidelines.[25]

With respect to evaluation of abnormal cytology, any immunocompromised patient with an abnormal Pap smear should be evaluated by colposcopy. Treatment of cervical dysplasia is similar in immunocompromised patients compared with the general population. Massad and colleagues described that women with HIV are less likely to have regression of CIN 1, but there was not a significant difference in progression to high-grade dysplasia when compared with controls.[26] Thus observation with colposcopy and cytology at 6-month intervals is a reasonable option for the management of CIN 1. In women with CIN 2 or 3, treatment should be pursued with either an ablative or excisional procedure. There is a high rate of recurrence of low-grade dysplasia following treatment, but treatment of CIN 2 or 3 reduces the possible development of cervical cancer.

Case Scenario 4

A 35-year-old woman has been previously treated for CIN 3 with CO_2 laser ablation of the transformation zone. A recent Pap smear is reported as HSIL. Colposcopy and a cervical biopsy is performed and reported as carcinoma in situ (CIS) with endocervical gland involvement.

What are the pros and cons for ablative and excisional procedures?

The choice in treatment of CIN varies based on multiple factors, including the patient's wishes, desire for future fertility, anatomy, and extent of disease. Outcomes of ablative and excisional procedures are comparable, especially with respect to cancer-free survival.[27] Prior to any treatment, the cervix is visualized either with colposcopy after application of acetic acid or "painted" with Lugol's solution to outline the lesion. Treatment modalities that ablate abnormal tissue include electrocautery, cryotherapy, and CO_2 laser therapy. These may be preferred in patients who are young and nulliparous, as there is less chance of impacting pregnancy outcomes.[28]

Although electrocautery appears to yield similar results, it is an older technique used prior to the advent of the other ablative procedures. It is preformed by cauterizing cervical tissue with sufficient depth to destroy disease in the cervical glands. The procedure itself is rather cost-effective; however, the depth of the burn can cause significant pain, requiring the patient to be anesthetized in an operating room, thus offsetting the cost savings.

Cryotherapy is achieved by freezing the cervical epithelium, usually with nitrous oxide, through a probe. Typically there is minimal pain and no anesthesia is required, making this procedure an ideal choice for an office setting. The outcomes of cryotherapy depend upon the preoperative workup in addition to operator experience. Prior to any ablative procedure, endocervical curettage must be preformed to exclude the possibility of dysplasia within the cervical canal. A "double-freeze" is the recommended approach, first by freezing until a 4 to 5-mm ice ball extends along the outer edge of the probe, followed by a 5-minute thaw, and then refreezing in the same fashion. This method has minimal surgical risk compared with the excisional methods. After the procedure there is typically significant drainage for up to 2 weeks as the cervical bed heals. Follow-up includes a repeat Pap smear and ECC in 6 months to assure adequate treatment. Cervical stenosis is a possible outcome, which is why the endocervical canal should be assessed. If the initial Pap smear post-procedure is positive, it is more likely associated with persistent disease, rather than recurrence.

Laser therapy is accomplished with the use of a CO_2 laser beam, typically attached to the colposcope. The laser desiccates cervical tissue, thus destroying abnormal cells. It is usually carried to a depth of 5 to 7 mm and a width of 4 to 5 mm beyond the visible lesion. Although it is a costly modality, one benefit of laser therapy is that the transformation zone tends to remain visible post-treatment, which is not the case with the other ablative therapies.

The benefit of an excisional procedure is that it is both diagnostic and can be curative. Just as with ablative procedures, it is helpful to use Lugol solution to outline the abnormal area or to perform colposcopy to define the outer limits of the lesion prior to the procedure. A loop electrosurgical excisional procedure (LEEP) is performed using a wire loop with electrodiathermy to excise the transformation zone. Typically the cervix is infiltrated first with a local anesthetic and dilute epinephrine, allowing the procedure to be done in the office. This is the major benefit of a LEEP over the more traditional cold knife conization of the cervix, making it more cost-effective and convenient for both the patient and the provider. It is important to tag the specimen with suture for orientation, especially in the event that a margin is found to be positive.

There are certain situations where a cold knife cone (CKC) biopsy is superior to LEEP. First and foremost, the CKC is done with a scalpel in the operating room as an outpatient procedure. As such, the margins of the specimen are not cauterized, which helps the pathologist to determine if the entire lesion has been removed. If there is any concern for carcinoma in-situ or atypical glandular cells preoperatively, a CKC is the procedure of choice over LEEP. In the past, hysterectomy was preferred to CKC for CIN 3, but studies show that conization is just as effective as hysterectomy, with similar rates of recurrence and invasive cancer.[29]

Is there evidence that these treatment methods might compromise fertility or increase the risk of poor obstetrical outcomes?

The majority of literature investigating pregnancy outcomes after treatment of cervical neoplasia looks at results in small groups of women and in a retrospective fashion. A true large prospective randomized control trial has not been preformed. Despite this, most studies show an increased risk of poor obstetrical outcomes, such as preterm delivery and preterm premature rupture of membranes, following excisional procedures. A meta-analysis showed an increased risk of preterm delivery and low birth-weight in patients treated with cold knife conization, laser conization, and radical diathermy.[30] There was not a significant risk increase with cryotherapy, laser ablation, or LEEP. Other studies have found an association between LEEP and poor obstetrical outcomes, although statistically significant results varied.[31, 32] There is also concern that all of the treatment options for CIN can cause cervical stenosis; however, it is unclear if this has a significant impact on fertility.

Because of these potential risks, we advocate observation for low-grade lesions in young nulliparous patients and ablative therapy when appropriate for the treatment of higher-grade dysplasia. In all circumstances the patient should be counseled as to the potential risks and benefits of the different treatment modalities.

Pathology notes

Most patients with a diagnosis of HSIL are managed with LEEP. Histologic evaluation of LEEP specimens allows confirmation of the diagnosis of HSIL and evaluation for the presence or absence of invasive carcinoma. Reported success rates in treating dysplasia by LEEP range from 60% to 95%, depending on the criteria used to define failure. LEEP specimens showing positive margins for HSIL, multiple quadrant involvement by HSIL, and extension of HSIL into endocervical glands have been shown to have higher recurrence rates.[35] Pathology reports from LEEP specimens should at a minimum comment on margin status, specifically designating the positive margin (endocervical, deep radial, or ectocervial) when appropriate. On rare occasion, a patient with biopsy-confirmed HSIL may have a LEEP specimen negative for dysplasia. These patients still need follow-up similar to those with a positive LEEP. Although cytology is good at evaluating cure post-LEEP, HPV testing appears better, with a sensitivity of approximately 95% in identifying patients with recurrent/persistent disease.

---

the need for close follow-up. Cautery from the LEEP is thought to summon an immune response

A LEEP is performed. Pathologic interpretation is somewhat compromised in that there is a thermal artifact at a margin with "microinvasive" squamous cell carcinoma.

How would you manage this patient with a positive surgical margin?

A positive margin of carcinoma in-situ on a LEEP specimen increases the risk for persistent disease. Re-excision can be offered, but expectant management with cytology and endocervical curettage at 6-month intervals is a reasonable option. Reich and associates looked at a large group of patients with positive margins of CIN 3 after excision. Seventy-eight percent remained disease free.[33] Of those with recurrence, the majority occurred within the first year, emphasizing to heal the cervical bed, which may effectively clear the abnormal cells. Therefore, a repeat excision is not necessary if the patient is compliant with follow-up Pap smears.

If microinvasive squamous cell carcinoma is diagnosed on a LEEP specimen, the patient can be offered two options. In general, microinvasive squamous cell carcinoma can be treated with either a CKC or hysterectomy. The decision to treat with an excisional procedure versus hysterectomy is influenced by multiple factors such as tumor size, age, parity, and the patient's wishes. In this clinical scenario, as the surgical margin is positive but obscured, it is necessary to repeat an excisional procedure with a cold knife conization. The extent of invasion is important to determine the cancer stage as well as treatment.

Pathology notes

If the cone excision contains invasive carcinoma, including those meeting criteria for microinvasion, the pathology report should include the histologic type of carcinoma, greatest depth of invasion, greatest horizontal extent of tumor, regions of the cervix involved (for oriented specimens), presence/absence of lymphovascular space invasion, and margin status. Small invasive tumors should be measured with an ocular micrometer to ensure accuracy.

Pathology notes (*continued*)

The depth of invasion is measured from the base of the overlying surface epithelium, or from the closest endocervical gland for tumors arising from CIN 3 that have replaced an endocervical gland (Fig. 4.1). Identification of early invasive squamous lesions is typically straightforward for the pathologist, but recognition of early invasion within endocervical glandular neoplasia is more difficult. The patterns of invasion for glandular lesions are variable and often subtle resulting in problems for pathologists to consistently and accurately identify and measure early invasive (microinvasive) adenocarcinoma of the cervix. Recognition of alternative invasive patterns including cribriform architecture (Plate 4.1) and glandular confluence with irregular borders by the pathologist are essential in accurately classifying the difficult lesions. Most cases of endocervical adenocaricnoma fall into the "usual-type" group and are associated with high-risk HPV subtypes, especially subtypes 18 and 16. The typical immunophenotype of these tumors, p16 strong positive, CEA positive, vimentin negative, and estrogen receptor negative, can be helpful in ex-cluding an endometrial primary for tumors detected in curettage specimens.

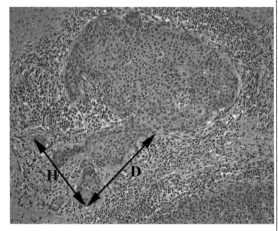

Figure 4.1 Measurement of invasive squamous cell carcinoma. Microinvasive squamous cell carcinoma of the cervix arising within CIN 3 replacing an endocervical gland. The depth of invasion is measured from the edge of the endocervical gland to the greatest depth of invasion (D) and the greatest horizontal extent of tumor (H) is also measured.

What is the treatment for a patient with an excisional specimen that shows microinvasive squamous cell carcinoma of the cervix?

If the surgical specimen has clear margins, and the patient wishes to preserve fertility, the patient is effectively treated. In a retrospective review of 166 patients with microinvasive squamous cell carcinoma, surgical treatments with conization, simple hysterectomy, and radical hysterectomy were compared. Of the patients who underwent conization, none developed recurrent invasive cancer, but 3 out of 30 developed CIN 3.[34] A conization could be offered as a fertility-sparing treatment option if indeed microinvasive squamous cell carcinoma is present. Gaducci and colleagues looked retrospectively at patients treated with conization for a stage IA1 squamous cell carcinoma. Of 143 cases, none had recurrent invasive disease after 45-month follow-up.[36] These decisions warrant a referral to a gynecologic oncologist, as the extent of invasion dictates the appropriate surgery and factors such as age and parity influence patient counseling.

If adenocarcinoma in-situ (AIS) is diagnosed on biopsy or excisional specimen, what is the next step in management?

If AIS is diagnosed on biopsy done at the time of colposcopy, it is necessary that the patient be evaluated further with a CKC to exclude the possibility of invasive disease. This is an important step in determining the correct treatment for the patient. Any lesion that contains abnormal glandular cells on biopsy should be evaluated with conization rather than LEEP because adenocarinoma in-situ is not a contiguous lesion and the ability to evaluate the surgical margin is crucial. If there is no evidence of invasion, the patient can undergo a simple hysterectomy to complete treatment

As many patients with AIS are of childbearing age, a conization can be done to preserve fertility. If margins are clear, the patient should then be followed closely as she is at high risk for persistent and recurrent disease.[37] Once childbearing is complete, the patient should undergo hysterectomy as long as she has not had recurrent disease.

References

1. Wright TC Jr., Massad LS, Dunton CJ, Spitzer M, Wilkinson EF, Solomon D. 2006 ASCCP-sponsored consensus conference. 2006 consensus guidelines for the management of women with abnormal cervical screening tests. *J Low Genit Tract Dis.* 2007;11:201–222.
2. Wright TC Jr., Massad LS, Dunton CJ, Spitzer M, Wilkinson EF, Solomon D. 2006 ASCCP-sponsored consensus conference. 2006 consensus guidelines for the management of women with cervical intraepithelial neoplasia or adenocarcinoma in situ. *J Low Genit Tract Dis.* 2007;11:223–239.
3. Ries LAG, Melbert D, Krapcho M, et al., eds. *SEER Cancer Statistics Review, 1975-2005.* National Cancer Institute, Bethesda. http://seer.cancer.gov/csr/1975_2005/, based on November 2007 SEER data submission, posted to the SEER website 2008.
4. Dunne EF, Unger ER, Sternberg M, et al. Prevalence of HPV infection among females in the United States. *JAMA.* 2007;297:813–819.
5. Franco EL, Villa LL, Sobrinho JP, et al. Epidemiology of acquisition and clearance of cervical human papillomavirus infection in women from a high-risk area for cervical cancer. *J Infect Dis.* 1999;180:1415–1423.
6. Bosch FX, de Sanjose S. The epidemiology of human papillomavirus infection and cervical cancer. *Dis Markers.* 2007;23:213–227.
7. Rodriguez AC, Schiffman M, Herrero R, et al.; Proyecto Epidemiologico Guanacaste Group. Rapid clearance of human papillomavirus and implications for clinical focus on persistent infections. *J Natl Cancer Inst.* 2008;100:513–517.
8. Results of a randomized trial on the management of cytology interpretations of atypical squamous cells of undetermined significance. ASCUS–LSIL Triage Study (ALTS) Group. *Am J Obstet Gynecol.* 2003;188:1383–1392.
9. Nobbenhuis MA, Walboomers JM, Helmerhorst TJ, et al. Relation of human papillomavirus status to cervical lesions and consequences for cervical cancer screening: a prospective study. *Lancet.* 1999;354:20–25.
10. ACOG practice bulletin. Clinical management guidelines for obstetricians and gynecologists. No. 45, Aug 2003. Cervical cytology screening. *Obstet Gynecol.* 2003;102:417–427.
11. ACOG practice bulletin. Clinical management guidelines for obstetricians and gynecologists. No. 66, Sept 2005. Management of abnormal cervical cytology and histology. *Obstet Gynecol.* 2005;106:645–664.
12. Cuzick J, Clavel C, Petry KU, et al. Overview of the European and North American studies on HPV testing in primary cervical cancer screening. *Int J Cancer.* 2006;119:1095–1101.
13. Mayrand MH, Duarte-Franco E, Rodrigues I, et al.; Canadian Cervical Cancer Screening Trial Study Group. Human papillomavirus DNA versus Papanicolaou screening tests for cervical cancer. *N Engl J Med.* 2007;357:1579–1588.
14. Human papillomavirus testing for triage of women with cytologic evidence of low-grade squamous intraepithelial lesions: baseline data from a randomized trial. The Atypical Squamous Cells of Undetermined Significance/Low-Grade Squamous Intraepithelial Lesions Triage Study (ALTS) Group. *J Natl Cancer Inst.* 2000;92:397–402.
15. ACOG practice bulletin. Clinical management guidelines for obstetricians and gynecologists. No. 61, April 2005. Human papillomavirus. *Obstet Gynecol.* 2005;105;905–918.
16. Bansal N, Wright JD, Cohen CJ, Herzog TJ. Natural history of established low grade cervical intraepithelial (CIN 1) lesions. *Anticancer Res.* 2008;28:1763–1766.
17. McCredie MR, Sharples KJ, Paul C, et al. Natural history of cervical neoplasia and risk of invasive cancer in women with cervical intraepithelial

neoplasia 3: a retrospective cohort study. *Lancet Oncol.* 2008;9:425–434.

18. Haidopoulos D, Voulgaris Z, Protopapas A, et al. Cervical intraepithelial neoplasia in young women. *J Obstet Gynaecol.* 2007;27:709–712.

19. Fuchs K, Weitzen S, Wu L, Phipps MG, Boardman LA. Management of cervical intraepithelial neoplasia 2 in adolescent and young women. *J Pediatr Adolesc Gynecol.* 2007;20:269–274.

20. Moore K, Cofer A, Elliot L, Lanneau G, Walker J, Gold MA. Adolescent cervical dysplasia:histologic evaluation, treatment, and outcomes. *Am J Obstet Gynecol.* 2007;197:141.e1–141.e6.

21. Hunter MI, Monk BJ, Tewari KS. Cervical neoplasia in pregnancy. Part 1: screening and management of preinvasive disease. *Am J Obstet Gynecol.* 2008;199:3–9.

22. Kane S, Khatibi B, Reddy D. Higher incidence of abnormal Pap smears in women with inflammatory bowel disease. *Am J Gastroenterol.* 2008;103:631–636.

23. Malouf MA, Hopkins PM, Singleton L, Chhajed PN, Plit ML, Glanville AR. Sexual health issues after lung transplantation: importance of cervical screening. *J Heart Lung Transplant.* 2004l;23:894–897.

24. Wright TC Jr., Ellerbrock TV, Chiasson MA, Van Devanter N, Sun XW. Cervical intraepithelial neoplasia in women infected with human immunodeficiency virus: prevalence, risk factors, and validity of Papanicolaou smears. New York Cervical Disease Study. *Obstet Gynecol.* 1994;84:591–597.

25. Harris TG, Burk RD, Palefsky JM, et al. Incidence of cervical squamous intraepithelial lesion associated with HIV serostatus, CD4 cell counts, and human papillomavirus test results. *JAMA.* 2005;293:1471–1476.

26. Massad LS, Evans CT, Minkoff H, et al. Natural history of grade 1 cervical intraepithelial neoplasia in women with human immunodeficiency virus. *Obstet Gynecol.* 2004;104:1077–1085.

27. Kalliala I, Nieminen P, Dyba T, Pukkala E, Anttila A. Cancer free survival after CIN treatment: comparisons of treatment methods and histology. *Gynecol Oncol.* 2007;105:228–233.

28. Crane JM, Delaney T, Huchens D. Transvaginal ultrasonography in the prediction of preterm birth after treatment for cervical intraepithelial neoplasia. *Obstet Gynecol.* 2006;107:37–44.

29. DiSaia. *Clin Gynecol Oncol.* 2002.

30. Arbyn M, Kyrgiou M, Simoens C, et al. Perinatal mortality and other severe adverse pregnancy outcomes associated with treatment of cervical intraepithelial neoplasia: meta-analysis. *BMJ.* 2008;337:a1284.

31. Sadler L, Saftias A, Wang W, Exeter M, Whittaker J, McCowan L. Treatment for cervical intraepithelial neoplasia and risk of preterm delivery. *JAMA.* 2004;291:2100–2116.

32. Samson SL, Bentley JR, Fahey TJ, McKay DJ, Gill GH. The effect of loop electrosurgical excision procedure on future pregnancy outcome. *Obstet Gynecol.* 2005;105:325–332.

33. Reich O, Lahousen M, Pickel H, Tamussino K, Winter R. Cervical intraepithelial neoplasia III: long-term follow-up after cold-knife conization with involved margins. *Obstet Gynecol.* 2002;99:193–196.

34. Creasman WT, Zaino RG, Major FJ, DiSaia PJ, Hatch KD, Homesley HD. Early invasive carcinoma of the cervix (3 to 5 mm invasion): risk factors and prognosis. A Gynecologic Oncology Group study. *Am J Obstet Gynecol.* 1998;178:62–65.

35. Livasy CA, Maygarden SJ, Rajaratnam CT, Novotny DB. Predictors of recurrent dysplasia after a cervical loop elecrosurgery excision procedure for CIN 3: a study of margin, endocervical gland, and quadrant involvement. *Mod Pathol.* 1999;12:233–238.

36. Gadducci A, Sartori E, Maggino T, et al. The clinical outcome of patients with stage Ia1 and Ia2 squamous cell carcinoma of the uterine cervix: a Cooperation Task Force (CTF) study. *Eur J Gynaecol Oncol.* 2003;24:513–516.

37. Young JL, Jazaeri AA, Lachane JA, et al. Cervical adenocarcinoma in situ: the predictive value of conization margin status. *Am J Obstet Gynecol.* 2007;197:195.e1–195.e7.

CHAPTER 5

Endometrial Hyperplasia and Endometrial Cancer

Aaron Shafer, MD
Department of Obstetrics and Gynecology, University of North Carolina School of Medicine, Chapel Hill, NC, USA

Linda Van Le, MD, FACOG
Department of Obstetrics and Gynecology, University of North Carolina School of Medicine, Chapel Hill, NC, USA

Pathology Notes: Chad Livasy, MD
Associate Professor, Department of Pathology and Laboratory Medicine, University of North Carolina School of Medicine, Chapel Hill, NC, USA

Endometrial hyperplasia is a common clinical problem that all gynecologists will encounter in their practice. By definition, endometrial hyperplasia is an abnormal proliferation of both the glandular and stromal elements of the endometrium, with the glandular component being the most prominent.[1,2] In addition to causing abnormal uterine bleeding, endometrial hyperplasia can predispose a woman to developing endometrioid adenocarcinoma. It is for this reason that hyperplasia warrants proper evaluation and management. Endometrial hyperplasia classification is based on two main histologic descriptions: architectural and cytologic. Architectural appearance refers to the amount of glandular crowding, and is classified as simple or complex.[2] The presence or absence of cellular atypia is the most important prognostic factor in a woman with endometrial hyperplasia and will most often determine the treatment. It should be understood that only those patients with cytologic atypia are at significant risk of developing endometrial cancer.[1,3]

Gynecological Cancer Management: Identification, Diagnosis and Treatment, Edited by Daniel L. Clarke-Pearson and John T. Soper. Published 2010 by Blackwell Publishing, ISBN: 978-1-4051-9079-4.

Pathogenesis

Endometrial hyperplasia is a result of estrogen excess in the absence of adequate progesterone.[2,4,5] Often this estrogen excess is due to obesity, polycystic ovarian disease, or prolonged anovulation in a perimenopausal woman.[4-6] The exact mechanism that leads from estrogen overexposure to endometrial hyperplasia is not fully understood. The endometrial estrogen receptor is involved as is demonstrated by the effect that tamoxifen, a selective estrogen receptor modulator (SERM), has on the endometrium. Tamoxifen and other SERMs are competitive inhibitors of estrogen for the estrogen receptor (ER). Depending on the site, tamoxifen binding to the ER can have either a stimulatory (pro-estrogenic) or inhibitory (anti-estrogenic) effect.[7] In the uterus, as opposed to the breast, tamoxifen has a pro-estrogenic effect. Up to 40% to 50% of patients using tamoxifen will develop some form of endometrial hyperplasia or polyp.[4] Further evidence of the link between unopposed estrogen and endometrial hyperplasia is the data from the PEPI trial, which showed that patients taking estrogen alone developed simple hyperplasia, complex hyperplasia, and atypical hyperplasia more frequently than those taking placebo or estrogen + progesterone.[8] These women were given 0.625 mg of conjugated equine estrogen (CEE) per day. In a subsequent study, when the dose of CEE was dropped to 0.3 mg/day, the rates of endometrial hyperplasia were no different than those taking placebo.[9] This suggests that not only is estrogen without progesterone needed for the development of endometrial hyperplasia, but also that the dose of estrogen is a key in the development of hyperplasia. It should be noted that the longest follow-up in this and other low-dose estrogen trials is only 24 months. Additionally, other studies have shown a trend, though not statistically significant, towards higher rates of endometrial hyperplasia in patients taking low-dose unopposed estrogen when compared to placebo.[10] The addition of progesterone to estrogen in HRT for postmenopausal women reduces the risk of hyperplasia to that of placebo, even at moderate to high doses of estrogen.[10]

Tamoxifen use increases the risk of endometrial cancer.[5,11] The risk of endometrial cancer is greatest in women over the age of 50. Patients diagnosed with endometrial cancer while on tamoxifen are likely to have stage I disease and have an excellent prognosis.[11] Women who are on tamoxifen should be queried as to any abnormal bleeding and prompt evaluation should be initiated.

It is important to keep in mind that estrogen-secreting tumors such as granulosa cell tumors can present as abnormal uterine bleeding. Between one-quarter and one-half of women with granulosa cell tumors will have endometrial hyperplasia at the time of hysterectomy for their ovarian tumor.[6,12,13] This is especially important in women of child-bearing age, in whom endometrial hyperplasia, specifically atypical hyperplasia, is more uncommon. A pelvic ultrasound looking for adnexal masses is important to help rule out an estrogen-secreting tumor. In a younger woman without a history of anovulation, who is not obese, and has an adnexal mass on imaging, granulosa cell tumors should be high on the differential.[12] (See Chapter 11 for a more in-depth discussion of granulosa cell tumors).

Presentation/Diagnosis

The most common presenting symptom of endometrial hyperplasia is abnormal uterine bleeding.[5,14] In working up a patient with abnormal uterine bleeding, it is important to first decide whether the patient is premenopausal or postmenopausal, as this will raise or lower the suspicion for endometrial hyperplasia or carcinoma. In postmenopausal women with vaginal bleeding, endometrial hyperplasia and carcinoma must always be at the top of the differential diagnosis list. Even so, most abnormal uterine bleeding in these women (60–80%) is due to endometrial atrophy. Endometrial hyperplasia is found about 15% of the time and carcinoma in approximately 7% to 10% of these menopausal patients who have uterine bleeding.[4,5] Other causes of postmenopausal uterine bleeding can be estrogen replacement therapy and endometrial polyps.[4] Any perimenopausal or postmenopausal woman with uterine bleeding should be evaluated with endometrial biopsy via pipelle or D&C (Box 1). If possible, endometrial pipelle in the office is preferred, as it is less invasive, cheaper, and has equal if not superior sensitivity to D&C, especially for the diagnosis of a diffuse process involving the endometrium in the postmenopausal woman.[15]

Women taking tamoxifen who still have a uterus are at a higher risk of developing endometrial hyperplasia and endometrial carcinoma, with a risk ratio of 2.53 of developing endometrial carcinoma compared to those who took placebo. Even so, the

---

Box 1 Who needs endometrial sampling (endometrial biopsy or D&C)?

- Postmenopausal women with spotting or bleeding
- Postmenopausal women on tamoxifen with vaginal bleeding
- Premenopausal women taking tamoxifen with abnormal uterine bleeding
- Women over the age of 35 with an AGUS Pap smear
- Premenopausal women with abnormal uterine bleeding who are obese or have a long-tanding history of anovulation

absolute risk of endometrial cancer in a woman on tamoxifen is less than 1 in 1000.[11] As such, women on tamoxifen should be counseled that they have an increased risk of both endometrial hyperplasia and carcinoma. Any woman taking tamoxifen should be instructed to report vaginal bleeding if she is postmenopausal.[12] Premenopausal women appear to have no difference in the rates of endometrial hyperplasia or carcinoma while on tamoxifen, and therefore do not need any care other than routine gynecologic care.[11, 16] Women who do present to a gynecologist complaining of abnormal uterine bleeding while on tamoxifen should have prompt histologic evaluation with either an endometrial biopsy or dilatation and curettage. Based on the current literature and recommendations, there is no benefit to routinely performing ultrasounds or endometrial biopsies on women who are taking tamoxifen and are asymptomatic. Only women who had abnormal bleeding patterns while taking tamoxifen were shown to have significant endometrial hyperplasia or carcinoma.[5, 16]

In a premenopausal woman, abnormal uterine bleeding is less likely to be caused by endometrial hyperplasia or carcinoma. There are certain risk factors, however, which put younger women at higher risk for atypical hyperplasia or carcinoma, and these are important to keep in mind when evaluating a premenopausal woman with abnormal uterine bleeding. A personal history of anovulation, polycystic ovarian syndrome (PCOS), diabetes, or obese patients, should be considered for endometrial sampling in the presence of abnormal uterine bleeding.[4] PCOS and anovulation, which often coexist, predispose patients to a relative state of unopposed estrogen. In addition, women with PCOS have higher levels of circulating androgens, which can undergo peripheral conversion to estrogen via aromatase in adipose tissue.[5, 6] ACOG recommends endometrial sampling in women with suspected anovulatory bleeding if they are over the age of 35.[17]

Pap smears are not designed to screen for endometrial pathology and should not be used for this purpose; however, certain findings on directed or screening cervical cytology may lead to a diagnosis of endometrial hyperplasia. In postmenopausal women with uterine bleeding, the presence of endometrial cells or histiocytes on Pap smear is associated with a three- to fourfold increased risk of having concurrent endometrial carcinoma.[5] Atypical glandular cells (AGUS) may be indicative of endometrial pathology, including hyperplasia. In younger women an AGUS Pap smear is still most often associated with a squamous cervical lesion; however, in older women (>50 years old), the chances of a non-squamous lesion (glandular lesion) increase significantly.[5] Therefore, endometrial biopsy is recommended for women over the age of 35 with an AGUS Pap smear (in addition to colposcopy and endocervical sampling). Women under age 35 with "atypical endometrial cells" on their Pap smear, or an AGUS Pap smear with obesity, oligomenorrhea, or abnormal bleeding, should also have endometrial sampling.[18]

While the pathologic criteria for simple, complex, and atypical hyperplasia are generally agreed upon, there is a large subjective component to the actual pathologic interpretation (Box 2). The Gynecological Oncology Group (GOG) undertook a study to examine the reliability of the diagnosis of atypical endometrial hyperplasia (AEH). A total of 302 women with AEH diagnosed at "referring" institutions had their endometrial biopsies or curettings reviewed by the three experts. Only 38% of the time did the expert panel agree with the outside pathologists' interpretation of AEH, and only 15% of the time did all three experts agree with the outside diagnosis of AEH. In 25% of the cases, the

---

Box 2 Key features of hyperplasia

Simple architecture
Dilated cystic glands with abundant intervening stroma
Occasional irregular glandular borders

Complex architecture
Crowded glands with little intervening stroma
Variable and irregular glandular borders

Cellular atypia
Loss of cellular polarity
High nuclear-to-cytoplasmic ratio
Vesicular nuclei
Prominent nucleoli
Presence of mitotic figures

expert panel downgraded the diagnosis to either normal endometrium or hyperplasia without atypia, and 29% of the time they upgraded the specimen to a diagnosis of endometrial carcinoma. Speaking to the point of variation in interpretation, it should be noted that there was also a fair amount of discordance between the "expert pathologists" as well. All three experts agreed on the diagnosis in only 40% of the 302 cases. Most often, all three agreed on a diagnosis of normal (57%) or carcinoma (44%).[19] This study demonstrates the difficulty and subjectivity of a diagnosis of atypical hyperplasia even among "expert" gynecologic pathologists. Therefore, if a clinician has questions regarding the diagnosis of hyperplasia, referral of slides for a review by a gynecologic pathologist is a reasonable option.

Endometrial hyperplasia and endometrial carcinoma

The abnormal uterine bleeding that accompanies endometrial hyperplasia can be bothersome and impact on a woman's life. For this reason, treatment of hyperplasia is important. As mentioned earlier, however, the more pressing concern when a patient is diagnosed with endometrial hyperplasia is the predisposition to developing endometrial cancer that hyperplasia confers. The chance that a particular patient will develop or be diagnosed with endometrial carcinoma depends on the type of hyperplasia. The most important feature on endometrial biopsy or curettings is the presence or absence of cytologic atypia. In a study of 170 women who were diagnosed with endometrial hyperplasia and did not undergo hysterectomy for at least 1 year, the risk of finding endometrial carcinoma at the time of hysterectomy increased dramatically with the presence of cytologic atypia. Specifically, almost 30% of women with complex atypical hyperplasia had endometrial cancer at the time of their hysterectomy.[3]

In the time since the publication by Kurman and associates in 1985[3] much work has been done to examine the relationship between complex atypical hyperplasia and endometrial cancer. The question is whether complex hyperplasia with atypia (CAH) is a precursor lesion to carcinoma, whether they are coexistent lesions, or possibly a combination of both. The 29% risk of carcinoma found in the study by Kurman and colleagues has been the classic rate of cancer quoted by gynecologists and has directed much of our care, specifically the recommendation for hysterectomy. A subsequent study by the Gynecologic Oncology Group (GOG), however, revealed that the risk of endometrial cancer in women with CAH may be higher than previously thought.[20] In a prospective study of 289 women diagnosed with atypical hyperplasia in the "community," 42.6% had endometrial cancer in their hysterectomy specimens. All patients had hysterectomies within 12 weeks of their endometrial biopsy or curettage and none of these women had intervening treatment. The diagnosis of cancer in the hysterectomy specimens was made by a panel of three gynecologic pathologists; these experts reviewed the original biopsies as well. This study is the second part of the GOG study described above. Nineteen percent of the carcinomas were found in patients whose biopsies were read by the expert panel as "less than atypical hyperplasia."[20] In the hysterectomy specimens, 65% of the cancers were confined to the endometrium (stage IA). However, 10.6% of the carcinomas were invasive into the outer half of the myometrium (stage IC). None of the cancers were more advanced than stage I. [20] This study demonstrates the high risk of coexistent endometrial cancer when a patient has atypical hyperplasia. It is important to note that these patients all had hysterectomies within 3 months of their diagnosis as opposed to those in the study by Kurman and associates, who were followed for at least 1 year after their diagnosis of hyperplasia. This underscores the importance of treatment for CAH.

The historic risk of endometrial cancer quoted to patients with atypical hyperplasia (either simple or complex) was between 17% and 25%.[5] Two retrospective studies in combination with the prospective GOG study suggest that this incidence is higher, probably at least 40%.[5,20] This is important when counseling a patient with CAH and deciding on treatment.

Pathology notes

Endometrial hyperplasia

The main reason that many endometrial biopsies are performed is to identify the cause of abnormal bleeding, and the expectation is that the pathologist will help to determine whether the bleeding is organic in nature (eg, endometrial hyperplasia or carcinoma) or functional. When endometrial hyperplasia is identified, it is further subcategorized based on histopathology to predict the risk for progression to adenocarcinoma. The exact classification and nomenclature used for endometrial hyperplasia remains controversial to this day. Before discussing the specifics of endometrial hyperplasia, we will first focus on two potential problem areas related to excluding endometrial neoplasia—atrophic endometrium and disordered proliferative-type endometrium.

Many endometrial biopsies are performed on postmenopausal women. These patients will often have atrophic endometrium where the lining is particularly thin (<1 mm). It is typical that only scant material is obtained in biopsy specimens from these patients. The biopsies may contain only tiny strips of surface epithelium with absent to minimal stroma. The scant material indicates the condition of the endometrium, atrophy, and such biopsies should not be diagnosed as "insufficient for diagnosis." If you are having a high rate of unsatisfactory cases in your postmenopausal patients, you may want to have the pathologist clarify what tissue, if any, was present in the biopsy.

The term disordered proliferative-type endometrium is used in cases of abnormal endometrium showing focal irregular branching and dilation of glands, often in association with glandular and stromal breakdown. Although the glandular architecture is abnormal, the gland-to-stroma ratio in these cases is not increased as would be seen in endometrial hyperplasia. This disordered pattern is typically due to persistent unopposed estrogen stimulation in patients experiencing chronic anovulation. Simple hyperplasia without atypia is the main other diagnostic consideration for patients with disordered proliferative-type endometrium.

The most widely used classification of endometrial hyperplasia, the WHO classification, divides hyperplasia into the following four types: simple hyperplasia without atypia, complex hyperplasia without atypia, simple hyperplasia with atypia, and complex hyperplasia with atypia. The diagnosis of simple hyperplasia with atypia is exceedingly rare, and this diagnosis should probably be confirmed by a second pathologist to ensure accuracy before a patient is treated. The WHO classification system is based on configuration and number of glands, degree of glandular crowding, and presence/absence of nuclear atypia. Nuclear atypia is the feature that determines whether hyperplasia is classified as atypical or not. The presence of atypia is associated with increased risk for progression to adenocarcinoma (approximately 25–30%) as compared to cases lacking atypia (1–3%). Problem areas in the pathologic evaluation of hyperplasia include defining the presence or absence of nuclear atypia and separating extreme cases of complex atypical hyperplasia from well-differentiated endometrioid adenocarcinoma. Critics of the WHO classification system point to studies showing poor interobserver agreement among pathologists in the diagnosis of atypia in hyperplasia cases.[21] An alternative classification system has been proposed.

The endometrial intraepithelial neoplasia (EIN) terminology proposed by Mutter and associates to classify hyperplasia is based on morphometric analysis of endometrial neoplasia and supported by molecular analysis of endometrial hyperplasia and carcinomas.[22–24] The EIN system is a two-tier system consisting of (1) endometrial hyperplasia and (2) EIN. Hyperplasia, which is not associated with significant risk for progression to adenocarcinoma, results from estrogenic stimulation of endometrium and tends to be a

Pathology notes (*continued*)

diffuse process with uniform cytology. EIN lesions start from a single cell or gland, showing loss of PTEN expression in model studies, and are therefore commonly focal lesions with volume percent stroma <50% and cytology dissimilar to the background non-neoplastic endometrium. Mimics such as polyps or basalis need to be excluded. The main diagnostic feature in EIN is glandular crowding, with gland/stroma ratio >50%. Atypia in this system is not defined relative to an absolute standard, but relative to the benign non-neoplastic glands in the same specimen (Fig. 5.1). Approximately 30% of cases with EIN will progress to adenocarcinoma. The management of patients with EIN lesions follows the same guidelines long established for complex atypical hyperplasia. EIN is not to be confused with endometrial intraepithelial carcinoma (EIC), the precursor lesion for serous carcinoma.

Biopsy sampling errors have been well documented in patients with complex atypical hyperplasia/EIN undergoing hysterectomy. Approximately 25% to 40% of these patients will be upgraded to endometrioid adenocarcinoma following thorough sampling of the endometrium from the hysterectomy specimen.[25] Frozen section evaluation, although imperfect, can help identify the few patients with adenocarcinoma showing significant myometrial invasion such that staging lymph node dissection should be performed. Simple gross inspection is accurate in most cases in determining the presence or absence of significant myometrial invasion, but frozen section is preferred to identify the rare cases with subtle myometrial invasion that may not be identified on gross exam.

Endometrial intraepithelial carcinoma (EIC) is occasionally detected in endometrial biopsies for bleeding, usually in postmenopausal women, and should clearly be distinguished from regular endometrial hyperplasia. EIC is the precursor of serous carcinoma of the endometrium. EIC is characterized by high-grade malignant cells, often scant to moderate in volume when present in biopsy specimen, seen in a background of atrophy (Plate 5.1). Immunohistochemical staining

A

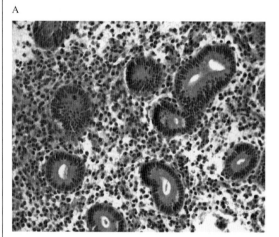

B

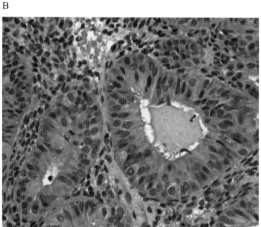

Figure 5.1 Endometrial intraepithelial neoplasia (EIN)/atypical hyperplasia. **A.** Endometrial biopsy showing background non-neoplastic glands to be used as reference in determining cytologic atypia. **B.** Region of the same biopsy showing a gland/stroma ratio > 50% reveals glands comprised of larger cells with larger round nuclei containing nucleoli, supporting the diagnosis of EIN.

Pathology notes (*continued*)

for p53 can be confirmatory for problematic cases, as these lesions show diffuse strong immunore-activity for p53. EIC is important to recognize in biopsies and separate from regular hyperplasia because it alters surgical management. If a diagnosis of EIC is made on endometrial biopsy, the patient should undergo TAH/BSO with surgical staging. Extrauterine tumor can be found in patients with EIC or minimal uterine serous carcinoma, even if the lesion is confined to a polyp. Hysterectomy specimens from patients with EIC should be thoroughly sectioned to evaluate for subtle myometrial invasion or lymphovascular space invasion.

Pathology reports from hysterectomy specimens showing carcinoma should include the following information, preferably in a template fashion: tumor type, FIGO grade, depth and percentage of myometrial invasion, presence/absence of cervical involvement, presence/absence of cervical stromal invasion and depth for cases with cervix involvement, presence/absence of lymphovascular space invasion, lymph node count (# positive and # identified), and AJCC pathologic TNM stage. Given that most gynecologists use the FIGO stage, the FIGO stage should also be reported next to the AJCC TNM stage.

Clinical Scenario 1

A 30-year-old G0 woman presents to your office with a 4-year history of menorrhagia. Over the past 6 months, the patient states that her menses have become more irregular as well. She is obese (5 ft 4 in, 130 kg) with a body mass index (BMI) of 49 kg/m^2. Her hemoglobin has been as low as 7.5 g/dL and she is currently on iron sulfate for her anemia, which has raised her hemoglobin to 8.5 g/dL. She undergoes a dilatation and curettage (D&C) and the pathology shows complex hyperplasia without atypia.

What are the different types/classifications of endometrial hyperplasia and their significance with regard to prognosis and natural history?

Endometrial hyperplasia is an abnormal proliferation of endometrial glands. These glands exhibit an abnormal shape and size, and there is an increase in the amount of glands compared to intervening stroma.[2] Hyperplasia is classified based on two pathologic descriptions: simple versus complex architecture and the presence or absence of cytologic atypia.[1,2] In simple hyperplasia without atypia, or simple hyperplasia, the endometrial glands are dilated, irregular, and

more numerous but there is abundant intervening stroma (Fig. 5.2). The glandular epithelium is similar to that found in proliferative endometrium.[1] In contrast to simple hyperplasia, complex hyperplasia is characterized by back-to-back glands with little intervening stroma. The glands appear more "complex" with more outpouchings and infoldings than in simple hyperplasia. There is an increase in the number of glands, but they are often less dilated than in simple hyperplasia

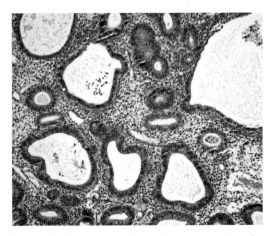

Figure 5.2 Simple hyperplasia without atypia. Note the large, dilated glands with abundant stroma between glands.

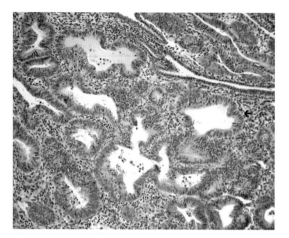

Figure 5.3 Complex hyperplasia without atypia. Note the back-to-back glands with little intervening stroma. The glands have irregular infoldings but retain their cellular polarity.

and there is less intervening stroma than in simple hyperplasia, with a gland-to-stroma ratio of 2 to 1 (Fig. 5.3).[1] In both simple and complex hyperplasia without atypia, there may be pseudostratification of the glandular epithelial cells, but the cells retain their polarity.

Hyperplasia with atypia, both simple and complex, is characterized by an increase in the nuclear to cytoplasmic ratio, nuclear stratification with loss of polarity in the glandular epithelial cells, an increase in the nuclear size and pleomorphism, and the presence of prominent nucleoli.[1-3] One may even see mitotic figures and irregular nuclear chromatin. While the WHO classification includes "simple hyperplasia with atypia" as a type of hyperplasia, this diagnosis is rarely if ever seen. Most, if not all, hyperplasia with cytologic atypia is complex atypical hyperplasia.[1] What distinguishes early endometrial carcinoma from complex atypical hyperplasia is stromal invasion, confluence of glands into a cribiform pattern, a surrounding desmoplastic reaction, an extensive papillary pattern, or replacement of the normal stromal cells with a squamous epithelium.[2,3]

In the current WHO classification system, hyperplasia is described both by its architecture (simple versus complex) and its cytologic appearance (presence or absence of atypia). Therefore, all endometrial hyperplasia can be classified into one of four categories using this system: simple hyperplasia without atypia, complex hyperplasia without atypia, simple hyperplasia with atypia, and complex atypical hyperplasia.[1] This is the preferred nomenclature, but occasionally one will see other descriptive terms such as "cystic" or "glandular" hyperplasia instead of simple hyperplasia, or the term "adenomatous" hyperplasia, which refers to complex hyperplasia.[1,5,14] Even if these terms are used, there should still be some mention of the presence or absence of cytologic atypia.

Some advocate for a new classification of endometrial hyperplasia based on the risk of concomitant or progression to endometrial carcinoma.[1,3] Hyperplasia without atypia would be replaced by "endometrial hyperplasia" and lesions usually considered atypical hyperplasia would be classified as "endometrial intraepithelial hyperplasia" or EIN. Under this classification system, the diagnosis of EIN specifies a precancerous lesion measuring at least 1 mm in size that has a high gland-to-stroma ratio (>1), and the glands in the lesion would demonstrate cytologic characteristics of atypia that are different from the surrounding endometrium.[1,4] EIN lesions are usually focal, but can diffusely involve the endometrium in up to 20% of cases. In addition to histologic characteristics, EIN takes into account genetic alterations such as PTEN and k-ras mutations. The argument for using the EIN classification instead of the WHO classification is that EIN is thought to better predict the progression to endometrial carcinoma. Over 40% of patients with EIN will develop carcinoma within 1 year, and those that do not are at a 45-fold greater risk of developing endometrial cancer than the general population.[4] This is a somewhat new concept, however, and the WHO classification is still the standard definition/classification for endometrial hyperplasia.[1]

The type of hyperplasia and the presence or absence of atypia are very important for prognosis for the patient in terms of their possible risk of developing endometrial carcinoma.

Patients with simple or complex hyperplasia without atypia have a 1% to 5% chance of developing endometrial cancer, whereas those with simple or complex hyperplasia with atypia have from a 15% to 40% chance of endometrial carcinoma.[3, 20] In addition, the type of hyperplasia will guide therapeutic options for the patient, are dictate whether conservative medical treatment or surgical therapy is warranted.

What are the treatment options for this 30-year-old woman with complex hyperplasia without atypia?

The presence or absence of cytologic atypia is the most important factor for risk of uterine carcinoma. Anovulatory young women of reproductive age who are diagnosed with endometrial hyperplasia without atypia and wish to preserve fertility should usually be treated with progestins. They can be placed on combined estrogen-progesterone oral contraceptives if there are no contraindications. Women of child-bearing age could also be placed on cyclic progestins for 12 to 14 days every month. Progestins such as medroxyprogesterone acetate (MPA) 10 mg/day or megestrol acetate 40 mg/day are very effective for hyperplasia without atypia.[5] The endometrium should be sampled again in 3 to 6 months to assess response to therapy. If the repeat endometrial biopsy is normal, then the patient may discontinue treatment. If the patient continues to be anovulatory, however, she should be given a progestin every 3 months to induce withdrawal bleeds to prevent the subsequent development of hyperplasia.[14] Placement of a progesterone-containing IUD (Mirena) or using Depo-provera may be considered if the woman does not want to conceive for an extended period of time.

For perimenopausal and postmenopausal women who have hyperplasia without atypia, a D&C should be preformed to confirm the diagnosis if initially only an endometrial biopsy was done. If the diagnosis of hyperplasia without atypia is confirmed, then continuous or cyclic (10–14 days out of the month) progestin therapy

with medroxyprogesterone acetate (MPA) 10 mg daily or norethindrone 5 mg daily for 3 months should be initiated, followed by repeat endometrial biopsy in 3 months. This will cause regression of hyperplasia in 80% to 90% of patients.[5] If the woman is on hormonal replacement therapy, it should either be discontinued, the estrogen dose lowered, the progestin dose raised, or MPA 10 mg, or some other oral progestin, daily for 12-14 days out of the month should be added to the regimen. [26]

Case Scenario 2

A 46-year-old woman is referred to you by her primary care doctor for abnormal bleeding. The patient says that she has never stopped having periods but that over the past few months they have become more irregular and she occasionally has "two periods a month."

How should this patient be evaluated?

As stated earlier, the most common presenting symptom of endometrial hyperplasia and endometrial carcinoma is abnormal uterine bleeding.[5, 14] In this perimenopausal patient, nonhyperplastic causes such as anovultory bleeding, uterine fibroids, or endometrial polyps are likely reasons for her abnormal bleeding. However, endometrial hyperplasia should always be in the differential, and 5% to 15% of patients will have some form of hyperplasia.[4, 5] Therefore, all perimenopausal and postmenopausal woman with uterine bleeding should be evaluated with endometrial biopsy or D&C. Office endometrial pipelle, if possible, is preferable, as it is less invasive, cheaper, avoids anesthesia, and has equal if not superior sensitivity to D&C for the diagnosis of diffuse endometrial pathology.[15] The possible advantage of a D&C in a patient like this is that it can be therapeutic as well as diagnostic if the cause is endometrial polyp or submucosal fibroid.

The use of ultrasound or saline-infused sonohysterography (SIS)—where saline is injected into the endometrial cavity while transvaginal ultrasound is performed—can help with the evaluation of abnormal uterine bleeding. SIS can often help identify endometrial polyps and submucosal fibroids[4] but is poor for diagnosing hyperplasia or carcinoma.[5] Ultrasound may be used in a postmenopausal woman with uterine bleeding to assist in the identification of endometrial pathology including hyperplasia and carcinoma. An endometrial stripe thickness of less than 5 mm is rarely associated with endometrial cancer. Combining ultrasound evaluation of endometrial thickness and an endometrial biopsy has a sensitivity of over 90% compared to hysteroscopy with D&C.[4,5] Endometrial thickness greater than 5 mm does not necessarily indicate endometrial hyperplasia or carcinoma, and an endometrial stripe greater than 5 mm has a positive predictive value of only 9% in an asymptomatic population.[5]

An endometrial biopsy is done in the office and returns complex hyperplasia with atypia. What are the treatment options?

For the perimenopausal or postmenopausal woman with hyperplasia of any type with atypia, the treatment of choice is hysterectomy with bilateral salpingo-oophorectomy (BSO). Given the fact that approximately 40% of these women will have endometrial carcinoma at the time of hysterectomy,[20] patients should be strongly encouraged to undergo hysterectomy with possible surgical staging if medically suitable.

What specific surgical procedure should be performed? Given that endometrial carcinoma may be discovered in the uterus, how should the general gynecologist proceed?

A hysterectomy and bilateral salpingo-oophorectomy should be performed. We believe that all methods of performing a hysterectomy are equally effective (abdominal, vaginal or laparoscopic). In nearly all cases (except in very

young women), we recommend removal of tubes and ovaries. The cervix should be removed in all circumstances and we advise against morcellation of the uterus. It is also recommended that peritoneal washings be obtained at the time of hysterectomy, because peritoneal cytology is an important component for staging endometrial carcinoma.

A decision to perform surgical staging (pelvic and para-aortic lymphadenectomy) would then await return of final pathology. Alternatively, frozen section could be performed at the time of hysterectomy and if there were evidence of carcinoma with myometrial invasion, immediate formal staging with pelvic and para-aortic lymphadenectomy could be performed. The strategy chosen may be dictated by the availability of a gynecologic oncologist, but patients should be counseled about the possible need for staging with lymphadenectomy if significant myometrial invasion or a high-grade lesion is identified.

Are there any treatments that could be used instead of surgery?

For women with atypical hyperplasia who are of child-bearing age (and desire preservation of fertility) or who are poor surgical risk, progestin therapy should be offered. Oral progestin therapy with high-dose progestins such as megestrol acetate 40 to 80 mg daily should be given and a repeat endometrial biopsy performed in 3 months. If at 3 months the hyperplasia persists, then the patient is kept on the oral progestins for another 3 months. If there is progression to carcinoma, then hysterectomy is recommended. If there is resolution of the hyperplasia, the patient should be encouraged to conceive right away, or placed on combined OCPs until she is ready to attempt conception. For patients in whom compliance may be an issue, Depo-provera given IM every 3 months is an option. Most data on the efficacy of progestin therapy for endometrial hyperplasia and carcinoma are retrospective.[5,27] However, a recent prospective, multi-institutional trial in Japan examined the efficacy of oral medroxyprogestrone acetate (MPA) for atypical hyperplasia or grade 1 endometrial cancer. Of the 45 eligible patients, 17 had atypical hyperplasia. On a regimen of oral MPA over a treatment period of 26 weeks, 82% of patients had complete resolution of the hyperplasia. None progressed to cancer.[28] Of note, after initial treatment, these patients were maintained on combined OCPs after the 26-week trial period. Likewise, older patients who are treated with progestins rather than surgery should be encouraged to continue progestins indefinitely after there has been regression of their hyperplasia.

Clinical Scenario 3

A 58-year-old G3P3 who was diagnosed with stage I breast cancer 4 years ago is referred to you by her medical oncologist after she complained of some vaginal spotting. She is in remission from her breast cancer and has been on tamoxifen for the past 4 years.

What should her workup include? What are her risks for endometrial pathology?

Women taking tamoxifen who still have a uterus are at a higher risk of developing endometrial hyperplasia and endometrial carcinoma (risk ratio of 2.53) compared to patients who took placebo in a randomized trial.[8] Other case-controlled studies have also shown an increased risk of developing endometrial hyperplasia while on tamoxifen, especially for postmenopausal women.[29] Despite this, the absolute risk of endometrial cancer in a woman on tamoxifen is less than 1 in 1000.[11] Therefore, women on tamoxifen should be counseled about their increased risk of both endometrial hyperplasia and carcinoma, and any woman taking tamoxifen should be instructed to report any abnormal vaginal bleeding, especially if she is postmenopausal.[16] Premenopausal women appear to have no difference in the rates of endometrial hyperplasia or carcinoma while on tamoxifen and therefore do not need any care other than routine gynecologic care.[11, 16] Women who present to a gynecologist complaining of abnormal uterine bleeding while taking tamoxifen should have prompt histologic evaluation with either an endometrial biopsy or dilatation and curettage. Some advocate hysteroscopy with D&C for these women as these hyperplastic endometrial lesions can often be focal as opposed to diffuse.[29] Based on the current literature and recommendations, there is no reason to routinely do ultrasounds or endometrial biopsies on women who are taking tamoxifen and are asymptomatic. Only women who had abnormal bleeding patterns while taking tamoxifen were shown to have significant endometrial hyperplasia or carcinoma.[5, 16]

There is evidence to suggest that women with pretreatment endometrial pathology, specifically polyps, who are placed on tamoxifen have an 18 times greater risk for developing atypical hyperplasia compared to those without endometrial polyps while on tamoxifen. Therefore, sonohysterogram should be considered for a woman with a past history of endometrial polyps before instituting tamoxifen therapy. If she has polyps, then she should be counseled about her higher risk of developing endometrial hyperplasia and the need to be more vigilant in reporting symptoms such as vaginal bleeding.[16]

Clinical Scenario 4

A 33-year-old G0 woman presents with menometrorrhagia. She states that she has not had regular periods since her early 20s. She says that she bleeds 15 to 20 days out of the month. Some of these days, her bleeding is quite heavy. D&C reveals complex hyperplasia with atypia. The patient is not married and wishes to retain her fertility.

What are her options for treatment other than hysterectomy?

As noted above, systemic progestins may be used to treat endometrial hyperplasia. For patients with CAH, oral megestrol acetate in doses of 40 to 80 mg daily is an acceptable regimen. Intramuscular medroxyprogesterone acetate is also acceptable in patients in whom compliance might be an issue. Repeat endometrial biopsy should be done in 3 to 6 months. Systemic progestins have a success rate of eliminating hyperplasia in up to 80% of cases.[28]

Alternatively, there is a growing body of evidence that local progestin therapy with a progestin-containing IUD is effective in treating endometrial hyperplasia as well as early endometrial cancer.[27,30–34] In a comparative study, 26 patients with all grades of endometrial hyperplasia were treated with a levonorgestrel (LNG)-containing IUD and compared to a historic cohort of patients treated with an oral progestin. All 26 patients in the IUD group showed resolution of the hyperplasia by 3 months, while 14 of the 31 patients treated orally had persistent hyperplasia at 3 months. It should be noted, however, that only 4 of the 26 IUD patients had atypical hyperplasia, while 10 of the 31 oral progestin patients had atypical hyperplasia.[32] Another study of 20 women with hyperplasia, 8 with atypical hyperplasia, treated with an LNG-containing IUD, demonstrated that 19 had complete histologic resolution of their hyperplasia. One patient with atypical hyperplasia had persistent non-atypical hyperplasia 3 years after initiation of treatment with the LNG IUD. No one progressed to carcinoma.[34] A third retrospective study looked at 258 patients with hyperplasia (with and without atypia) treated with obsevation, oral progestins, or LNG IUD. One-hundred percent of patients with the IUD regressed to normal within 6 months, while 55% of those receiving oral progestins showed regression. Interestingly, patients with hyperplasia without atypia had a similar regression rate whether they received oral progestins or observation only.[27] In a large, prospective observational study in England, 105 women with hyperplasia were treated with an LNG IUD. There was regression in 90% of patients, but only 67% among patients with atypical hyperplasia. This study was limited because only 9 patients had atypical hy-

perplasia and 2 patients were identified with cancer.[31]

Additionally, there have been case reports of patients treated for hyperplasia with an LNG IUD progressing to endometrial carcinoma.[35] It appears that LNG-containing IUDs are very successful when treating hyperplasia without atypia, and generally have a good response among patients with atypia. Systemic effects of progestins should be limited during the duration of IUD use. Formal randomized trials are needed to determine if they have a better response rate than systemic progestins. However, careful surveillance in patients initially treated for atypical hyperplasia is necessary. Surveillance can include either transvaginal ultrasound or endometrial biopsy. It appears that patients with endometrial stripes that are thinking or are less than 5 to 6 mm while being treated for atypical hyperplasia will have resolution, while those who have thicker stripes (>10 mm) or whose endometrial stripe thickness increases during treatment are at higher risk of persistence or progression.[28,33,35] For evaluation of histologic regression after placement of an LNG IUD, office endometrial pipelle can be performed with the IUD in situ. Endometrial sampling should be done every 3 months until regression and then every 6 months after that, alternating with TVUS.

References

1. Horn LC, Meinel A, Handzel R, Einenkel J. Histopathology of endometrial hyperplasia and endometrial carcinoma: an update. *Ann Diagn Pathol.* 2007;11:297–311.
2. Ronnett BM, Kurman RJ. Precursor Lesions of Endometrial Carcinoma. In: Kurman RJ, ed. *Blaustein's Pathology of the Female Genital Tract.* 5th ed. New York: Springer-Verlag;2002:467–500.
3. Kurman RJ, Kaminski PF, Norris HJ. The behavior of endometrial hyperplasia. A long-term study of "untreated" hyperplasia in 170 patients. *Cancer.* 1985;56:403–412.
4. Espindola D, Kennedy KA, Fischer EG. Management of abnormal uterine bleeding and the pathology of

endometrial hyperplasia. *Obstet Gynecol Clin North Am.* 2007;34:717–737, ix.

5. Montgomery BE, Daum GS, Dunton CJ. Endometrial hyperplasia: a review. *Obstet Gynecol Surv.* 2004;59:368–378.

6. Boruban MC, Altundag K, Kilic GS, Blankstein J. From endometrial hyperplasia to endometrial cancer: insight into the biology and possible medical preventive measures. *Eur J Cancer Prev.* 2008;17:133–138.

7. Riggs BL, Hartmann LC. Selective estrogen-receptor modulators—mechanisms of action and application to clinical practice. *N Engl J Med.* 2003;348:618–629.

8. Writing Group for the PEPI trial. Effects of hormone replacement therapy on endometrial histology in postmenopausal women. The Postmenopausal Estrogen/Progestin Interventions (PEPI) trial. *JAMA.* 1996;275:370–375.

9. Genant HK, Lucas J, Weiss S, et al. Low-dose esterified estrogen therapy: effects on bone, plasma estradiol concentrations, endometrium, and lipid levels. Estratab/Osteoporosis Study Group. *Arch Intern Med.* 1997;157:2609–2615.

10. Lethaby A, Suckling J, Barlow D, Farquhar CM, Jepson RG, Roberts H. Hormone replacement therapy in postmenopausal women: endometrial hyperplasia and irregular bleeding. *Cochrane Database Syst Rev.* 2004: CD000402.

11. Fisher B, Costantino JP, Wickerham DL, et al. Tamoxifen for prevention of breast cancer: report of the National Surgical Adjuvant Breast and Bowel Project P-1 study. J Natl Cancer Inst. 1998;90:1371–1388.

12. Schumer ST, Cannistra SA. Granulosa cell tumor of the ovary. *J Clin Oncol.* 2003;21:1180–1189.

13. Zanagnolo V, Pasinetti B, Sartori E. Clinical review of 63 cases of sex cord stromal tumors. *Eur J Gynaecol Oncol.* 2004;25:431–438.

14. Disiai PJ. Endometrial hyperplasia/estrogen therapy. In: DiSiai PJ, Creasman WT, eds. *Clinical Gynecologic Oncology.* 6th ed. St. Louis: Mosby;2002:113–136.

15. Dijkhuizen FP, Mol BW, Brolmann HA, Heintz AP. The accuracy of endometrial sampling in the diagnosis of patients with endometrial carcinoma and hyperplasia: a meta-analysis. *Cancer.* 2000;89:1765–1772.

16. ACOG committee opinion no. 336. Tamoxifen and uterine cancer. *Obstet Gynecol.* 2006;107:1475–1478.

17. ACOG practice bulletin: management of anovulatory bleeding. *Int J Gynaecol Obstet.* 2001;72:263–271.

18. ACOG practice bulletin number 66, September 2005. Management of abnormal cervical cytology and histology. *Obstet Gynecol.* 2005;106:645–664.

19. Zaino RJ, Kauderer J, Trimble CL, et al. Reproducibility of the diagnosis of atypical endometrial hyperplasia: a Gynecologic Oncology Group study. *Cancer.* 2006;106:804–811.

20. Trimble CL, Kauderer J, Zaino R, et al. Concurrent endometrial carcinoma in women with a biopsy diagnosis of atypical endometrial hyperplasia: a Gynecologic Oncology Group study. *Cancer.* 2006;106:812–819.

21. Zaino RJ, Kauderer J, Trimble CL, et al. Reproducibility of the diagnosis of atypical endometrial hyperplasia. *Cancer.* 2006;106:804–811.

22. Mutter GL, Baak JP, Crum CP, et al. Endometrial precancer diagnosis by histopathology, clonal analysis, and computerized morphometry. *J Pathol.* 2000;190:462–469.

23. Mutter GL. Diagnosis of premalignant endometrial disease. *J Clin Pathol.* 2002;55:326–331.

24. Mutter GL; the Endometrial Collaborative Group. Endometrial intraepithelial neoplasia (EIN): will it bring order to chaos? *Gynecol Oncol.* 2000;76:287–290.

25. Trimble CL, Kauderer J, Zaino RJ, et al. Concurrent endometrial carcinoma in women with a biopsy diagnosis of atypical endometrial hyperplasia: a Gynecologic Oncology Group study. *Cancer.* 2006;106:812–819.

26. Figueroa-Casas PR, Ettinger B, Delgado E, Javkin A, Vieder C. Reversal by medical treatment of endometrial hyperplasia caused by estrogen replacement therapy. *Menopause.* 2001;8:420–423.

27. Orbo A, Arnes M, Hancke C, Vereide AB, Pettersen I, Larsen K. Treatment results of endometrial hyperplasia after prospective D-score classification. A follow-up study comparing effect of LNG-IUD and oral progestins versus observation only. *Gynecol Oncol.* 2008.

28. Ushijima K, Yahata H, Yoshikawa H, et al. Multicenter phase II study of fertility-sparing treatment with medroxyprogesterone acetate for endometrial carcinoma and atypical hyperplasia in young women. *J Clin Oncol.* 2007;25:2798–2803.

29. Cohen I. Endometrial pathologies associated with postmenopausal tamoxifen treatment. *Gynecol Oncol.* 2004;94:256–266.

30. Varma R, Sinha D, Gupta JK. Non-contraceptive uses of levonorgestrel-releasing hormone system (LNG-IUS)—a systematic enquiry and overview. *Eur J Obstet Gynecol Reprod Biol.* 2006;125:9–28.

31. Varma R, Soneja H, Bhatia K, et al. The effectiveness of a levonorgestrel-releasing intrauterine system (LNG-IUS) in the treatment of endometrial hyperplasia-A long-term follow-up study. *Eur J Obstet Gynecol Reprod Biol.* 2008.

32. Vereide AB, Arnes M, Straume B, Maltau JM, Orbo A. Nuclear morphometric changes and therapy monitoring in patients with endometrial hyperplasia: a study comparing effects of intrauterine levonorgestrel and systemic medroxyprogesterone. *Gynecol Oncol.* 2003;91:526–533.

33. Wildemeersch D, Dhont M. Treatment of nonatypical and atypical endometrial hyperplasia with a levonorgestrel-releasing intrauterine system. *Am J Obstet Gynecol.* 2003;188:1297–1298.

34. Wildemeersch D, Janssens D, Pylyser K, et al. Management of patients with non-atypical and atypical endometrial hyperplasia with a levonorgestrel-releasing intrauterine system: long-term follow-up. *Maturitas.* 2007;57:210–213.

35. Kresowik J, Ryan GL, Van Voorhis BJ. Progression of atypical endometrial hyperplasia to adenocarcinoma despite intrauterine progesterone treatment with the levonorgestrel-releasing intrauterine system. *Obstet Gynecol.* 2008;111:547–549.

CHAPTER 6
Unusual Neoplasms of the Uterus

Alberto A. Mendivil, MD
Department of Obstetrics and Gynecology, University of North Carolina School of Medicine, Chapel Hill, NC, USA

Daniel L. Clarke-Pearson, MD, FACOG, FACS
Department of Obstetrics and Gynecology, University of North Carolina School of Medicine, Chapel Hill, NC, USA

Pathology Notes: Chad Livasy, MD
Associate Professor, Department of Pathology and Laboratory Medicine, University of North Carolina School of Medicine, Chapel Hill, NC, USA

An enlarged symptomatic uterus or abnormal bleeding is a common indication for performing a hysterectomy. Often the presumptive preoperative diagnosis is a benign uterine leiomyoma (fibroid), which in fact is the most common reason for performing a hysterectomy. Despite appropriate preoperative evaluation, the final pathology report will on occasion return with an unwelcome diagnosis such as a uterine sarcoma. While some sarcomas portend a grave prognosis, others will have been adequately treated by the hysterectomy. This chapter will review these unusual uterine neoplasms (sarcomas) and give guidelines as to appropriate preoperative, intraoperative, and postoperative management.

Neoplasms of the uterus can originate in the endometrial cavity (endometrium), the smooth muscular (myometrium) or connective tissue (stromal) layers. Uterine sarcomas arise from the mesenchymal layer of the uterine body and represent a broad spectrum of neoplasms (Table 6.1). They account for 3% to 9% of all uterine cancers and are divided into two groups: a pure form in which only mesenchymal elements are present (leiomyosarcoma, endometrial stromal sarcoma), and a mixed type that involves malignant epithelial and mesenchymal elements (carcinosarcoma). There are also benign and "borderline" counterparts of these tumors.

Even though these tumors are a common cause of abnormal uterine bleeding, many are not diagnosed by endometrial biopsy or D&C; this is especially true of leiomyosarcomas and endometrial stromal sarcomas.

Risk factors

Uterine sarcomas generally arise in postmenopausal women. The known risk factors for developing cancer of the endometrium (obesity, hypertension, diabetes, nulliparity) are not present in sarcomas. One of the rare causes of uterine sarcoma may be related to pelvic ionizing radiation (5–10% of cases). History of tamoxifen therapy has also been implicated in the development of uterine carcinosarcoma. Tamoxifen-related uterine carcinosarcomas present in advanced stage and tend to occur about 5 years after initiation of tamoxifen therapy.[1] Because these tumors are relatively rare, epidemiologic studies have not been able to elucidate underlying risk factors for uterine sarcomas.

Gynecological Cancer Management: Identification, Diagnosis and Treatment, Edited by Daniel L. Clarke-Pearson and John T. Soper. Published 2010 by Blackwell Publishing, ISBN: 978-1-4051-9079-4.

Table 6.1 Classification of uterine sarcomas

Non-Epithelioid Neoplasms

    Leiomyosarcoma
        Epithelioid
        Myxoid
    Endometrial stromal neoplasms
        Stromal nodule
        Low-grade stromal sarcoma
        Undifferentiated stromal sarcoma
    Smooth muscle tumor of uncertain malignant potential
    (STUMP)
    Mixed endometrial stromal and smooth muscle tumor
    Leiomyoma
        Histologic variants
            Mitotically active variant
            Cellular variant
            Hemorrhagic cellular variant
            Epithelioid variant
            Myxoid
            Atypical variant
            Lipoleiomyoma variant

Mixed Epithelial and Non-Epithelial Tumors

    Adenosarcoma
        Homologous
        Heterologous
    Carcinosarcoma
        Homologous
        Heterologous
    Adenofibroma
    Carcinofibroma
    Adenomyoma

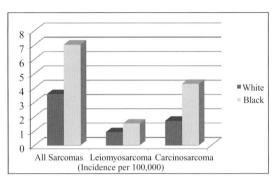

Figure 6.1 Incidence rates per 100,000 women by race; age-adjusted incidence of all sarcomas, leiomyosarcoma, and carcinosarcoma. (From Jeffers MD, Farquharson MA, Richmond JA, McNicol AM. p53 immunoreactivity and mutation of the p53 gene in smooth muscle tumours of the uterine corpus. *J Pathol.* 1995;177:65–70.)

life; and for endometrial stromal sarcoma (ESS), in the fourth decade of life.

The incidence of carcinosarcoma increases with increasing age. The incidence of all sarcomas also varies among races. While the absolute numbers of cases of sarcoma are greater for white women than black women, the age-adjusted incidence of uterine sarcomas is almost two times greater for black women than white women (Fig. 6.1), largely because of an increased prevalence of carcinosarcomas. For all other uterine sarcomas, the incidence of disease is similar across races.[3]

Incidence

Uterine sarcomas represent a small fraction of all uterine malignancies. (Carcinosarcomas account for 4% and leiomyosarcomas account for 1.5% of all uterine cancers.) The incidence of all uterine sarcomas ranges from 0.5 to 3.3 cases per 100,000 women (compared to the incidence of endometrial adenocarcinoma of 25 per 100,000 women).[2] The most common sarcoma is uterine carcinosarcoma (50%), followed by leiomyosarcoma (30%) and endometrial stromal sarcoma (10–15%). The peak incidence of carcinosarcoma is in the sixth decade of life; for leiomyosarcoma, in the fifth decade of

Leiomyosarcomas

Leiomyosarcomas are distinct from leiomyomas (fibroids), and in general it is not felt that a leiomyoma will "transform" into a leiomyosarcoma. The reported incidence of leiomyosarcoma found in a uterus that also contains fibroids is only 0.13% to 0.29%.[4]

Etiology/Histologic findings

Malignant smooth muscle neoplasms of the uterus (leiomyosarcomas) differ from the benign smooth muscle tumors (leiomyomas) in their histologic composition and molecular biology.

Leiomyosarcomas have increased cellularity, presence of coagulative necrosis, high mitotic index, and the degree of nuclear pleomorphism. There are other "borderline" smooth muscle tumors that require careful pathologic evaluation. These include smooth muscle tumors of uncertain malignant potential (STUMP), and "variants" of leiomyomas that are mitotically active, cellular hemorrhagic, epithelioid myxoid, atypical, or lipoleiomyoma. These are discussed in the "Pathology Notes" section later in the chapter.

In patients with leiomyosarcoma, for example, extensive cellular atypia is present, along with a high mitotic index (reported as mitoses per 10 high-power fields [hpfs]). From a molecular genetics perspective one may distinguish leiomyosarcomas from leiomyomas in several ways. p16 is a cell cycle mediator that is highly active in leiomyosarcomas but much less active in leiomyomas. P53, a tumor suppressor gene, has been found to be mutated in malignant smooth muscle tumors of the uterus.[5] Mutations in mismatch repair genes are seen in 15% to 30% of endometrial cancers but are uncommon in uterine sarcomas (5%).[6] Finally, mutations in the c-myc proto-oncogene have not only been found in uterine sarcomas but also in ovarian, endometrial, and cervical cancers.[7] These findings are currently not useful in the management of these malignancies, but in the future may help to develop "targeted therapies."

Pathology Notes

Smooth muscle tumors of the uterus

Pathologic evaluation of smooth muscle neoplasms of uterus is typically straightforward, with most tumors being classified simply as benign leiomyoma. The discussion here will focus on leiomyoma variants, problematic uterine smooth muscle tumors, and leiomyosarcoma. Regardless of the various terms applied to describe unusual uterine smooth muscle tumors, the pathologist's chief role is to classify these tumors as benign, of uncertain malignant potential, or malignant. The expected biological behavior of the tumor should be clearly communicated in the pathology report. If there is any uncertainty about the terminology used in the pathology report, direct communication between the gynecologic surgeon and the pathologist is valuable.

There are several benign variants of leiomyoma including cellular, symplastic, and epithelioid. A **cellular leiomyoma** shows increased cellularity relative to the usual leiomyoma and must be distinguished from an endometrial stromal nodule by the pathologist (Fig. 6.2). **Symplastic leiomyomas** typically show clusters of bizarre, pleomorphic, large, multinucleated smooth muscle and an absence of other concerning features for malignancy including increased mitotic activity or coagulative necrosis. **Epithelioid leiomyomas** are comprised predominantly of rounded cells rather than the usual spindled cells of a typical leiomyoma. Each of these benign variants is distinguished from leiomyosarcoma through the pathologic evaluation of multiple histologic features including degree/extent of cytologic atypia, mitotic index, invasiveness of tumor margins, and presence/absence of coagulative necrosis. Thorough histologic sampling, 1 section/cm of tumor, is important for problematic cases with equivocal histopathologic findings.

Leiomyosarcomas are malignant sarcomas derived from smooth muscle and are the most common malignant mesenchymal tumor of the uterus. Most present as a solitary large (>5 cm) myometrial mass. These tumors show diversity in both morphology and grade, with some tumors being low grade and difficult to distinguish from benign leiomyoma and others being high grade and difficult to distinguish from undifferentiated uterine sarcoma (Fig. 6.3). There is no

Pathology notes (*continued*)

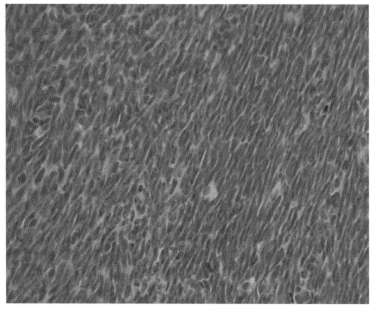

Figure 6.2 Cellular leiomyoma. High-power magnification of a section from a circumscribed myometrial nodule shows extreme hypercellularity of the smooth muscle cells. In the absence of other concerning features—including cytologic atypia, increased mitotic activity, or coagulative necrosis—these tumors behave in a completely benign fashion.

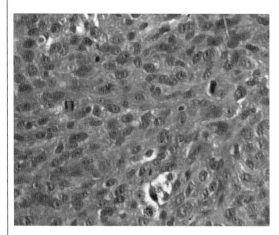

Figure 6.3 Leiomyosarcoma. Section from a large solitary yellow myometrial mass with irregular margins shows a high-grade sarcoma with markedly elevated mitotic figures (58 mitoses/10 high-power fields). Immunohistochemical stains for smooth muscle actin and desmin confirmed the presence of smooth muscle differentiation.

universally accepted grading system for uterine leiomyosarcoma to divide these tumors into low and high grade.

Pathology reports for leiomyosarcoma should include tumor size, mitotic count reported as mitotic figures per 10 high-power fields (on average), pattern of invasion (pushing versus infiltrative), and margin status. Tumor mitotic index has been shown to be of prognostic importance for uterine leiomyosarcoma.[8] Tumors with high mitotic rates and infiltrative margins have been associated with poorer prognosis. Several tumor biomarkers have also been evaluated for prognostic significance in uterine leiomyosarcoma, including Ki-67, but none of these markers appear ready for widespread clinical application. Variants of leiomyosarcoma include **myxoid leiomyosarcoma** and **epithelioid leiomyosarcoma.** Most myxoid leiomyosarcomas have low-grade histologic features.

Pathology notes (*continued*)

A small minority of smooth muscle neoplasms are particularly problematic for pathologists to characterize the expected biological behavior and are diagnosed as **smooth muscle tumors of uncertain malignant potential (STUMP).** These smooth muscle tumors usually either have some worrisome features of malignant behavior but do not meet criteria for an unequivocal diagnosis of sarcoma, or have an unsusual constellation of atypical histologic findings such that there are few clinical outcome data to predict biological behavior. The diagnosis of STUMP should be used judiciously, and some of these cases may benefit from an expert opinion from a pathologist with special expertise in evaluating problematic uterine smooth muscle tumors. Patients with a pathologic diagnosis of uterine STUMP should undergo long-term follow-up, as some of these tumors may recur years after the primary diagnosis.

Carcinosarcoma

Uterine **carcinosarcoma** is the term used to describe tumors that display both malignant epithelium and malignant stroma. Carcinosarcomas are the most common type of uterine sarcoma and comprise about 43% of all uterine sarcomas. There are benign forms of mixed neoplastic tumors such as **adenofibroma** and **adenomyoma.** A term previously used to describe uterine carcinosarcomas was **mixed Müllerian mesodermal tumors (MMMT).** The tumor may be composed of obvious carcinoma that may be mucinous, squamous, endometrioid, clear cell, papillary serous, and a component of malignant spindle cells. In general, the carcinomatous portion of the tumor predominates the histology, and thus the clinical behavior of the disease typically resembles high-risk adenocarcinomas of the endometrium. Papillary serous cell type is the most common epithelial component.

Carcinosarcomas are derived from a single stem cell. Recent studies have shown that 85% to 95% of tumors are actually metaplastic carcinomas—a tumor with the pathologic features of a carcinoma but with cells transforming along sarcomatous lines derived from the carcinomatous cells. The sarcomatous component may be homologous or heterologous. Homologous tumors are present in just over half the cases and consist of high-grade spindle-cell tumors such as leiomyosarcoma or fibrosarcoma. Heterologous tumors are present in just under half the cases and contain components of rhabdomyosarcoma, chondrosarcoma, osteosarcoma, or liposarcoma. Carcinosarcomas typically grow as fleshy, necrotic, and hemorrhagic masses that fill the endometrial cavity.[9] On gross inspection, most tumors are polypoid, often protruding through the endocervical canal. Carcinosarcomas commonly present with abnormal uterine bleeding, an enlarged uterus, and a prolapsing "leiomyoma" or "polyp" filling the upper vagina. Myometrial invasion and retroperitoneal and intra-abdominal tumor metastases are present in about 78% of cases.

Both carcinosarcomas and endometrial adenocarcinomas share similar risk factors: obesity, nulliparity, and exogenous estrogen use. The disease typically affects women their 60s. In a study of 424 women, Zelmanowicz and colleagues found that uterine carcinosarcomas were seven times more likely to be found in black women than in white women. Women with carcinosarcomas were also three times more likely to be morbidly obese. Oral contraceptive therapy appears to be protective against both endometrial adenocarcinoma and carcinosarcoma.[10]

Tamoxifen, an anti-estrogenic agent, is used for the treatment and prevention of breast cancer due to its ability to compete with estrogen for receptor-binding sites on breast epithelium and breast cancer cells. The anti-estrogenic properties of tamoxifen are active in the breast and ovary. However, in contrast, tamoxifen acts like an "estrogen" in the bone and endometrium. Tamoxifen causes estrogenic changes in the vagina and cervix and increases the rate of uterine polyps Uterine carcinosarcomas may occur as a result of tamoxifen therapy. A twofold to threefold increased risk of uterine carcinosarcoma has been reported in patients who use long-term tamoxifen. There have been multiple case reports demonstrating the association of tamoxifen use and the development of uterine carcinosarcomas, which have been reported to occur after 5 to 7 years of therapy. McCluggage and colleagues studied 19 patients with uterine carcinosarcoma associated with tamoxifen use and found that stage distribution was evenly divided between early and advanced-stage disease; other studies have reported a trend toward early-stage disease.[11,12]

The development of uterine carcinosarcomas is also associated with previous abdominopelvic radiation therapy. In locally advanced stage cervical cancer, the uterus is left in situ and treatment consists of pelvic radiation. While an effective treatment of cervical cancer, radiation therapy appears to increase the subsequent occurrence of uterine carcinosarcomas by as much as three times when compared to the general population.[13]

Pathology notes

Endometrial carcinosarcoma

Endometrial carcinosarcomas are aggressive neoplasms comprised of mixed malignant carcinomatous and sarcomatous elements. Most of these tumors are thought to arise from a progenitor-type cell that shows divergent differentiation. These tumors show tremendous histopathologic diversity in both the carcinomatous and sarcomatous elements. The quantity of carcinomatous and sarcomatous components is also highly variable emphasizing the need for thorough pathologic sampling of high-grade endometrial cancers to properly categorize the tumor. Studies have evaluated several variables of the sarcomatous component including sarcoma type, presence of heterologous elements (skeletal muscle, cartilage, bone, etc.), grade, and mitotic count, but none of these factors has been shown to correlate with prognosis. The histology of the carcinomatous component has been shown to correlate with prognosis. Tumors containing serous and clear cell carcinomatous components have been shown to be at increased risk for metastasis. Pathology reports should document the histology of the carcinomatous component in carcinosarcoma cases. Endometrial carcinosarcomas should be staged using the same FIGO surgical/pathologic staging system as that used for endometrial adenocarcinoma.

Müllerian adenosarcoma

Müllerian adenosarcoma must be distinguished from carcinosarcomas as the treatment and prognosis are significantly different. Uterine adenosarcoma is a rare tumor comprised of benign epithelium admixed with a malignant low-grade stromal component. The diagnosis of adenosarcoma in endometrial biopsies/curettings may be challenging for pathologist due to the subtle histologic features of this tumor; the differential diagnosis includes adenofibroma, endometrial polyp, and atypical polypoid adenomyoma. Pathology reports for hysterectomy specimens containing Müllerian adenosarcoma should report depth of myometrial invasion and presence/absence of sarcomatous overgrowth, as myometrial invasion and sarcomatous overgrowth are both risk factors for recurrence. The sarcomatous component within adenosarcomas often shows expression of estrogen receptor and progesterone receptor, suggesting tumor hormonal sensitivity. These tumors are usually confined to the uterus and surgical resection (hysterectomy) is the cornerstone of treatment.

Stromal sarcomas

Endometrial stromal lesions are typically well-differentiated, low-grade tumors that contain proliferative endometrial stromal cells with lush vasculature. The cells lack any of the features of aggressive tumors such as prominent atypia or pleomorphism. They grow in a compact pattern and are stratified according to two groups: stromal nodules or stromal sarcomas. Stromal sarcomas have infiltrating, angioinvasive margins and are further subdivided into low-grade stromal sarcomas or undifferentiated endometrial sarcomas based on the cytologic appearance of the tumor cells. Stromal nodules have extremely close ("pushing") margins between tumor and normal myometrium (Table 6.2).

Table 6.2 Comparison of Low-Grade and undifferentiated stromal sarcomas

Characteristic	Low-Grade ESS	Undifferentiated ESS
Growth rate	Indolent	Aggressive
5-year survival	80–100%	25–55%
Recurrence	37–60%	50–85%
Sites of recurrence	Local, distant (rare)	Local, distant
Cellular atypia	Absent	High-grade

From Gadducci A, Sartori E, Landoni F, et al. Endometrial stromal sarcoma: analysis of treatment failures and survival. *Gynecol Oncol*. 1996;63:247–253.

Pathology notes

Endometrial stromal tumors

Endometrial stromal tumors are rare neoplasms comprised of cells that morphologically resemble proliferative-phase endometrial stromal cells. The current WHO classification of endometrial stromal tumors recognizes three categories: endometrial stromal nodule (benign), low-grade endometrial stromal sarcoma, and undifferentiated endometrial sarcoma (Fig. 6.4) Historically, endometrial stromal sarcomas have been divided into low grade (<10 mitotic figures/10 high-power fields) and high grade (≥10 mitotic figures/10 high-power fields) groups based solely on mitotic count.[14] The main previous study of these high-grade sarcomas included both conventional endometrial stromal sarcomas with an increased mitotic count and the aggressive tumors now called high-grade undifferentiated sarcomas.[14] The poor outcomes observed in the high-grade sarcoma group were largely attributable to inclusion of the high-grade undifferentiated sarcoma cases. More recent studies have not shown the same prognostic significance of mitotic count in endometrial sarcoma once the undifferentiated sarcomas are excluded.[15,16]

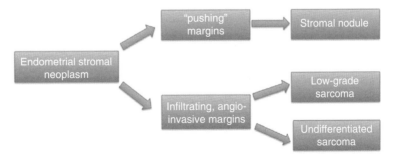

Figure 6.4 Classification of endometrial stromal neoplasm subtypes.

Pathology notes (*continued*)

The division of endometrial sarcoma into low- and high-grade categories based on mitotic count has fallen out of favor. The current WHO grouping is based on tumor cytology rather than mitotic count. Infiltrative tumors with cytology resembling normal proliferative-phase stromal cells are classified as low-grade endometrial stromal sarcomas. Infiltrative tumors with marked cytologic atypia, dissimilar to normal endometrial stromal cells, are classified as undifferentiated endometrial sarcomas once leiomyosarcoma and carcinosarcoma have been excluded by the pathologist. The very rare tumors that show mixed features of conventional endometrial stromal sarcoma and undifferentiated sarcoma should still probably be classified as high-grade endometrial stromal sarcomas.

Stromal nodule

Stromal nodule lesions are the least common form of endometrial stromal tumors. They are benign tumors that can be small and clinically insignificant or grow to a very large size and cause bleeding. Microscopically they have well-circumscribed margins and lack infiltrating margins or vascular involvement of tumor. Endometrial stromal nodules are commonly confused with cellular leiomyomas.[17] Once removed, patients are considered cured; and recurrence has not been reported.

Stromal sarcoma

Endometrial stromal sarcomas (ESS) can be either low grade or undifferentiated. They make up 0.2% of all uterine cancers and 7% to 15% of uterine sarcomas. Clinically, low-grade EES is

a slow-growing tumor and the third most common form of uterine sarcoma. The use of the term "high-grade ESS" is not part of the current standard nomenclature for these tumors. Tumors with high-grade cytologic atypia, not resembling normal proliferative-phase endometrial stromal cells, should be classified as undifferentiated stromal sarcomas.[15, 18] The average patient is in her 40s and typically presents with abnormal uterine bleeding and an enlarged uterus. It is often challenging to make a definitive diagnosis based on endometrial curettings alone, and thus careful pathologic evaluation is required of the entire uterus

Low-grade ESS is a clinically indolent tumor and commonly presents with abnormal uterine bleeding. Women with this disease are usually either perimenopausal or have completed child-bearing, making hysterectomy the definitive treatment. Microscopically they have cells resembling proliferative-phase endometrial stromal cells that infiltrate myometrial vessels and lymphatics. These tumors rarely metastasize or recur, and when they do, they are usually limited to the pelvis. However, pulmonary metastases are recognized in 10% of those with metastatic disease. The 5-year survival rate is excellent (80–100%), particularly for early-stage disease.[1]

Undifferentiated stromal sarcoma is a clinically more aggressive endometrial sarcoma characterized by relatively high rates of metastases and recurrence. It has marked cellular atypia with high mitotic index and commonly presents in an advanced stage. The most significant prognostic factor for these tumors is stage.[19]

Clinical Scenario 1

A 43-year-old P3003 presents with increasingly heavy menses, pain, and uterine enlargement to 14 weeks gestational size. The uterine fundus is irregular, and a 6 cm lower uterine fi-

broid is tender to palpation. Imaging shows multiple fibroids, some which appear heterogeneous and necrotic. Endometrial biopsy shows proliferative endometrium, and hysteroscopy and D&C show no additional abnormalities. The patient does not respond to progestin therapy and total abdominal hysterectomy is performed. Final pathology reports: "atypical smooth muscle tumor with central coagulative necrosis, multinucleate and bizarre cells, and a mitotic count of 4 mitoses/10 high-power fields."

How often are leiomyosarcomas diagnosed in fibroid uteri?

On the surface, it appears easy to make the assumption that leiomyosarcomas "evolve" from leiomyomas. However, both entities are completely independent and can coexist. The incidence of leiomyosarcoma in fibroids is only 0.13% to 0.29%.[4] "Rapidly growing leiomyoma" has been considered an indication for hysterectomy as it is presumed to possibly indicate a leiomyosarcoma. In truth, the concept of rapidly growing leiomyomas does not increase the risk of uterine sarcoma. Parker and colleagues studied 1332 patients who underwent surgery for leiomyomas. In 28% of the patients, the indication for surgery was for "rapidly growing" leiomyomas. Only one patient of 371 women in this group was subsequently diagnosed with a sarcoma, suggesting that the concept of "rapidly growing" fibroids does not increase the risk for leiomyosarcoma.[20]

What techniques can be used to diagnose LMS preoperatively?

A large pelvic mass and/or abnormal uterine bleeding can be clues to an evolving neoplastic process. Unfortunately, imaging studies and clinical findings are not specific for sarcomas. Magnetic resonance imaging (MRI) and computed tomography (CT) may be used, but their specificity is low. While endometrial adenocarcinoma develops a mass arising from the endometrium, leiomyosarcomas often will have masses arising from the myometrial bed. Evidence of necrosis, hemorrhage, and cystic changes in a uterine mass may potentially indicate a leiomyosarcoma, but a necrotic leiomyoma may appear very similar. The most worrisome imaging finding would be evidence of other solid intraperitoneal masses (metastases to peritoneal surfaces; Fig. 6.5).[10]

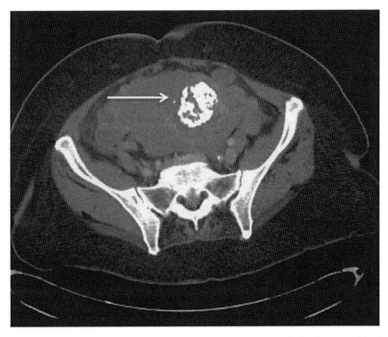

Figure 6.5 Computed tomography image of a uterine leiomyosarcoma; large calcification noted in the central portion of a separate leiomyoma (*arrow*).

Lymphadenopathy should be considered concerning, although leiomyosarcomas rarely metastasize to lymph nodes. Positron emission tomography (PET) scan can be suggestive of malignancy, especially if there are metabolically active masses with areas of central necrosis.[21] Since imaging does not distinguish "benign" from "malignant" uterine tumors, the value of performing imaging studies prior to surgery is limited to the identification of metastatic disease. Certainly there is no reason that most patients with presumed leiomyomas should undergo imaging.

What are histologic criteria for leiomyosarcoma?

Leiomyosarcoma is a malignant neoplasm made up of cells showing smooth muscle differentiation. The diagnosis of leiomyosarcomas is made based on any of the following histologic criteria: (1) moderate to severe cytologic atypia with coagulative necrosis, (2) diffuse moderate to severe cytologic atypia and mitotic index >10/10 high-power fields, or (3) coagulative necrosis and mitotic index >10/10 high-power fields. Hypercellularity is often present in these tumors but is not used as part of the criteria to define leiomyosarcoma.

In contrast, leiomyomas have uniform packed, spindle-shaped cells and a minimal number of mitotic figures. Hyaline degeneration is common in general with calcifications often seen in postmenopausal women. Cellular leiomyomas differ from leiomyomas and histologically are similar to leiomyosarcomas. Staining for desmin strongly favors a diagnosis of highly cellular leiomyoma versus that of a stromal tumor. Grossly, the masses are soft and may show focal extension into the adjacent myometrial tissue. They have increased cellularity microscopically but lack the nuclear atypia and coagulative tumor necrosis found in LMS. Mitotic figures are rare in cellular leiomyoma (< 5/HPF).[22]

Smooth muscle tumors of uncertain malignant potential (STUMP) are a heterogeneous group of smooth muscle tumors in which the histopathologic features (mitotic index, degree of cytologic atypia, and presence or absence of coagulative necrosis) do not clearly define the biologic behavior of the tumor. This classification was created to identify those tumors that had an unpredictable ability to behave clinically aggressively. Most STUMP tumors are clinically indolent and have a low risk of malignant potential.[23]

If only TAH is performed and leiomyosarcoma is diagnosed, what further surgical treatment is needed?

In general, leiomyosarcoma is a surgically staged disease and follows the FIGO surgical staging system (Table 6.3). The usual management of leiomyosarcoma consists of at least total hysterectomy; in postmenopausal women, bilateral salpingo-ophorectomy is also included. Omentectomy and pelvic washings are indicated if the diagnosis of leiomyosarcoma is known prior to surgery; however, the prognostic value of these procedures is unclear. (Furthermore, the diagnosis of leiomyosarcoma is often not established until full pathologic evaluation of the uterus.) Any extra-uterine disease should be removed, including enlarged bulky lymph nodes. The role of routine systemic lymphadenectomy in patients with leiomyosarcoma is unclear. Complete lymphadenectomy has not been shown to have a survival benefit. The incidence of lymph node involvement in clinical stage I leiomyosarcoma is only 2.4%.[13]

Table 6.3 Modified International Federation of Gynecology and Obstetrics (FIGO) staging of uterine cancer

FIGO stage	Description
I	Tumor confined to the uterus
II	Tumor invades the cervix but does not invade beyond uterus
III	Local and/or regional spread (positive lymph nodes)
IV	Distant metastases

Does a bilateral salpingo-ophorectomy need to be performed when treating a leiomyosarcoma?

In postmenopausal women, a bilateral salpingo-ophorectomy is usually perfomed. Given that leiomyosarcomas have a poor prognosis, one might think that removing sources of hormones might improve survival. However, in premenopausal women, consideration may be given to ovarian preservation, as the incidence of ovarian involvement is only 3%.[24] A study by physicians at the Mayo Clinic reviewed over 240 cases of leiomyosarcoma and evaluated a group of patients whose ovaries were preserved after hysterectomy. They observed no significant differences in the patients who underwent ovarian preservation or ovarian removal in terms of survival or recurrence.[25]

Clinical Scenario 2

A 58-year-old woman presents with post-menopausal bleeding while on tamoxifen adjuvant therapy for early breast cancer. An ultrasound shows a 3-cm endometrial mass, and an endometrial biopsy shows a carcinosarcoma (mixed Müllerian mesodermal tumor [MMMT]).

What are the subsequent steps in managing this patient?

Carcinosarcomas of the uterus are aggressive uterine malignancies and should be managed by a gynecologic oncologist who has the experience and treatment armentarium to obtain maximal treatment outcomes.

The initial step in evaluating the patient is to undertake a metastatic survey, which usually includes a physical exam, CXR, and CT scan of the abdomen and pelvis. Medical evaluation is important, as many of these women are older and have medical comorbidities that might complicate subsequent therapy.

The cornerstone to initial therapy is surgery.

Uterine carcinosarcomas behave similarly to high-grade endometrial adenocarcinomas and are staged according to the FIGO staging system (Table 6.3). Comprehensive staging includes total hysterectomy, bilateral salpingo-ophorectomy, pelvic and para-aortic lymphadenectomy, and pelvic washings. Omentectomy is not typically included in the staging for endometrial cancers. Surgical staging studies have shown that 38% of patients with uterine carcinosarcoma present with extra-uterine disease.[26] It is of interest that the portion of the tumor likely to metastasize is the carcinomatous component. While true sarcomas metastasize hematogenously, uterine carcinosarcomas commonly metastasize to the pelvic or para-aortic lymph nodes; lymph node metastases are found in from 16% to 31% of cases. Because survival is directly associated with stage at presentation, it is essential for patients to undergo comprehensive surgical staging.

Whether the procedure is performed as an "open" procedure through a laparotomy incision, laparoscopically, or with a surgical robot, there does not appear to be a difference in overall outcome (although the morbidity of minimally invasive procedures appears to be less than when performed by laparotomy).

Compared to endometrial adenocarcinoma, what is the prognosis of uterine carcinosarcoma?

Patients with uterine carcinosarcoma typically fare worse than those with grade 3 endometrioid adenocarcinoma and other aggressive subtypes such as serous and clear cell histologies. The 5-year survival rate for patients with uterine carcinosarcoma is about 53% to 74% for stage I disease. For patients with advanced-stage disease, 5-year survival decreases to 15% to 29%. This is compared to endometrial adenocarcinoma grade 3, where 5-year survival for stage I is 74% and for advanced-stage disease is 20% to 32%. Over half of patients will uterine carcinosarcoma will recur.[9, 26]

What are the factors that influence prognosis of patients with carcinosarcomas?

The single most important prognostic factor in uterine carcinosarcoma survival is stage at diagnosis. There are no differences in survival between tumors with homologous or heterologous sarcomatous elements. Other features that are prognostic in addition to stage are size of tumor (>5 cm = worse prognosis) and depth of myometrial invasion. Prognosis is also worse in patients where the carcinomatous element is serous or clear cell.[9] Lymphovascular space invasion (LVSI) was also found to be a prognostic indicator. In one study, patients with positive versus negative LVSI were noted to have 5-year survival rates of 50% and 27%, respectively. Curiously, histology, mitotic index, and tumor grade of the sarcomatous component were not associated with significant survival differences.[27]

Following surgery, adjuvant therapies might be considered. Pelvic radiation, extended field radiation (to include the para-aortic lymphnodes), and systemic chemotherapy have all been evaluated. Given the poor prognosis of patients with metastatic disease or other high-risk features, one is tempted to offer some sort of adjuvant therapy. To date, however, adjuvant therapy has not been shown to be of survival benefit. Therefore, patients should be encouraged to participate in clinical trials.

Clinical Scenario 3

A 45-year-old undergoes vaginal hysterectomy for "fibroid uterus." Normal ovaries are left in situ. Final pathology describes an invasive endometrial stromal sarcoma with histologically negative margins.

What further surgical therapy is advised? Should the patient have comprehensive surgical staging?

Comprehensive surgical staging may be more important for patients with undifferentiated ESS and of no value to those with low-grade ESS. The incidence of positive pelvic lymph nodes in one study is greater for undifferentiated disease than low grade disease (18% versus 9%); the incidence of para-aortic lymph nodes in undifferentiated disease versus low-grade disease is 15% versus 0%, respectively.[28] While cytoreductive surgery (debulking) has been shown to be prognostic in epithelial ovarian cancer and high-grade endometrial adenocarcinomas, the role of cytoreductive surgery in ESS has not been established. The removal of large-volume disease may be helpful for palliation of symptoms such as bowel obstruction or bleeding.

Should the ovaries be removed?

Removal of ovarian tissue in either presumed or confirmed early-stage low-grade ESS has not been shown to be of benefit. Li and colleagues showed that in stage I low-grade ESS, retention of ovarian tissue did not impact survival.[29, 30] Therefore, removal of the ovaries should be part of the informed consent process, particularly in premenopausal women. In contrast, patients with undifferentiated ESS should have both ovaries removed, especially in cases of receptor-positive disease.

What would management be if "endolymphatic stromal myosis" were diagnosed, with invasion into vessels at margins of the specimen?

Endolymphatic stromal myosis is an older nomenclature used to describe what is now called a "low-grade endometrial stromal sarcoma." The term was first used to describe a tumor with less than 10 mitoses per 10 high-power fields and frequently with less than 5 mitoses per 10 high-power fields. They were also described to have a more protracted clinical course.[31] While this term was ubiquitous in the past, it has largely been replaced by the diagnosis of "low-grade endometrial stromal sarcoma."

ESS expresses estrogen and progesterone receptors in over half of specimens studied. The presence or absence of steroid receptors does not seem to affect prognosis or survival. In a study of 60 patients, estrogen receptors were present in 48% of cases; progesterone receptors were present in 30% of cases. Less than 1% of recurrences showed any response to subsequent hormonal therapy.[32] Soper and others have noted there is no survival benefit with the presence of hormone receptors in ESS.[33, 34]

Treatment of persistent or recurrent disease with hormonal therapy has yielded mixed results. Nonetheless, treatment with megestrol acetate has been a widely accepted adjuvant therapy with relatively few side effects. Tamoxifen has also been used as adjuvant treatment and there are reports of the use of gonadotropin-releasing hormone (GnRH) analogs or aromatase inhibitors. While the doses for treatment are not universal, a reasonable starting dose of Megace is 40 mg twice daily and increasing to 160 mg per day, if tolerated. Duration of therapy can either be for 5 years or indefinitely.[35, 36]

What are the clinical and histologic features of parasitic leiomyomas, leiomyomatosis peritonalis disseminata, and intravenous leiomyomatosis?

Parasitic leiomyoma

Parasitic leiomyoma is a phenomenon in which a leiomyoma (typically subserosal or pedunculated) comes in contact with the adjacent peritoneum and eventually migrates away and becomes detached from the uterine corpus. The resultant tumor is solitary, with the blood supply coming from the parietal peritoneum. There are also case reports of parasitic leiomyomas arising from previous myomectomy or after morcellation from supracervical hysterectomy.[22, 37] Histologically, the tumors are similar to leiomyomas and lack any cytologic atypia or necrosis. The treatment of these tumors consists of surgical resection.

Pathology notes

Pathology reports for endometrial stromal tumors should include tumor type, mitotic count, description of growth pattern (infiltrative/circumscribed), presence/absence of lymphovascular space invasion, extent of myometrial involvement, presence/absence of extra-uterine spread, and stage. Patients with tumor confined to the uterus have an excellent prognosis. There are no reliable histopathologic features to predict which patients with stage I low-grade endometrial stromal sarcoma will develop recurrence. Low-grade endometrial stromal sarcomas often express progesterone receptor, which can be evaluated by the pathologist for potential hormonal therapy. Undifferentiated uterine sarcoma should be considered an aggressive neoplasm with consideration of adjuvant therapy for both local and systemic control following surgery.

Clinical Scenario 4

A 38-year-old undergoes an exploratory laparotomy for a 34 weeks–size fibroid uterus. At surgery, a 15-cm "fibroid" derives its blood supply from the mid-omentum, with no attachment to the uterus.

Leiomyomatosis peritonalis disseminata

Leiomyomatosis peritonealis disseminata (LPD) is extremely rare disease that on imaging studies appears similar to diffuse carcinomatosis. Grossly the lesions may be located on virtually any abdominopelvic organ such as the small intestine,

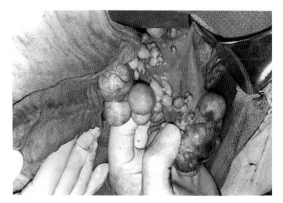

Figure 6.6 Leiomyomatosis peritonealis disseminata involving the pelvic peritoneum and broad ligament.

uterus, fallopian tubes, mesentery, parietal peritoneum, and ovaries (Fig. 6.6). Histologically the lesions lack cellular atypia or mitoses, and the cells appear arranged in a fashion similar to those seen in leiomyomas.[38] The tumors are found in women of reproductive age, during pregnancy, and in women with a history of prolonged use of oral contraceptives. There are also case reports of LPD found in postmenopausal women who had previous hysterectomies.[39] The masses are benign; however, there are rare cases of malignant transformation, particularly with recurrences. The etiology of LPD is unknown but the cells are thought to originate in the submesothelial mesenchymal cells of the subperitoneal mesenchyme. There are no formal treatment guidelines but patients are often treated with some form of hormonal agent such as GnRH analogs, megestrol acetate, and danazol. In a study of 11 patients with LPD, 10 were estrogen and progesterone receptor positive, justifying the use of hormonal treatments.[40]

Intravenous leiomyomatosis

Intravenous leiomyomatosis (IVL) is defined as the presence of benign smooth muscle tissue in the systemic vasculature either within or outside a leiomyoma. In 30% of cases, the tumor may be outside the pelvis and reach the heart via the inferior vena cava. These tumors typically have < 5 mitoses per 10 high-power field. The presence of morphologically benign smooth muscle tumor within solid organs excludes IVL and raises the possibility of benign metastasizing leiomyoma. Histologically, the intravascular tissues have worm-like collections of tumor. Clinically, the uterus is usually enlarged and replaced by multiple myomatous masses. The recommended management for IVL is complete resection of the intravenous tumor in addition to total hysterectomy and bilateral salpingo-oophorectomy. Preoperative consultation with cardiothoracic surgery is important for planning of possible cardiac bypass if necessary for intravascular or intracardiac surgery.[22, 41]

Clinical Scenario 5

A patient with a past history of a hysterectomy for uterine fibroids is found to have multiple solid pulmonary nodules. Figure 6.7 shows the findings on CT scan. The cytopathology report from a fine-needle aspiration biopsy is "fibrous tissue."

If this patient subsequently undergoes VATs resection of multiple pulmonary "benign" leiomyomas, what is the preferred management?

Benign metastasizing leiomyomatosis (BML) is a rare disorder that is typically found in perimenopausal women. It is regarded as the result of a monoclonal neoplasm that has undergone hematogenous spread. The disease is characterized by benign-appearing smooth muscle normally present in uterine leiomyomas. The tumors may spread to distant sites, most commonly the lung. Other sites of disease include retroperitoneal and mediastinal lymph nodes. The diagnosis of BML is made only when the diagnosis of leiomyosarcoma has been excluded. The tumors may be estrogen and progesterone receptor positive, often shrink with pregnancy, and stop growing after menopause or oophorectomy. As a result, BML is typically treated with hormonal agents.[22] In patients with a large pulmonary

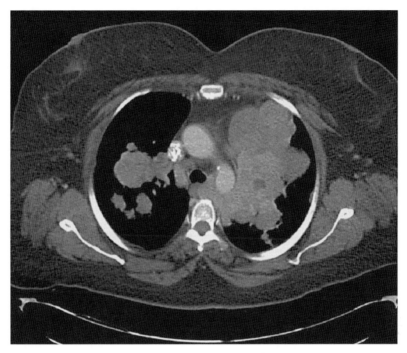

Figure 6.7 Chest CT image showing intrathoracic benign metastasizing leiomyomatosis.

tumor burden, parenchymal-sparing surgical excision is reasonable. Often, however, the size or number of lesions precludes aggressive surgical management.

Receptor studies in BML indicate that these tumors may be hormonally induced hyperplastic lesions. Removal of endogenous sex hormone production can be achieved via bilateral salpingo-oophorectomy, low-dose pelvic (ovarian) radiation, or using cytotoxic chemotherapy for a short course. GnRH analogs can also be used for the purposes of reversible chemical castration. Reduction of endogenous gonadotropins leads to a decrease in endogenous steroid production and secretion. The use of progesterone and estrogen receptor modulators has been justified by the fact that most case reports described in the literature confer a 90% to 95% estrogen and/or progesterone receptor presence. Megestrol acetate is commonly used, at a starting dose of 40 mg twice daily and increasing the dose to 160 mg daily if tolerated. Progesterone treatment is effective

in treating the disease as well as preventing recurrences. Aromatase inhibitors may also be effective in treating BML by blocking sex steroid synthesis.[42]

References

1. SEER Uterine Cancer Age-Adjusted Incidence. NCI, 2005. Accessed July 22, 2008.
2. Brooks SE, Zhan M, Cote T, Baquet CR. Surveillance, epidemiology, and end results analysis of 2677 cases of uterine sarcoma 1989–1999. *Gynecol Oncol.* 2004;93:204–208.
3. Leibsohn S, d'Ablaing G, Mishell DR Jr., Schlaerth JB. Leiomyosarcoma in a series of hysterectomies performed for presumed uterine leiomyomas. *Am J Obstet Gynecol.* 1990;162:968–974; discussion 974–976.
4. Jeffers MD, Farquharson MA, Richmond JA, McNicol AM. p53 immunoreactivity and mutation of the p53 gene in smooth muscle tumours of the uterine corpus. *J Pathol.* 1995;177:65–70.

5. Amant F, Dorfling CM, Dreyer L, Vergote I, Lindeque BG, Van Rensburg EJ. Microsatellite instability in uterine sarcomas. *Int J Gynecol Cancer*. 2001;11:218–223.

6. Jeffers MD, Richmond JA, Macaulay EM. Overexpression of the c-myc proto-oncogene occurs frequently in uterine sarcomas. *Mod Pathol*. 1995;8:701–704.

7. Moinfar F, Azodi M, Tavassoli FA. Uterine sarcomas. *Pathology*. 2007;39:55–71.

8. Jones MW, Norris HJ. Clinicopathologic study of 28 uterine leiomyosarcomas with metastasis. *Int J Gynecol Pathol*. 1995;14:243–249.

9. McCluggage WG. Uterine carcinosarcomas (malignant mixed Müllerian tumors) are metaplastic carcinomas. *Int J Gynecol Cancer*. 2002;12:687–690.

10. Zelmanowicz A, Hildesheim A, Sherman ME, et al. Evidence for a common etiology for endometrial carcinomas and malignant mixed mullerian tumors. *Gynecol Oncol*. 1998;69:253–257.

11. McCluggage WG, Abdulkader M, Price JH, et al. Uterine carcinosarcomas in patients receiving tamoxifen. A report of 19 cases. *Int J Gynecol Cancer*. 2000;10:280–284.

12. Kloos I, Delaloge S, Pautier P, et al. Tamoxifen-related uterine carcinosarcomas occur under/after prolonged treatment: report of five cases and review of the literature. *Int J Gynecol Cancer*. 2002;12:496–500.

13. Meredith RF, Eisert DR, Kaka Z, Hodgson SE, Johnston GA Jr., Boutselis JG. An excess of uterine sarcomas after pelvic irradiation. *Cancer*. 1986;58:2003–2007.

14. Norris HJ, Taylor HB. Mesenchymal tumor of the uterus. A clinical and pathological study of 53 endometrial stromal tumors. *Cancer*. 1966;19:755–766.

15. Evans HL. Endometrial stromal sarcoma and poorly differentiated endometrial stromal sarcoma. *Cancer*. 1982;50:2170–2182.

16. Chang KL, Crabtree GS, Lim-Tan SK, et al. Primary uterine endometrial stromal neoplasms. A clinicopathologic study of 117 cases. *Am J Surg Pathol*. 1990;14:415–438.

17. Tavassoli FA, Norris HJ. Mesenchymal tumours of the uterus. VII. A clinicopathological study of 60 endometrial stromal nodules. *Histopathology*. 1981;5:1–10.

18. Oliva E, Clement PB, Young RH. Endometrial stromal tumors: an update on a group of tumors with a protean phenotype. *Adv Anat Pathol*. 2000;7:257–281.

19. Gadducci A, Sartori E, Landoni F, et al. Endometrial stromal sarcoma: analysis of treatment failures and survival. *Gynecol Oncol*. 1996;63:247–253.

20. Parker WH, Fu YS, Berek JS. Uterine sarcoma in patients operated on for presumed leiomyoma and rapidly growing leiomyoma. *Obstet Gynecol*. 1994;83:414–418.

21. Giuntoli RL II, Bristow RE. Uterine leiomyosarcoma: present management. *Curr Opin Oncol*. 2004;16:324–327.

22. Clement PB. The pathology of uterine smooth muscle tumors and mixed endometrial stromal-smooth muscle tumors: a selective review with emphasis on recent advances. *Int J Gynecol Pathol*. 2000;19:39–55.

23. O'Neill CJ, McBride HA, Connolly LE, McCluggage WG. Uterine leiomyosarcomas are characterized by high p16, p53 and MIB1 expression in comparison with usual leiomyomas, leiomyoma variants and smooth muscle tumours of uncertain malignant potential. *Histopathology*. 2007;50:851–858.

24. Leitao MM, Sonoda Y, Brennan MF, Barakat RR, Chi DS. Incidence of lymph node and ovarian metastases in leiomyosarcoma of the uterus. *Gynecol Oncol*. 2003;91:209–212.

25. Giuntoli RL II, Metzinger DS, DiMarco CS, et al. Retrospective review of 208 patients with leiomyosarcoma of the uterus: prognostic indicators, surgical management, and adjuvant therapy. *Gynecol Oncol*. 2003;89:460–469.

26. Yamada SD, Burger RA, Brewster WR, Anton D, Kohler MF, Monk BJ. Pathologic variables and adjuvant therapy as predictors of recurrence and survival for patients with surgically evaluated carcinosarcoma of the uterus. *Cancer*. 2000;88:2782–2786.

27. Sartori E, Bazzurini L, Gadducci A, et al. Carcinosarcoma of the uterus: a clinicopathological multicenter CTF study. *Gynecol Oncol*. 1997;67:70–75.

28. Leath CA III, Huh WK, Hyde J Jr., et al. A multi-institutional review of outcomes of endometrial stromal sarcoma. *Gynecol Oncol*. 2007;105:630–634.

29. Berchuck A, Rubin SC, Hoskins WJ, Saigo PE, Pierce VK, Lewis JL Jr. Treatment of endometrial stromal tumors. *Gynecol Oncol*. 1990;36:60–65.

30. Li AJ, Giuntoli RL II, Drake R, et al. Ovarian preservation in stage I low-grade endometrial stromal sarcomas. *Obstet Gynecol*. 2005;106:1304–1308.

31. Piver MS, Rutledge FN, Copeland L, Webster K, Blumenson L, Suh O. Uterine endolymphatic stromal myosis: a collaborative study. *Obstet Gynecol*. 1984;64:173–178.

32. Wade K, Quinn MA, Hammond I, Williams K, Cauchi M. Uterine sarcoma: steroid receptors and response to hormonal therapy. *Gynecol Oncol*. 1990;39:364–367.

33. Soper JT, McCarty KS Jr., Hinshaw W, Creasman WT, McCarty KS, Clarke-Pearson DL. Cytoplasmic estrogen and progesterone receptor content of uterine sarcomas. *Am J Obstet Gynecol.* 1984;150:342–348.

34. Sutton GP, Stehman FB, Michael H, Young PC, Ehrlich CE. Estrogen and progesterone receptors in uterine sarcomas. *Obstet Gynecol.* 1986;68:709–714.

35. Chu MC, Mor G, Lim C, Zheng W, Parkash V, Schwartz PE. Low-grade endometrial stromal sarcoma: hormonal aspects. *Gynecol Oncol.* 2003;90:170–176.

36. Reich O, Regauer S. Hormonal therapy of endometrial stromal sarcoma. *Curr Opin Oncol.* 2007;19:347–352.

37. Moon HS, Koo JS, Park SH, Park GS, Choi JG, Kim SG. Parasitic leiomyoma in the abdominal wall after laparoscopic myomectomy. *Fertil Steril.* 2008.

38. Heinig J, Neff A, Cirkel U, Klockenbusch W. Recurrent leiomyomatosis peritonealis disseminata after hysterectomy and bilateral salpingo-oophorectomy during combined hormone replacement therapy. *Eur J Obstet Gynecol Reprod Biol.* 2003;111:216–218.

39. Herrero J, Kamali P, Kirschbaum M. Leiomyomatosis peritonealis disseminata associated with endometriosis: a case report and literature review. *Eur J Obstet Gynecol Reprod Biol.* 1998;76:189–191.

40. Bekkers RL, Willemsen WN, Schijf CP, Massuger LF, Bulten J, Merkus JM. Leiomyomatosis peritonealis disseminata: does malignant transformation occur? A literature review. *Gynecol Oncol.* 1999;75:158–163.

41. Moorjani N, Kuo J, Ashley S, Hughes G. Intravenous uterine leiomyosarcomatosis with intracardial extension. *J Card Surg.* 2005;20:382–385.

42. Rivera JA, Christopoulos S, Small D, Trifiro M. Hormonal manipulation of benign metastasizing leiomyomas: report of two cases and review of the literature. *J Clin Endocrinol Metab.* 2004;89:3183–3188.

CHAPTER 7

Management of Women at High Risk for Gynecologic Cancers

Lisa N. Abaid, MD, MPH
Gynecologic Oncology Associates, Newport Beach, CA, USA

Paola A. Gehrig, MD, FACOG, FACS
Department of Obstetrics and Gynecology, University of North Carolina School of Medicine, Chapel Hill, NC, USA

Pathology Notes: Chad Livasy, MD
Associate Professor, Department of Pathology and Laboratory Medicine, University of North Carolina School of Medicine, Chapel Hill, NC, USA

Background

Cancer develops as a result of genetic mutations that alter the normal mechanisms of cellular population control. This is usually due to a series of mutations in several different genes, which ultimately disrupts the processes of proliferation, apoptosis (cell death), or senescence (aging). These mutations may be inherited or acquired. Acquired mutations can result from carcinogenic exposures, or may occur endogenously due to intracellular mutagenic events.

The risk of most cancers increases with time (age) due to accumulating genetic damage over a person's lifetime. It is thought that at least three to six genetic mutations may be needed for a cell to undergo malignant transformation. While the majority of cancers are due to sporadic or acquired mutations, a significant minority of cancers result from inherited mutations. Characteristic features of a family with an inherited mutation include young age at onset, multiple affected family members with clusters of specific malignancies, and individuals with more than one primary malignancy. While many rare hereditary cancer syndromes have been identified, the most common mutations predispose affected individuals to breast/ovarian cancer (BRCA 1 and BRCA 2), colon/endometrial cancer (MSH2 and MLH1), and melanoma.[1]

Genes asociated with developing cancer

Three main classes of genes have been linked to the development of cancer: oncogenes, tumor suppressor genes, and mismatch repair genes. Although all of them occur relatively frequently, tumor suppressor genes have been those most associated with hereditary cancer syndromes, followed by DNA repair genes and oncogenes. Oncogenes, which are expressed as a dominant allele, encode proteins that promote cell growth in an uncontrolled fashion, thereby increasing the malignant transformation of cells. The nonmutated version of the gene, called a proto-oncogene, carries the code for proteins involved in various aspects of normal cell replication. The proto-oncogene can be transformed into an oncogene via amplification

Gynecological Cancer Management: Identification, Diagnosis and Treatment, Edited by Daniel L. Clarke-Pearson and John T. Soper. Published 2010 by Blackwell Publishing, ISBN: 978-1-4051-9079-4.

and overexpression, a point mutation, or by translocation and exposure to a promoter sequence that results in overexpression. HER-2/neu is an example of an oncogene that is found in a variety of cancers, but it has clinical relevance primarily in breast cancer.[1]

Tumor suppressor genes are recessive genes that encode factors that inhibit cell growth by inhibiting cellular division, initiating apoptosis (cell death) or promoting DNA repair. Loss of both alleles is necessary to promote malignant transformation. The "two-hit" mechanism applies to both inherited and acquired cancers. In hereditary cancers, one mutated allele may be inherited and the second acquired over time, while in sporadic cancers, both mutations are acquired. Similarly to oncogenes, tumor suppressor genes may be mutated by point mutations and deletions or additions of nucleotides. Examples of tumor suppressor genes include p53, p16, and the retinoblastoma (Rb) gene.[1]

Mismatch repair genes correct DNA damage that occurs during normal DNA replication. A malfunction in one of these genes can result in a buildup of errors, some of which may ultimately affect the genes involved in cell regulation. Some inherited cancers are a result of germline mutations in mismatch repair genes. One example is hereditary nonpolyposis colorectal cancer (HNPCC), which causes an increased risk of colorectal and endometrial cancer, in addition to several other cancers of the gastrointestinal (gastric and biliary) and reproductive tracts, including ovarian cancer.[2]

Genetics underlying gynecologic malignancies

Ovarian cancer

Among women in the United States, ovarian cancer is the eighth most prevalent cancer and the fifth leading cause of death from cancer. Approximately 12% of women with invasive ovarian cancer have an underlying BRCA1 or BRCA2 mutation. Women who carry a BRCA mutation are at a greatly increased risk for breast and ovarian cancer and at a moderately elevated risk of fallopian tube and primary peritoneal cancer. Patho-

logic types are similar to those women who are not BRCA carriers, except for low malignant potential and mucinous tumors, which are uncommon in BRCA mutation carriers. At the time of presentation, most tumors are stage III or IV, but early-stage ovarian and tubal cancers are being detected with increasing frequency with the use of screening methods and at the time of prophylactic salpingo-oophorectomy. In BRCA1 carriers, malignancy may originate in the fallopian tube or multifocal sites.[3]

BRCA testing may be offered to all women, or their first-degree female relatives, diagnosed with invasive, nonmucinous, epithelial ovarian cancer. Testing is generally recommended when the family pedigree suggests at least a 10% probability of finding a mutation. This correlates with two first- or second-degree family members with either ovarian cancer at any age or premenopausal breast cancer (age <50). Complete gene sequencing is the most accurate way to test for BRCA1 and BRCA2, but this is expensive and time consuming. Therefore, testing should first be performed on the affected patient, and only then, if positive, offered to her unaffected female relatives. In this fashion, the other family members can be tested for the specific mutation, thereby lowering the cost of testing. However, an unaffected relative may be tested if there are no living affected family members.[3]

Fallopian tube cancer

Primary cancer of the fallopian tube is extremely rare, but is more prevalent among BRCA mutation carriers. One population-based study found that 16% of women with fallopian tube cancer were BRCA positive, 11% for BRCA1 and 5% for BRCA2.[4] Additionally, occult malignancies may be present, often multifocally, in the fallopian tube at the time of prophylactic salpingo-oophorectomy. This underscores the importance of removing the entire fallopian tube when performing a prophylactic salpingo-oophorectomy.[3]

Endometrial cancer

Endometrial cancer can be divided into two broad categories, which have different clinical and biologic behavior. Type I endometrial cancer is related to prolonged, unopposed estrogen exposure, is typically associated with complex atypical hyperplasia, and is generally early-stage, low-grade, and has a lower mortality rate. Type II cancers are of a non-endometrioid histology, generally papillary serous or clear cell, are rarely estrogen dependent, and are more aggressive, with a higher risk of distant metastases and a poorer outcome.[1]

While all cancers are a result of some form of genetic alteration, 5% of endometrial cancers arise in the setting of hereditary nonpolyposis colorectal cancer syndrome (HNPCC). HNPCC is characterized by a loss of mismatch repair genes, which results in an increase in mutations found in repetitive DNA sequences, called microsatellites. The term "microsatellite instability" describes these accumulated mutations in microsatellite sequences. Women with HNPCC have been reported to have a 42% to 60% risk of endometrial cancer, usually type I, and a 40% to 60% lifetime risk of colon cancer.[5] In women with both types of cancer, endometrial cancer presents first in approximately half. Women with HNPCC also have an increased risk of ovarian cancer, approximately 5% to 12%, with a mean age at diagnosis in the early 40s. These cancers have a better prognosis, with a lower grade and earlier stage than sporadic ovarian cancers, and 20% are diagnosed with a synchronous endometrial cancer.[1] Genetic testing is recommended for women with family histories suggesting of HNPCC. The gold standard for testing is mutational analysis of the MSH2 and MLH1 genes.

Sporadic endometrial cancers have been associated with inactivation of the tumor suppressor genes PTEN and p53. PTEN (chromosome 10q) mutations are the most commonly identified mutation, found in 30% to 50% of endometrial cancers. They are associated with endometrioid histology, early stage, and higher survival.[6] Conversely, p53 mutations, which are found in 20% of endometrial cancers, are typically associated with non-endometrioid tumors (papillary serous and clear cell), and higher grade and stage tumors.[7] In addition to tumor suppressor genes, oncogenes have also been implicated in the development of endometrial cancer. Her-2/neu, which is most commonly associated with breast cancer, has been noted to occur in 10% to 15% of endometrial cancers. These malignancies are also more often papillary serous, of advanced stage, and associated with a poor prognosis.[8] The majority of these mutations are found only in tumor cells and are not germline mutations, which precludes genetic testing of unaffected individuals.

Clinical Scenario 1

A 22-year-old nulliparous white female seeks your consultation. Her mother has just died of advanced ovarian cancer at age 42. In addition, she has two maternal aunts who have had breast cancer and are survivors (Figure 7.1). Her

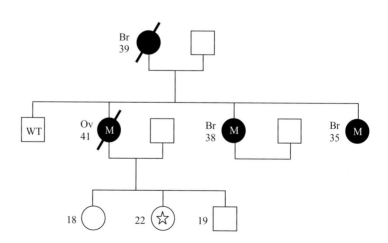

Figure 7.1 Hereditary breast and ovarian cancer perdigree. The star designates the patient described in the clinical scenario. M denotes the family members who have tested positive for BRCA1 and the solid circles represent those who have a cancer diagonis. The type of cancer and age at diagonis is indicated to the left, and slashes represent deaths from cancer. WT indicates negative testing for BRCA1 mutation.

maternal grandmother died of premenopausal breast cancer at age 40. The patient has a younger brother and a sister who are healthy. Her mother and her mother's sisters have all tested positive for BRCA1, but the patient and her siblings have not been tested. There is no Ashekenazi Jewish heritage on either the maternal or paternal side of the family and no significant cancer history on her father's side. She would like to know her risk of carrying a mutation.

BRCA1 and 2 mutations are inherited by an autosomal dominant pattern, though there are varying degrees of penetrance. The genetic mutation may be inherited from either the maternal or paternal side of the family tree. In the general population, BRCA mutations are carried by less than 0.1%.[9] This rate varies greatly depending on ethnic background, with the highest carrier rate of 2% seen in women of Ashkenazi Jewish descent.[10] With this patient's mother having a known mutation and no significant history on her paternal side, her risk of inheriting a BRCA1 mutation is 50%.

For this patient, what would the benefit of her undergoing genetic testing? What is her cancer risk should her testing be positive?

The benefit of testing would primarily be for cancer risk assessment and to allow the patient to make decisions regarding surveillance and prophylactic surgery if she were to test positive. A negative test would provide reassurance and allow her to receive routine screening. On the other hand, negative genetic testing does not completely exclude the possibility that the patient might develop breast or ovarian cancer. Unfortunately, misunderstanding by patients and some physicians has led to a false sense of reassurance in women who test negative for BRCA1/2. A possible negative consequence of testing is the potential for discrimination by medical insurers in the event of a positive test. However, there is currently little evidence of any widespread discriminatory practices based on genetic testing results.[11] "Survivor's guilt" commonly experienced by women who are negative for the mutation but have affected releatives,

may require counseling and support of the *unaffected* woman.

Women with BRCA1 or 2 mutations have a 50% to 85% lifetime risk of breast cancer, with some breast cancers diagnosed before the age of 30. BRCA1 is associated with a 30% to 40% ovarian cancer risk and BRCA2 with a 15% to 25% risk. In contrast, the baseline risk for sporadic breast cancer is 11% and for sporadic ovarian cancer is 1.6%. BRCA1 carriers are diagnosed with ovarian cancer at age 51, on average, compared with 57.5 years for BRCA2 carriers. After age 35, the risk of contracting ovarian cancer for BRCA1 carriers is 1% per year, compared with BRCA2 carriers, who are rarely diagnosed prior to age 50. Conflicting data exist regarding whether BRCA mutations increase the risk of endometrial cancer, but to date there is not an established association.[1] BRCA mutations also increase the risk of fallopian tube and primary peritoneal cancer. Up to one-third of patients with primary peritoneal cancer have also been found to harbor BRCA mutations.[1]

Men who carry a BRCA mutation are at increased risk for breast and prostate cancer, and may have a slightly higher risk of pancreatic and colon cancer. Unlike female carriers, male breast cancer is more common with a BRCA2 mutation. The lifetime risk of breast cancer is 0.2% to 2.8% in male BRCA1 carriers and 3% to 12% in male BRCA2 carriers. In contrast, the risk of sporadic male breast cancer is 0.1%. Male BRCA2 carriers also have a 35% to 40% risk of developing prostate cancer.[12]

If this patient's testing were negative, she would carry the baseline lifetime risks for breast and ovarian cancer.

What screening progam should this 22-year-old nulligravid female follow if she tests positive for a high-risk BRCA1 or BRCA2 mutation? What are the recommendations regarding prophylactic surgery?

The National Comprehensive Cancer Network (NCCN) recommends clinical breast exams at 6-month intervals with annual mammograms starting at age 25. NCCN guidelines for ovarian cancer screening include transvaginal ultrasound and CA-125 measurements every 6 months starting at age 35, or 5 to 10 years prior to the earliest age of first diagnosis of ovarian cancer in a relative.[13] Despite these guidelines, we recognize that there is no evidence that screening will result in early detection or improved survival from ovarian cancer.

Options and timing of prophylactic mastectomy and salpingo-oophorectomy should be discussed, with the inclusion of a genetic counselor and possibly a surgical oncologist/gynecologic oncologist. Risk-reducing salpingo-oophorectomy is recommended at age 35 to 40 or on completion of child-bearing, but may be individualized based on the earliest age of onset of ovarian cancer in the family.[13] Use of oral contraceptives may also reduce ovarian cancer risk if the patient's reproductive wishes are uncertain. However, oral contraceptives have been suggested to increase the risk of breast cancer in BRCA mutation carriers, so this decision must be individualized.[14]

Clinical Scenario 2

A 36-year-old has a family history of a maternal grandmother with colon cancer, a maternal first cousin with endometrial cancer, and a paternal aunt with premenopausal breast cancer.

Is this woman at an increased risk for cancer, and if so, should she see a genetic counselor?

High risk for breast/ovarian cancer
The NCCN has developed criteria to identify women at risk for harboring a genetic predisposition for breast or ovarian cancer, and for whom referral to a geneticist is recommended. The criteria include early-onset or multifocal breast cancer, breast cancer clustered with other primary cancers, a family member with a known mutation, any male relative with breast cancer, any

first-degree relative with ovarian, fallopian tube, or primary peritoneal cancer, and certain high-risk groups such as women of Ashekenazi Jewish descent and breast or ovarian cancer at any age.[13]

Women who meet these criteria should be evaluated by a genetic counselor in order to decide whether BRCA testing should be undertaken and who should be tested. A full family history including at least three generations should be obtained, as well as pathologic confirmation of cancer diagnoses in affected family members. Further discussions regarding surveillance or prophylactic surgery would be held depending on whether the individual elected for testing and, if so, the results of the test.

High risk for endometrial cancer
Endometrial cancer is the most common gynecologic cancer, affecting over 40,000 women in the United States each year. Approximately 5% of cases are due to hereditary factors, and of those, the majority are associated with HNPCC. HNPCC is transmitted in an autosomal dominant pattern and is characterized by defective DNA mismatch repair genes. The lifetime risk of endometrial cancer in HNPCC patients is in the range of 40% to 60%, with a 5% to 15% risk of ovarian cancer.[15, 16] Endometrial cancer presents earlier in patients with HNPCC, with mean age at the time of diagnosis in the early 40s, compared with the early 60s in sporadic endometrial cancer. The stage and histology as well as the prognosis are similar for HPNCC-associated and sporadic endometrial cancer. HNPCC-associated ovarian cancer also presents in the early 40s. The stage and grade are generally more favorable than in sporadic cases, and 20% are diagnosed with a synchronous endometrial cancer.[1]

No guidelines currently exist on endometrial cancer surveillance and management recommendations for women with HNPCC, although annual ultrasonographic measurement of the endometrial stripe thickness has been proposed. Colon cancer screening recommendations have been put forth by the NCCN and are reviewed later in this chapter. While no data exist to support prophylactic hysterectomy, there have been no documented failures of hysterectomy in preventing endometrial cancer. Given the high incidence in these patients, hysterectomy with bilateral salpingo-oophorectomy should be considered as a preventive measure, especially if child-bearing has been completed.[3]

Ninety-five percent of endometrial cancers are sporadic, and many of these are related to unopposed estrogen exposure. Three-quarters of women with endometrial cancer have type I cancer, which tends to be endometrioid histology, low grade, estrogen dependent (ER/PR positive), and has a relatively good prognosis. Risk factors include obesity (> 50 lbs overweight) and exogenous unopposed estrogen use, both of which increase the risk of endometrial cancer by 10-fold. Tamoxifen use is also associated with a 10% increase in endometrial cancer risk over baseline. Reproductive risk factors include nulliparity, early menarche, and late menopause. Despite identification of these risk factors, no screening recommendations currently exist for sporadic endometrial cancer.[17]

Clinical Scenario 3

A 44-year-old comes in for her annual exam. She reports that she has just been diagnosed with a hyperplasic colonic polyp. She underwent a colonoscopy because her father was recently diagnosed with colon cancer at the age of 75. She knows that one of his sisters had endometrial cancer and his first cousin also had colon cancer. She wonders if she is at any increased risk for cancer as all the cancers in the family are on her "father's side."

Given that the paternal side of her family tree appears to harbor the high-risk factors, is this patient at increased risk, and should she be evaluated by a genetic counselor?

HNPCC is transmitted in an autosomal dominant manner and accounts for 2% to 3% of all colorectal adenocarcinomas.[18,19] As previously discussed, HNPCC is caused by a defect in DNA mismatch repair genes and may be inherited from the maternal or paternal side. In addition to an increased risk of endometrial cancer, this defect results in a 40% to 60% risk of colon cancer. The diagnosis of colon cancer is made at a mean age of 48 years, but can be seen in the early 20s. Almost three-fourths of lesions are proximal to the splenic flexure and 10% will be diagnosed with synchronous or metachronous tumors.[20]

HNPCC was historically divided into Lynch syndrome I, which was hereditary site-specific colon cancer, and Lynch syndrome II, which was characterized by a high risk of extracolonic tumors, most commonly endometrial cancer. However, the lines between the two types are becoming blurred as more data are gathered on families with these genetic alterations.

The Amsterdam and Bethesda criteria have been developed to identify families who should be offered genetic testing. In general, families with multiple members affected by early-onset colon or endometrial cancer, or other HNPCC-associated cancers such as ovarian, gastric, hepatobiliary, small bowel, or transitional cell carcinomas, should be seen by a geneticist for further evaluation.

After seeing a genetic counselor and undergoing testing, she found out that she does carry a mutation of MSH2.

How is testing for HNPCC performed? What type of screening should she have for colon cancer? Would you recommend routine endometrial biopsy?

The mismatch repair (MMR) genes that are most commonly associated with HNPCC are MLH1, MSH2, MSH6, and PMS2. Testing for germline mutations in these genes can identify unaffected carriers. Affected individuals are tested first by performing microsatellite instability or immunohistochemical analysis on a colon cancer specimen to detect the protein expression of the MMR genes. Non-affected individuals who meet criteria for testing may have blood drawn for genetic testing (similar to BRCA1 and BRCA2 testing). Lack of protein expression denotes a mutation in that particular gene. False-negative rates range from 5% to 10%.[21]

Women with HNPCC syndrome should undergo colonoscopy between the ages of 20 to 25, or 10 years before the youngest relative at the time of diagnosis, according to NCCN guidelines. This should be repeated at 1- to 2-year intervals. While consideration can be given to annual endometrial evaluations with ultrasound or biopsy, no data exist to suggest that this reduces the risk of developing cancer. However, any clinically abnormal bleeding should be promptly investigated.[22]

Clinical Scenario 4

A 25-year-old gravida 2, para 2 was recently tested and is positive for a BRCA1 mutation. She and her husband may want more children.

What type of screening would you recommend until she is ready to have prophylactic (risk-reducing) surgery?

In women with BRCA1 or 2 mutations who do not undergo prophylactic mastectomy or salpingo-oophorectomy, close surveillance is recommended. The NCCN guidelines for breast cancer surveillance in BRCA-positive women include breast self-exam starting at age 18, clinical breast exam every 6 months starting at age 25, and annual mammogram or breast MRI starting at age 25, or earlier based on the earliest age of onset in a relative. Ovarian cancer surveillance recommendations include transvaginal ultrasound and CA-125 measurements at 6-month intervals starting at age 35, or 5 to 10 years before the age at which the youngest affected relative was diagnosed.[13] Close surveillance has not been found to impact mortality, and no data exist to show that 6-month intervals are superior to more or less frequent monitoring. However, given the high cancer incidence associated with these mutations, an elevated level of suspicion

and a low threshold for further evaluation seem advisable. An exciting field of study in the quest for improved screening strategies is that of proteomics. Proteomics is the evaluation of multiple serum protein markers to determine differences in protein patterns that can differentiate benign from malignant disease. There have been several promising studies, but this field requires validation in larger trials before being introduced into widespread clinical use.

Clinical Scenario 5

A 35-year-old with a family history concerning for a genetic predisposition for ovarian and breast cancer comes to your office. She is not sure if she wants to undergo testing as she fears losing her insurance.

She wants to know what the guidelines are for recommending prophylactic surgery to decrease her risk. What is your advice?

The Society of Surgical Oncology developed a position statement on potential indications for bilateral prophylactic mastectomies in patients without a cancer diagnosis. Individuals with BRCA mutations or other genetic susceptibility for breast cancer, strong family history with negative genetic testing, or histologic diagnosis such as atypical hyperplasia or lobular carcinoma-in-situ were considered candidates for surgery. Treatment decisions should be made using a multidisciplinary team approach, with consideration for patient age and full discussion of other risk-reduction options.[22]

Guidelines put forth by the Society of Gynecologic Oncologists in 2005 give recommendations on appropriate candidates for prophylactic salpingo-oophorectomy and optimal timing. Any woman with a known BRCA mutation should be offered prophylactic salpingo-oophorectomy, with management individualized for women with a highly suggestive family history who have not undergone testing or who have had negative testing. Women with BRCA1 mutations should be offered surgery after the completion of child-bearing, and are advised to undergo salpingo-oophorectomy by no later than the early 40s. Women with BRCA2 mutations have a 2% to 3% risk of ovarian cancer by age 50, but earlier salpingo-oophorectomy will reduce the risk of breast cancer, which approaches 26% to 34% by age 50. Therefore, women with BRCA2 mutations should likewise be offered salpingo-oophorectomy at the completion of child-bearing or by her early 40s in order to benefit from the reduction in both breast and ovarian cancer risks.[23]

No formal guidelines exist to recommend hysterectomy and salpingo-oophorectomy for women with HNPCC. However, consideration of laparoscopic salpingo-oophorectomy at the completion of child-bearing or by age 35 has been suggested by the National Institutes of Health (NIH) and the American College of Obstetricians and Gynecologists (ACOG).[24]

She undergoes genetic testing and she is a BRCA1 mutation carrier. She is considering prophylactic mastectomy and salpingo-oophorectomy.

How do you advise her?

Although it is not possible to eliminate the risk of developing breast cancer, prophylactic mastectomy will reduce the incidence by 90% in BRCA mutation carriers.[22, 25] However, with careful surveillance, it is possible to detect early breast cancer more readily than early ovarian cancer. For many women, this makes surveillance a more attractive option than prophylactic mastectomy. Drawbacks include both the physical and psychological consequences of the surgery. Advancements in surgical techniques have allowed women a wide range of options regarding the timing and type of breast reconstruction, with less disfigurement than women treated with older surgical techniques. Even so, a thorough evaluation and counseling by a multidisciplinary team, including surgical oncologists, geneticists, counselors, and medical oncologists, is recommended.

The benefits of prophylactic salpingo-oophorectomy are twofold: reduction in ovarian cancer risk and, by reducing estrogen levels, an attendant reduction in breast cancer risk. Additionally, it is a low-risk procedure that can usually be performed laparoscopically in an outpatient setting.

Prophylactic salpingo-oophorectomy performed before menopause has been shown to lower subsequent breast cancer risk by almost 50%. Salpingo-oophorectomies performed on women under age 40 were associated with a greater reduction in breast cancer than surgeries performed on women who were closer to age 50. Use of hormone replacement therapy did not negate the reduction in risk.[26] Additionally, salpingo-oophorectomy reduces the risk of ovarian or primary peritoneal cancer by 96%, but continued surveillance of these women is still recommended. Microscopic ovarian and fallopian tube cancers have been found in 2% to 10% of women undergoing prophylactic salpingo-oophorectomy, underscoring the need for careful and systematic pathologic examination of these specimens.[23] At the time of surgery, the surgeon should alert the pathologist to the patient's diagnosis (BRCA1, BRCA2, etc.), so that appropriate serial sectioning and processing of the ovary and fallopian tube can be conducted (see "Pathology Notes").

The surgical risks of salpingo-oophorectomy are low, but premenopausal women may suffer significant vasomotor symptoms from surgical menopause. Low-dose estrogen-replacement therapy can be used safely until around age 50, with no increase in breast or ovarian cancer risk.[26] Bone density should be monitored, especially in women at risk for osteoporosis, and in the absence of vasomotor symptoms, bisphosphonates can be used to prevent bone loss.

Would you recommend that she have a hysterectomy at the time of her prophylactic salpingo-oophorectomy?

Hysterectomy at the time of prophylactic oophorectomy is an individualized patient decision. If the patient has other indications for hysterectomy, such as symptomatic fibroids or dysfunctional bleeding, then performing a hysterectomy at the time of salpingo-oophorectomy is reasonable. In women who are planning to take tamoxifen for chemoprevention, there is a significant risk of developing endometrial polyps and a 10% increase in the risk of endometrial cancer over baseline.[27] In this setting, hysterectomy may also be considered. Drawbacks of hysterectomy are increased time of surgery and increased risk of complications. In the absence of a discrete indication for hysterectomy, it is unnecessary to remove the uterus. However, the tube and ovary should be removed in their entirety (see Box 1). While the short interstitial portion of the fallopian tube is not removed completely during a salpingectomy, there have been no reported cases of fallopian tube malignancy in this region following prophylactic salpingectomy.

Prophylactic salpingo-oophorectomy can be performed laparoscopically depending on the comfort level of the surgeon. Washings should be obtained and a thorough peritoneal survey done, with a biopsy of any suspicious lesions. If an adequate assessment cannot be carried out laparoscopically, then a laparotomy should be performed. The surgeon must alert the pathol-

---

Box 1 Surgical steps of a prophylactic salpingo-oophorectomy in a BRCA carrier

Obtain peritoneal washings, submit to cytopathology
Thorough inspection of pelvic and abdominal peritoneal surfaces, diaphragm and omentum
Thorough inspection of uterus, ovaries, fallopian tubes
Enter the retroperitoneal space and identify the ureter
Isolate and divide the infundibulopelvic ligament (ovarian vessels) proximally, to remove all ovarian tissue
Divide the fallopian tube at the uterine cornua and divide the remaining mesosalpinx
Label pathology specimen to indicate BRCA mutation status

---

ogist as to the patient's genetic mutation and request special pathologic processing (see "Pathology Notes").

She has read that sometimes you may find a "small" cancer at the time of prophylactic surgery, She would like to know if her ovaries will be evaluated differently than someone who does not have a genetic mutation.

What do the pathologists at your institution do to avoid missing a "small" cancer?

Pathology notes

While the majority of patients undergoing risk reducing salpingo-oophorectomy (RRSO) will have negative pathology, detailed pathologic evaluation will occasionally uncover small significant lesions. Patients with a germ-line mutation in BRCA1 or 2 have a lifetime risk of developing ovarian cancer ranging from 15% to 40%. The tubal fimbria have also emerged as a site of carcinoma origin in these patients.[28] Given the lack of effective screening methods to detect early ovarian or tubal carcinoma, most patients opt for RRSO.

From a pathology viewpoint, it is important that these specimens are handled differently than routine BSO specimens so as not to miss early small carcinomas arising in the ovary or within the fimbriated portion of the fallopian tube. If a patient has a confirmed BRCA mutation, this should be communicated to the pathologist on the surgical pathology request slip.

The protocol for gross dissection of these high-risk specimens is as follows. The ovaries are sectioned in 2.0-mm intervals along the medial-lateral plane and submitted entirely for histologic evaluation. The fallopian tubes are bisected near the fimbriated end to isolate the fimbriated portion of the tube. The fimbriated end is then sectioned longitudinally and combined with the

Pathology notes (*continued*)

remainder of the tube sectioned in 2-mm to 3-mm intervals. Microscopic evaluation of the fallopian tube focuses on the fimbriated tubal epithelium, and for the ovary on the surface epithelium. When early tubal and ovarian carcinomas are detected in these patients, the histology is typically high-grade with serous features. Immunohistochemical stains for p53 and Ki-67 are helpful in confirming small foci of carcinoma. The tumor foci typically show strong nuclear p53 overexpression and an increased *Ki-67* index relative to adjacent nonneoplastic epithelium.

References

1. Maxwell GL, Berchuck A. Biology and genetics. In: Berek JS, Hacker NF, eds. *Practical Gynecologic Oncology*. 4th ed. Philadelphia: Lippincott Williams & Wilkins; 2005:3–42.
2. DiSaia PJ, Creasman WT. Genes and cancer. In: DiSaia PJ, Creasman WT. *Clinical Gynecologic Oncology*. 6th ed. St. Louis: Mosby; 2002:563–587.
3. Narod SA. Clinical genetics of gynecologic cancer. In: Hoskins WJ, Perez CA, Young RC, Barakat RR, Markman M, Randall ME, eds. *Principles and Practice of Gynecologic Oncology*. 4th ed. Philadelphia: Lippincott Williams & Wilkins; 2005:33–38.
4. Aziz S, Kuperstein G, Rosen B, et al. A genetic epidemiological study of carcinoma of the fallopian tube. *Gynecol Oncol*. 2001;80:341–345
5. Lancaster JM, Powell CB, Kauff ND, et al. Society of Gynecologic Oncologists Education Committee Statement on Risk Assessment for Inherited Gynecologic Cancer Predispositions. *Gynecol Oncol*. 2007;107:159–162.
6. Risinger JI, Hayes K, Maxwell GL, et al. PTEN mutation in endometrial cancers is associated with favorable clinical and pathologic characteristics. *Clin Cancer Res*. 1998;4:3005–3010.
7. Kohler MF, Berchuck A, Davidoff AM, et al. Overexpression and mutation of p53 in endometrial carcinoma. *Cancer Res*. 1992;52:1622–1627.
8. Slomovitz BM, Broaddus RR, Burke TW, et al. Her-2/neu overexpression and amplification in uterine papillary serous carcinoma. *J Clin Oncol*. 2004;22:3126–3132.
9. Ford D, Easton DF, Peto J. Estimates of the gene frequency of *BRCA1* and its contribution to breast and ovarian cancer incidence. *Am J Hum Genet*. 1995;57:1457.
10. Struewing JP, Hartge P, Wacholder S, et al. The risk of cancer associated with specific mutations of *BRCA1* and *BRCA2* among Ashekenazi Jews. *N Engl J Med*. 1997;336:1401.
11. ACOG Committee Opinion: Ethical Issues in Genetic Testing, no. 410, June 2008.
12. Tai YC, Domchek S, Parmigiani G, Chen S. Breast cancer risk among male *BRCA1* and *BRCA2* mutation carriers. *J Natl Cancer Inst*. 2007;99:1811.
13. NCCN Genetic/Familial High-Risk Assessment Clinical Practice Guidelines in Oncology, version 1, 2008. Available at: http://www.nccn.org. Accessed August 11, 2008.
14. Brohet RM, Goldgar DE, Easton DF et al. Oral contraceptives and breast cancer risk in the international BRCA1/2 carrier cohort study: a report from EMBRACE, GENEPSO, GEO-HEBON, and the IBCCS Collaborating Group. *J Clin Oncol*. 2007;25:3831–3836.
15. Watson P, Vasen HF, Mecklin JP, et al. The risk of extra-colonic, extra-endometrial cancer in the Lynch syndrome. *Int J Cancer*. 2008;123:444–449
16. Aarnio M, Mecklin JP, Aaltonen LA, Nystrom-Lahti M, Jarvinen HJ. Life-time risk of different cancers in hereditary non-polyposis colorectal cancer (HNPCC) syndrome. *Int J Cancer*. 1995;64:430–433.
17. Trope CG, Alektiar KM, Sabbatini PJ, Zaino RJ. Corpus: epithelial tumors. In: Hoskins WJ, Perez CA, Young RC, Barakat RR, Markman M, Randall ME, eds. *Principles and Practice of Gynecologic Oncology*. 4th ed. Philadelphia: Lippincott Williams & Wilkins; 2005:823–872.
18. Mecklin JP. Frequency of hereditary colorectal carcinoma. *Gastroenterology*. 1987;93:1021–1025.
19. Samowitz WS, Curtin K, Lin HH, et al. The colon cancer burden of genetically defined hereditary nonpolyposis colon cancer. *Gastroenterology*. 2001;121:830–838.
20. Lynch HT, Smyrk TC, Watson P, et al. Genetics, natural history, tumor spectrum, and pathology

of hereditary nonpolyposis colorectal cancer: an updated review. *Gastroenterology.* 1993;104:1535–1549.

21. NCCN Clinical Practice Guidelines in Oncology Colorectal Cancer Screening, version 2, 2008. Available at: http://www.nccn.org. Accessed August 11, 2008.

22. Society of Surgical Oncology Position Statement on Prophylactic Mastectomy. Updated March 2007. Available at http://www.surgonc.org. Accessed August 13, 2008.

23. Society of Gynecologic Oncologists Clinical Practice Committee Statement on Prophylactic Salpingo-oophorectomy. *Gynecol Oncol.* 2005;98:179–181.

24. Prophylactic Oophorectomy. ACOG Practice Bulletin Clinical Management Guidelines for Obstetrician-Gynecologists, no. **7**, September 1999.

25. Hartmann LC, Schaid DJ, Woods JE, et al. Efficacy of bilateral prophylactic mastectomy in women with a family history of breast cancer. *N Engl J Med.* 1999;340:77–84.

26. Rebbeck TR, Levin AM, Eisen A, et al. Breast cancer risk after bilateral prophylactic oophorectomy in BRCA1 mutation carriers. *J Natl Cancer Inst.* 1999;91:1475–1479.

27. Fisher B, Costantino JP, Redmond CK, Fisher ER, Wickerham DL, Cronin WM. Endometrial cancer in tamoxifen-treated breast cancer patients: findings from the National Surgical Adjuvant Breast and Bowel Project (NSABP) B-14. *J Natl Cancer Inst.* 1994;86:527–537.

28. Crum CP, Drapkin R, Kindelberger D, et al. Lessons from BRCA: the tubal fimbria emerges as an origin for pelvic serous cancer. *Clin Med Res.* 2007;5:35–44.

CHAPTER 8

Evaluation and Management of the Adnexal Mass

Lisa N. Abaid, MD, MPH
Gynecologic Oncology Associates, Newport Beach, CA, USA

Daniel L. Clarke-Pearson, MD, FACOG, FACS
Department of Obstetrics and Gynecology, University of North Carolina School of Medicine, Chapel Hill, NC, USA

Pathology Notes: Chad Livasy, MD
Associate Professor, Department of Pathology and Laboratory Medicine, University of North Carolina School of Medicine, Chapel Hill, NC, USA

Background

Adnexal masses arise primarily from the ovary, fallopian tube, uterus, cervix, or from within the broad ligament. Alternatively, they may originate from an adjacent gastrointestinal, genitourinary, or retroperitoneal structures. Masses may be of benign or malignant etiology, or may be a site of metastasis. Clinical decision-making and interventions are greatly impacted by factors such as patient age and risk factors, physical examination, characteristics of the mass on imaging, and serum tumor marker measurements. While the negative repercussions of delaying a cancer diagnosis are apparent, the harms of overly aggressive surgical intervention should not be minimized. Important decisions regarding whether or not to proceed with surgery, the route of surgical approach, and the decisions made in the operating room are equally important. A thorough discussion of options should be held with the patient prior to making a management plan.

Gynecological Cancer Management: Identification, Diagnosis and Treatment, Edited by Daniel L. Clarke-Pearson and John T. Soper. Published 2010 by Blackwell Publishing, ISBN: 978-1-4051-9079-4.

While the lifetime risk of ovarian cancer is 1.4% for U.S. women, up to 10% will undergo surgical intervention for an adnexal mass. Of those receiving surgery, 13% to 21% will be diagnosed with ovarian cancer.[1] The most important factor in predicting malignancy risk is increasing age, with nearly 70% of ovarian cancers diagnosed in women over age 55 years.[2] However, girls less than 15 years of age with an adnexal mass are also at an increased risk of malignancy. In addition to overall cancer risk, the prevalence of various benign and malignant neoplasms changes with age.

Types of adnexal mass by developmental stage

Ovarian cysts can occasionally develop during fetal life due to ovarian stimulation by maternal hormones. The cysts are follicular in origin and usually regress by 3 to 6 months of age. Premenarchal gynecologic neoplasms are rare; more common abdominal tumors in this age group include Wilms tumors or neuroblastomas.[3] Ovarian tumors in infancy and childhood are almost exclusively germ cell tumors, primarily teratomas and dysgerminomas, with rates of malignancy ranging from 21% to 35%.[4]

During adolescence, defined as menarche through age 19, the onset of menses may unmask previously undiagnosed abnormalities of the genital tract. Some of these may cause outflow obstruction, such as vaginal agenesis or imperforate hymen, which can present as a pelvic or abdominal mass. However, most adnexal masses in this age group are self-resolving functional cysts, which usually measure from 3 to 10 cm in size. Germ cell tumors are the most common neoplasm, and the majority of these are benign cystic teratomas (dermoid). Other less common causes of an adnexal mass in this age group include cysts that arise from mesonephric remnants and produce paratubal or paraovarian cysts. These are simple and thin-walled in nature, but can grow to a large size.[3]

Pelvic masses in reproductive-aged women are usually benign. They can arise from almost any gynecologic structure, in addition to adjacent non-gynecologic organs. Pregnancy-associated processes should always be considered and can be ruled out rapidly with a negative serum pregnancy test. In premenopausal women, the risk of malignancy with any adnexal mass is 6% to 11%.[5] The most common ovarian mass in women of this age group is a functional cyst, specifically a follicular or corpus luteum cyst. Other common non-neoplastic cysts include endometriomas and multiple follicular cysts associated with polycystic ovarian syndrome. The most common benign cystic neoplasms are serous and mucinous cystadenomas and benign cystic teratomas. Serous cystadenomas are more common than mucinous, and are more often bilateral (20–25% versus 5%). Other etiologies include inflammatory or infections processes, benign solid tumors such as Brenner tumors or fibromas, and malignancies. These will be discussed later in the chapter.[3]

Pregnant women are at the same age-related risks for benign and malignant adnexal masses as nonpregnant women. They are also at risk for several neoplasms that are unique to pregnant women; these include ectopic pregnancy, theca lutein cysts, corpus luteum of pregnancy, and lu-

teoma. Additionally, a molar gestation may present as a rapidly enlarging pelvic mass. These conditions are discussed in subsequent chapters.

Though the majority of adnexal masses diagnosed in perimenopausal and postmenopausal women are benign, 29% to 35% will be malignant.[5] Presence of ascites, bilaterality, and advancing age are risk factors for malignancy. Large size is associated with a higher probability of cancer in this age group, as two-thirds of ovarian masses greater than 10 cm are malignant. While endometriomas are far more common among reproductive-age women, 5% of cases occur in postmenopausal women, especially those using hormone replacement therapy. The most common benign tumors are epithelial in origin, typically serous, followed by germ cell and stromal tumors. It is important to consider diverticular disease in this age group, as 30% of women over age 60, and 65% of women over age 85, have diverticulosis.[3]

Women with non-gynecologic cancers are at risk for ovarian metastases (breast, colorectal, stomach, and pancreatic cancers). Approximately 50% to 90% of non-gynecologic ovarian metastases arise from a primary breast or gastrointestinal tract malignancy.[6] Additionally, one in five women with a history of nongynecologic cancer who present with an adnexal mass will have a malignancy, 60% of which are metastatic from other primaries.[7]

Imaging of pelvic masses

Women with an adnexal mass should undergo imaging, and high-frequency, gray-scale transvaginal ultrasonography is the modality of choice due to availability, tolerability, safety, and cost-effectiveness.[2] Abdominal ultrasonography should be a standard part of the assessment of a pelvic mass, as large masses may not be fully characterized transvaginally. The addition of color Doppler to assess blood flow in and around a mass can increase the sensitivity and specificity of ultrasound in detecting a malignancy.

When using strict diagnostic criteria, ultrasonography has a negative predictive value of up to 99%

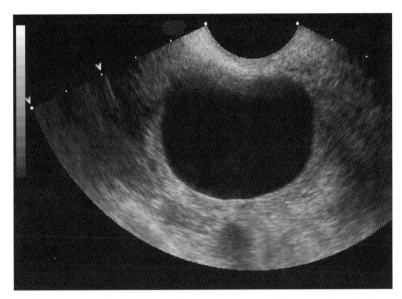

Figure 8.1 Ultrasound of smooth-walled simple ovarian cyst. (Image compliments of Glenn T. Yamagata, MD, Interventional Radiologist, Greensboro Radiology PA, Greensboro, NC.)

in excluding malignancy. Ultrasound findings that indicate a benign etiology include smooth cyst walls (Fig. 8.1), thin septations, absence of solid components or mural nodularity, and homogenous echotexture (Fig. 8.2). Endometriomas or hemorrhagic cysts may have increased echogenicity but should still have a smooth cyst wall (Fig. 8.3). Benign teratomas have a variety of sonographic appearances, but most have a uniformly increased echogenicity with highly echogenic mural nodules, representing calcifications, and fluid layering inside the cyst with or without floating debris.[8]

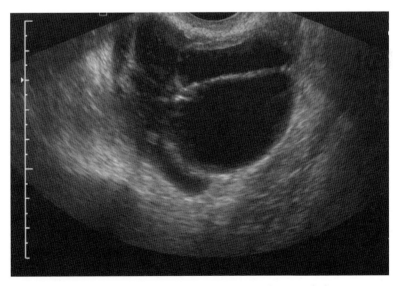

Figure 8.2 Ultrasound of ovarian cyst with thin sepatations. (Image compliments of Glenn T. Yamagata, MD, Interventional Radiologist, Greensboro Radiology PA, Greensboro, NC.)

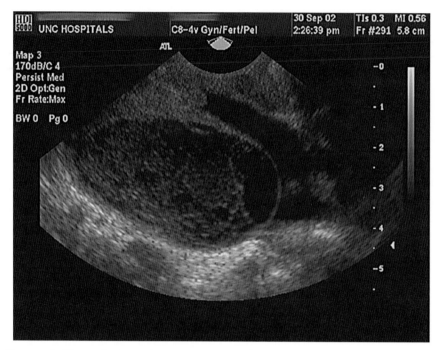

Figure 8.3 Ultrasound of hemorrhagic ovarian cyst. (Image compliments of Alice Chuang, MD, Department of Obstetrics and Gynecology, University of North Carolina.)

Sonographic hallmarks of malignancy include mural thickening or nodules, thick septations, and papillary projections into the cyst cavity. Increased blood flow within the septations or the solid areas is also concerning for cancer. Other associated suspicious findings are ascites, cul-de-sac nodules, lymphadenopathy, peritoneal implants, or hydronephrosis. Increasing size generally also correlates with increasing malignancy risk.[8]

Several ultrasound scoring systems have been formulated in an attempt to standardize the evaluation of an adnexal mass. Examples include the DePriest, Sassone, Lerner, and Ferrazzi systems, which assign risk based on a combination of factors such as presence and character of septations, papillary projections, and solid components, as well as overall size. The DePriest scoring system is shown in Table 8.1 and has been validated in

Table 8.1 Ultrasound scoring system to differentiate benign from malignant ovarian tumors[a]

Morphology	0	1	2	3	4
Cyst wall structure	Smooth (< 3 mm thick)	Smooth (> 3 mm thick)	Papillary projection (< 3 mm)	Papillary projection (≥ 3 mm)	Predominately solid
Volume (cm³)	< 10	10–50	50–200	200–500	> 500
Septum structure	No septa	Thin septa (< 3 mm)	Thick septa (3–10 mm)	Solid area (≥ 10 mm)	Predominately solid

[a] A morphology score > 5 is very suggestive of cancer (sensitivity 89%, specificity 70%, positive predictive value 46%). From DePriest PD, van Nagell Jr JR, Gallion HH, *et al.* Ovarian cancer screening in asymptomatic postmenopausal women. *Gynecol Oncol.* 1993;51:205–209.

Table 8.2 Test characteristics of various diagnostic methods in predicting ovarian malignancy

Method	Sensitivity (%)	Specificity (%)
Pelvic examination	45	90
CA-125	78	78
Ultrasound morphology	86–91	68–83
Doppler ultrasound	86	91
Computed tomography	90	75
Magnetic resonance imaging	91	88
Positron emission tomography	67	79

From Myers ER, Bastian LA, Havrilesky LJ, et al. *Management of Adnexal Mass.* Evidence Report/Technology Assessment no.130. AHRQ pub. no. 06-E004. Rockville, MD: Agency for Healthcare Research and Quality; February 2006.

multi-institutional trials. A morphology index (MI) score of 5 or more is 89% sensitive and 70% specific for ovarian cancer. The mean MI for malignant ovarian tumors is 7.3 and for benign lesions is 3.3. However, the positive predictive value is 46%, meaning that half of the masses with a score of 5 or greater are actually benign.[9]

Other imaging methods such as computed tomography (CT), magnetic resonance imaging (MRI), and positron emission tomography (PET) have a limited role in evaluating an adnexal mass, as they rarely provide additional useful information over an ultrasound (Table 8.2). However, one or more of these modalities may be indicated in certain situations. A CT scan of the abdomen and pelvis is often obtained preoperatively to search for distant metastases when ultrasound or clinical examination is highly suspicious for malignancy. A chest CT is usually added when the chest X-ray is abnormal. CT findings that are highly suspicious for malignancy include ascites, omental caking, lymphadenopathy, peritoneal thickening or implants, hepatic or lung metastases, and ureteral obstruction. MRI is useful in distinguishing adnexal from uterine pathology, and assessing the size, consistency, and location of leiomyomas. PET scan is not an appropriate modality for initial evaluation of a pelvic mass, but can have an important role in clinical management once a malignancy has been diagnosed.[2]

Tumor markers

CA-125 is a serum tumor marker that is elevated in 80% of women who present with epithelial ovarian cancer. It is less predictive of early-stage disease and is normal in 50% of women with stage I ovarian cancer.[1] CA-125 is usually used in the management of women with known ovarian cancer. In that circumstance, it is a good indicator of response to chemotherapy and may also be used to follow women who are in remission Recurrent ovarian cancer is often suspected because of an increasing CA-125 value and may precede clinical appearance of cancer by several months.

On the other hand, CA-125 has not been found to be of use in ovarian cancer screening or in the diagnosis of an adnexal mass. A number of benign, inflammatory, and infectious conditions can cause elevated CA-125 (Table 8.3). Other gynecologic malignancies such as serous endometrial cancer, fallopian tube carcinoma, and cervical adenocarcinoma can also be associated with

Table 8.3 Benign conditions associated with an elevated CA-125

Gynecologic causes	Non-gynecologic causes
Benign ovarian cysts or neoplasms	Pericarditis/pleuritis/peritonitis
Ovarian hyperstimulation	Ascites/pleural effusion
Meigs' syndrome	Liver disease/cirrhosis
Adenomyosis	Recent surgery
Leiomyomata	Radiation therapy
Endometriosis/ endometrioma	Congestive heart failure
Pregnancy (intrauterine or ectopic)	Renal disease
Menstruation	Mesothelioma
Pelvic inflammatory disease	Tuberculosis
Tubo-ovarian abscess	Sarcoidosis
	Lupus
	Polyarteritis nodosa
	Colitis/diverticulitis
	Diabetes

elevated CA-125. Non-gynecologic cancers that may cause elevated CA-125 include breast, colon, lung, and pancreatic cancer, and virtually any primary malignancy that results in widespread pleural or peritoneal-based metastases.[10] Furthermore, 1% of healthy women will have an unexplained elevation in CA-125.[11]

CA-125 testing is most clinically useful in conjunction with ultrasonographic findings in postmenopausal women. A postmenopausal woman with an elevated CA-125 in the setting of a sonographically suspicious pelvic mass has a high risk of malignancy. CA-125 is less accurate for predicting ovarian cancer in premenopausal women, who have a low prevalence of malignancy and a high rate of benign conditions that are associated with elevated CA-125. Sensitivity and specificity for cancer detection in premenopausal women are 50% to 74% and 26% to 92%, respectively, while for postmenopausal women they are 69% to 87% and 81% to 100%. The greatest difference is in positive predictive value, which is 5% to 67% in premenopausal women and 73% to 100% in postmenopausal women.[12]

The American College of Obstetricians and Gynecologists (ACOG) recommends CA-125 testing in all postmenopausal women who present with a pelvic mass. Testing in premenopausal women is less clinically useful with a simple ovarian cyst and no other associated findings, as the chance of malignancy approaches zero. Obtaining a CA-125 level is advisable for a woman of any age who has a complex or solid mass, a first-degree relative with breast or ovarian cancer, or evidence of ascites or metastatic disease.[2]

Carcinoembryonic antigen (CEA) is a serum marker that is primarily used to monitor colorectal cancer. It is often elevated in women with mucinous benign, malignant, and low malignant–potential tumors, which are clinically indistinguishable preoperatively from serous neoplasms.[13] Additionally, an elevated preoperative CEA in the setting of a pelvic mass may indicate metastatic ovarian disease from a gastrointestinal primary, and should prompt endoscopic evaluation prior to gynecologic surgery. CEA testing should be considered in addition to obtaining a CA-125 level in postmenopausal women with an adnexal mass.

Clinical Scenario 1

A 45-year-old woman presents for an annual exam and is found to have a palpable 6-cm left adnexal mass. She is asymptomatic and has no family history of breast or ovarian cancer. She is very concerned, as a close friend of hers was recently diagnosed with ovarian cancer. On closer questioning she reveals some reflux symptoms and a 3-pound weight gain over the last 12 months. She would like to know what your assessment is of her cancer risk and what are the next steps in her evaluation.

What are common presentations and physical findings in patients with an adnexal mass? How do presentations differ in those with benign or malignant masses?

Adnexal masses may present with a wide spectrum of symptoms, or may be completely asymptomatic. When symptoms are present, the character and timing of pain, vaginal bleeding, and gastrointestinal or genitourinary symptoms may provide helpful information as to the etiology. Mid-cycle pain suggests ovulation or presence of a follicular cyst, whereas chronic dysmenorrhea or dyspareunia may suggest endometriosis. Acute, severe pain, with or without nausea and vomiting, may indicate ovarian torsion, infarction, or hemorrhage into an ovarian mass. It may also be associated with degenerating fibroids, or a host of non-gynecologic etiologies. Inflammatory or infectious processes may present with pain and fever, such as ovarian torsion, degenerating fibroids, pelvic inflammatory disease, tuboovarian abscesses, appendicitis, or diverticulitis.[14]

Amenorrhea should always be evaluated first with a pregnancy test, as an ectopic pregnancy can cause pain with or without a mass. Heavy or painful menses can be associated with fibroids, and hormonally active tumors may provoke prepubescent or postmenopausal bleeding. While endometrial cancer is the most common malignancy associated with postmenopausal bleeding, fallopian tube cancer classically presents as vaginal bleeding or watery "tea-colored" vaginal discharge accompanied by an adnexal mass.[8]

Gastrointestinal symptoms of bloating, early satiety, or nonspecific discomfort are the most common complaints in advanced ovarian cancer, but may also be associated with a benign mass or a primary gastrointestinal process. Compression of the bladder by an adjacent adnexal mass can result in urinary frequency, urgency, and diminished bladder capacity.

The ability to evaluate the uterus and adenexae on physical examination is highly dependant on examiner experience and the patient's habitus. Even among experienced examiners, the pelvic examination has poor sensitivity to detect an adnexal mass in women with a body mass index (BMI) greater than 30.[15] Clinical characteristics of a mass that are suspicious for, but not diagnostic of, malignancy include irregularity, nodular or solid consistency, cul-de-sac nodularity, mass fixation or bilaterality, and ascites. Benign etiologies that can have similar findings include endometriosis, uterine fibroids, and chronic pelvic infections.[2]

What imaging should be performed in this case?

Ultrasound (transvaginal and abdominal) would be our initial recommendation for the evaluation of this palpable pelvic mass. The sonographer should describe the details of the mass characteristics including the following characteristics: solid versus cystic; presence and thickness of septations; solid nodules; surface excresences; and the presence of fluid in the cul de sac. The contralateral ovary and uterus should be imaged and described. Areas of the mass that are solid may be evaluated with color-flow Doppler. With this information in hand, the gynecologist may use a scoring system (such as described by De Priest and associates,[16] shown in Table 8.1).

Other imaging such as CT or MRI may be useful when attempting to determine if there are metastases in the upper abdomen or in lymph nodes; but we would always initiate our evaluation with ultrasound.

What laboratory studies should be obtained, and how should they be interpreted?

Initial laboratory testing should include a complete blood count to evaluate for anemia or leukocytosis, and a urine or serum beta-human chorionic gonadotropin (β-hCG) measurement to exclude a pregnancy-related etiology. Elevated hCG can also indicate gestational trophoblastic disease or a gem cell tumor. Assessment of germ cell tumor markers, including β-hCG, alpha-fetoprotein (AFP), and lactate dehydrogenase (LDH), is indicated when imaging shows a solid or complex adnexal mass in an adolescent or young woman. In a 45-year-old patient, obtaining germ cell tumor markers would be inappropriate.

If this patient has ovarian cancer, it is most likely epithelial in origin. CA-125 and CEA would be the two tumor markers that might be considered useful in the evaluation of this patient. It must always be remembered that only 80% of ovarian cancers will have an elevated CA-125 value (20% false negative), and that CA-125 is only elevated in from 25% to 50% of stage I ovarian cancers. Conversely, there are a host of benign conditions that will "falsely" elevate CA-125 (Table 8.3). Therefore, the CA-125 value must be interpreted in the context of the patient's age, symptoms, and ultrasound characteristics of the mass.

The patient's serum CA-125 is 12 U/mL (normal is < 35 U/mL) and her ultrasound shows a 5-cm cystic left adnexal mass that is predominantly cystic but has a solid area without increased flow on Doppler (Fig. 8.4). Ascites is not present, and the right ovary and uterus are normal. Given these findings, the patient would like to know the probability that she has cancer.

What findings on imaging increase or decrease the risk of malignancy?

This patient's ultrasound is indicative of a benign cystic teratoma. With a normal CA-125 value

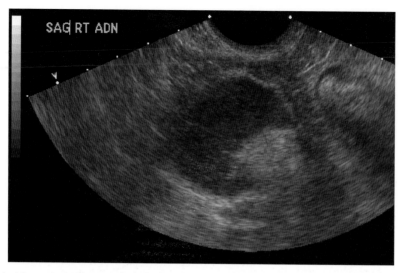

Figure 8.4 Clinical Scenario 1. Ultrasound of of pelvic mass. Note the smooth-walled cystic component and solid component, consistent with a mature teratoma (dermoid). (Image compliments of Glenn T. Yamagata, MD, Interventional Radiologist, Greensboro Radiology PA, Greensboro, NC.)

and a lack of other abnormalities on exam and ultrasound, her risk of malignancy is low. Her symptoms of occasional reflux and a 3-pound weight gain can be seen with ovarian cancer, but given the overall scenario are likely unrelated. Teratomas do not resolve spontaneously, and surgical removal is indicated in this case.

Clinical Scenario 2

A 25-year-old nulliparous woman is referred by her family physician for an 8-cm right ovarian mass. On ultrasound, the mass is primarily cystic with a thin septation, but there is a small excrescence that has increased blood flow (Fig. 8.5). She has some occasional cramping but is otherwise asymptomatic, with regular menses. Her CA-125 is 47 U/mL. She has no first-degree relatives with breast or ovarian cancer, but has a maternal great-aunt with postmenopausal breast cancer. She would like to attempt conception as soon as possible, once this mass is addressed.

Should this patient have surgery for the adnexal mass, or may she be followed conservatively? Should she be referred to a gynecologic oncologist?

Determining whether a woman should undergo surgery for an adnexal mass involves weighing several factors, the most important of which is risk of malignancy. Any mass suspected to be malignant should be evaluated surgically, unless surgery is contraindicated due to the patients' comorbidities. Even when a mass is most likely benign, symptoms such as pain or pressure, and risk of rupture or torsion, are indications for surgical removal.

Conservative management is reasonable when the clinical picture is consistent with benign disease or when the diagnosis is unclear, but surgical intervention would pose a substantial risk to the patient. Benign findings include functional cysts in premenopausal women, asymptomatic endometriomas, and simple cysts.[2]

Simple ovarian cysts (thin-walled and simple or with thin septations) that are stable or resolve over time are virtually always benign. One study

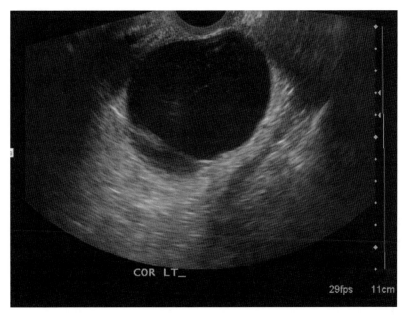

Figure 8.5 Clinical Scenario 2. Ultrasound of ovarian mass with thin septation and small nodule with increased blood flow. (Image compliments of Glenn T. Yamagata, MD, Interventional Radiologist, Greensboro Radiology PA, Greensboro, NC.)

of 2763 women with isolated unilocular ovarian cysts up to 10 cm found that 70% resolved spontaneously. Ten of these women went on to develop cancer, but all ten developed another morphologic abnormality, had resolution of the cyst prior to developing cancer, or developed cancer in the contralateral ovary. Monitoring in this study consisted of transvaginal ultrasounds at intervals of 3 to 6 months until resolution of the cyst or worsening sonographic appearance.[17] Though malignancy risk in cysts up to 10 cm is low, the risk of other problems such as torsion, rupture, or pain lead many to recommend surgical intervention for cysts that are larger than 5 cm.

Women who do not meet the criteria for conservative management should be offered surgical removal of the mass. ACOG and the Society of Gynecologic Oncologists have established referral guidelines to identify women who should be evaluated by a gynecologic oncologist (Box 1). It is important that women with ovarian cancer undergo initial surgery with a gynecologic

---

Box 1 Referral guidelines for women with a pelvic mass

- Ascites
- Evidence of metastatic disease
- Breast or ovarian cancer in a first-degree relative
- Nodular or fixed mass in a woman over 50 years
- Elevated CA-125 in a woman over 50 years
- CA-125 greater than 200 units/mL in a woman under 50 years
- Ultrasound findings suspicious for malignancy at any age
- Young women with elevated germ cell tumor markers (hCG, AFP, LD)

Data taken from ACOG/Society of Gynecologic Oncologists Committee Opinion no. 280: *The Role of the Generalist Obstetrician-Gynecologist in the Early Detection of Ovarian Cancer*. December 2002; and Society of Gynecologic Oncologists Practice Guidelines. Referral Guide: When to refer to gynecologic oncologists. *Gynecol Oncol.* 2000;78, S1–S13.

oncologist, as this is associated with improved surgical staging, optimal debulking, and overall survival.[18]

After a discussion of her options, your patient decides to proceed with surgery. She would like to know which surgical approach you recommend and the advantages and disadvantages of an open and laparoscopic approach. In the event that the mass is malignant, she would like to know if fertility preservation is an option.

What are surgical options and how do you decide which approach to take?

The surgical approach for an adnexal mass is dictated by mass characteristics, patient characteristics, patient preferences, and surgeon experience. The ideal approach would minimize recovery time, postoperative pain, blood loss, and risk, without compromising surgical technique or oncologic outcome in the event of a malignancy.

Minimally invasive surgery, which includes laparoscopic and robotic approaches, has the advantages of less postoperative pain, lower blood loss, shortened hospital stay, and reduced adhesion formation. Technical expertise in using the specialized equipment is required, and most training programs currently incorporate some types of minimally invasive procedures. Limitations occur with increasing mass size, adhesions, and predominantly solid masses. Depending on surgeon experience, cystic masses up to 10 cm in size can usually be safely decompressed and removed laparoscopically with steps taken to avoid tumor spill (Box 2). Several large series describe safe laparoscopic removal of large ovarian cysts measuring more than 10 cm.[19,20] The decision to attempt laparoscopic removal of a large cyst is surgeon and patient dependent, and must be individualized.

The primary concern regarding the use of laparoscopy is the risk of tumor rupture, which is felt to be greater when using a laparoscopic approach. Rupturing a malignant mass upstages the patient, necessitating chemotherapy when it otherwise may not have been indicated. Tumor spill

---

> **Box 2   Techniques to avoid spillage during laparoscopic decompression and removal of a cystic mass**
>
> - Open umbilical entry or needle insufflation in the left upper quadrant to avoid puncture of the mass.
> - Place additional trocars under direct visualization.
> - Obtain washings.
> - Lyse any adhesions.
> - Isolate and divide the ovarian blood supply (after identifying the ureter).
> - Place mass into a laparoscopic bag. (Note: large bags are available that can be placed through a 15-mm trocar. They are often used for laparoscopic splenectomy or nephrectomy.)
> - Remove one of the 10-mm trocars and bring the bag up to the skin.
> - Taking care not to perforate the bag, incise the cyst capsule and aspirate the contents.
> - Morcellate the cyst capsule.

has been associated with a shortened disease-free survival, even controlling for age, histology, lymphadenectomy, and adjuvant chemotherapy.[21] However, three randomized trials that included 394 women with clinically benign pelvic masses showed equivalent rupture rates, with conversion rates of 0% to 1.5%. All three trials demonstrated that laparoscopy resulted in significant reductions in operative time, morbidity, length of hospital stay, and postoperative pain.[2]

Robotic or laparoscopic pelvic surgery requires the patient to tolerate insufflation of the abdomen and steep Trendelenburg positioning. Lung disease, pulmonary hypertension, and morbid obesity may preclude a minimally invasive approach due to problems with ventilation. However, the majority of patients are able to withstand insufflation and positioning, often with some ventilatory adjustments, making collaboration and communication with the anesthesiologist throughout the surgery essential.

In this clinical scenario, the mass has some features suspicious for malignancy, specifically the excrescence. However, the patient's young age, minimally elevated CA-125, and lack of associated findings make her overall risk of invasive malignancy low, although this may be consistent with a tumor of low malignant potential. Her family history does not change her ovarian cancer risk. A laparoscopic approach would be reasonable. In all cases, peritoneal washings should be obtained and submitted to cytopathology, and a thorough visual inspection of the pelvis and entire upper abdomen should be performed, before removal of the cystic ovary.

Laparotomy should be performed if there are any findings suspicious for an invasive ovarian cancer, and a gynecologic oncologist should be available to perform debulking or staging surgery. Given the size and characteristics of the mass, a salpingo-oophorectomy would be preferable over cystectomy, with a frozen section obtained. Further decision-making should be discussed preoperatively, to include her options for fertility-conserving surgery in the event of an early-stage invasive cancer. This would consist of salpingo-oophorectomy, pelvic and para-aortic lymphadenectomy, omentectomy, and peritoneal biopsies. If the frozen section is consistent with a benign mass or clinical stage I low malignant–potential tumor, no further surgery is indicated. (See Chapters 9 and 10 for more discussion of LMP tumors and ovarian cancer.)

Clinical Scenario 3

You are performing an open oophorectomy on a 38-year-old woman, gravida 1, para 0010, with a 10-cm right adnexal mass. The mass was complex on ultrasound but there was no evidence of ascites and the contralateral ovary and uterus were normal. Her CA-125 was 67 U/mL. She would like to retain her uterus and left ovary unless there is a concern for cancer, as she may want to attempt conception in the future. Inspection of her peritoneal cavity reveals a smooth 10-cm cystic ovarian mass with no other abnormalities. You obtain washings and perform a right salpingo-oophorectomy. Upon bivalving the mass in the specimen container, you encounter several cysts containing serous fluid with some frond-like projections from the wall of the largest cyst.

When is a frozen section appropriate? How accurate is it and what are some of the potential pitfalls?

Obtaining a frozen section of an adnexal mass is indicated when the result could influence surgical decision-making. Although the positive predictive value of frozen section in identifying malignancy approaches 100%, treatment planning should still be based on the final pathology results. Simple cysts that contain clear fluid and have smooth walls can be considered benign, and a frozen section would be highly unlikely to provide useful clinical information. Conversely, even though we usually feel comfortable in making the diagnosis of ovarian cancer when widely metastastatic disease is found to involve the the omentum and peritoneum, we would obtain a frozen section to identify metastatic cancer which may have originated in the gastrointestinal or other nongynecologic sites.

Benign cystic teratomas typically contain hair and sebum, and a frozen section is not required in the absence of elevated tumor markers or findings suspicious for malignant disease. However, pathologic evaluation of benign-appearing teratomas is still necessary to rule out immature components.

Pathology notes

Frozen section evaluation of adnexal masses shows high accuracy for most ovarian lesions and is an essential part of intraoperative management for patients with an adnexal mass.

Pathology notes (*continued*)

Studies evaluating the accuracy of frozen section diagnosis have shown a sensitivity of 93% to 98% and a positive predictive value of 92% for benign lesions, and a sensitivity of 84% to 98% and a positive predictive value of 98% to 100% for malignant lesions.[22–24] Errors related to frozen section diagnosis are typically related to sampling issues (more common) or diagnostic interpretation. The pathologist has only limited tissue to evaluate at frozen section, as it is practical to only take 1 or 2 sections of an adnexal mass, in contrast to the usual 10 to 20 permanent sections evaluated for large ovarian masses. Due to technical issues with freezing of the tissue and rapid staining, the histologic quality of the frozen section slides is poorer than the permanent formalin-fixed, paraffin-embedded sections. Also, special stains cannot be used at frozen section to aid in the diagnosis or characterize cell types. Despite these limitations, frozen section evaluation correctly classifies most ovarian masses. Pathologists are particularly accurate in classifying the most common ovarian masses including carcinoma, cystadenoma, mature cystic teratoma, endometrioma, and follicular/luteal cysts.

The expectations of frozen section evaluation include characterization of the behavior of the lesion (benign vs. malignant vs. borderline) and classification of tumor type (surface-epithelial vs. germ cell vs. sex cord stromal). For carcinomas, a determination should be made whether the tumor likely represents an ovarian primary or a metastatic carcinoma. Integration of several factors including patient age, past medical history, gross appearance of mass, and histology is needed to provide the most accurate and complete frozen section diagnosis. For example, there are several gross and microscopic clues to raise suspicion of the more common metastatic tumors to the ovary including gastric, colorectal, and appendix. The gross appearance of ovarian masses often provides clues to the tumor type. For surface epithelial neoplasms, frozen section evaluation is focused on areas of solid nodules or excrescences. Intraoperative gross evaluation of the ovarian mass is a good time to evaluate for ovarian surface involvement (for carcinoma cases) or to document capsular rupture of neoplasm.

The following is a brief discussion of the more common problem areas in the frozen section evaluation of ovarian masses. A more complete list is provided in Box 3. Most frozen section errors represent sampling errors resulting in upgrading of benign or LMP tumors to higher-grade lesion after more extensive sampling. A common example is a tumor with borderline features at frozen section being upgraded to carcinoma on the final diagnosis. Large mucinous tumors diagnosed as mucinous cystadenoma may be upgraded to mucinous borderline tumor after further sampling on permanent sections. The changes meeting criteria for LMP can be extremely focal, present in only a few slides. For mucinous borderline neoplasms and mucinous adenocarcinomas, the possibility of metastasis may be raised in the final report after complete pathologic evaluation including immunohistochemical studies. Other common problems are related to not being able to perform special stains at the time of frozen section. Malignant undifferentiated tumors are problematic because they typically cannot be further classified until special stains are performed. Carcinomas with unusual growth patterns may mimic other tumors including certain sex cord stromal neoplasms precluding definitive distinction until special stains are performed. Rare tumors, particularly germ cell neoplasms and unusual sex cord stromal tumors, may cause problems for the pathologist due to the limitations of frozen section evaluation (diagnosis requires special stains) or unfamiliarity with histopathologic variants of certain unusual ovarian neoplasms. Lastly, distinguishing adult granulosa cell tumor from cellular fibroma/thecoma, carcinoid tumor, or poorly differentiated carcinoma may not be possible in some cases until special stains are performed.

Pathology notes (*continued*)

Despite the focus here on the problem areas, frozen section evaluation is generally an accurate test to determine which patients need intraoperative staging. The quality of the frozen section diagnosis depends in large part on the experience of the pathologist. Many large pathology groups have at least one person designated to have expertise in gynecologic pathology. It may be beneficial to have particularly challenging frozen sections evaluated by that person if possible. Unusual tumors in reproductive-age patients should be managed conservatively until the tumor can be definitively classified (on permanent section evaluation). Communication of diagnostic uncertainty in problematic cases is essential and a more lengthy intraoperative discussion between the pathologist and the surgeon is often helpful for these cases at the time when the pathologist renders his or her frozen section diagnosis.

Box 3 Problem areas in the frozen section evaluation of adnexal masses

- Borderline tumor upgraded to carcinoma on final
- Mucinous cystadenoma upgraded to mucinous borderline tumor on final
- Primary ovarian neoplasm versus metastasis
- Classification of undifferentiated malignant neoplasms
- Carcinomas with unusual architecture pattern mimicking another neoplasm
- Recognition of unusual patterns of clear cell carcinoma (eg, tubulocystic)
- Distinguishing adult granulosa cell tumor from its mimics
- Serous borderline tumor downgraded to serous cystadenofibroma on final
- Rare tumors
- Immature teratoma (immature foci may not be sampled at frozen)
- Corpus luteum or luteoma of pregnancy misinterpreted as steroid cell tumor
- Lymphomas involving ovary misdiagnosed as carcinoma

The frozen section is consistent with a serous tumor of low malignant potential. There is no gross evidence of metastatic spread.

What steps are appropriate when an unanticipated malignancy is found at the time of surgery?

Ideally, women who have a high risk of malignancy, as outlined in Box 1, would be referred to a gynecologic oncologist for surgery. However, not all women will be appropriately referred, and some women who do not meet referral criteria will have low malignant–potential tumors or invasive cancer.

Surgical management of unsuspected ovarian cancer is discussed in detail in Chapter 10. However, basic considerations when performing surgery for an adnexal mass include taking washings upon entry into the peritoneal cavity, conducting a careful survey of the entire peritoneal cavity, and making an adequate incision. A Pfannensteil incision may be adequate when removing presumed benign ovarian neoplasms that are small enough and where extensive adhesions are not suspected. In many cases a vertical incision is preferable so that the mass may be removed intact and, in case of an unanticipated malignancy, exploration of the upper abdomen, omentectomy and para-aortic lymphadenectomy can be accomplished. If a malignancy is unexpectedly found, and a surgeon with oncologic experience is not available, obtaining washings and removing the affected adnexa is recommended. In the case of obviously advanced disease, obtaining an adequate tissue specimen for diagnostic purposes and documenting disease volume and location is beneficial. Postoperatively, the patient should be immediate referred to a gynecologic oncologist who will then plan to complete the debulking procedure.

In this clinical scenario, the patient would like to preserve fertility. Lymphadenectomy and staging of low–malignant potential tumors may upstage a small number of women with clinical stage I disease, but unlike invasive ovarian cancer, does not alter prognosis, which is overall excellent. This patient should undergo a right salpingo-oophorectomy, with continued monitoring of her left ovary as her recurrence risk is greater if she retains an ovary. If fertility were not a consideration, a total hysterectomy and bilateral salpingo-oophorectomy would be indicated.[25] (See Chapter 9 for a more detailed discussion of LMP tumors; including the role of ovarian cystectomy in selected cases.)

References

1. National Institutes of Health Consensus Development Conference Statement. Ovarian cancer: screening, treatment, and follow-up. *Gynecol Oncol.* 1994; 55:S4–14.
2. *Management of Adnexal Masses.* ACOG Practice Bulletin. Clinical Management Guidelines for Obstetrician-Gynecologists: no. 83, July 2007.
3. Stenchever MA. Differential diagnosis of major gynecologic problems by age groups. In: Mishell DR. Stenchever MA, Droegemueller W, Herbst AL, eds. *Comprehensive Gynecology.* 3rd ed. St. Louis: Mosby-Year Book; 1997:149–170.
4. The adnexal mass and early ovarian cancer. In: DiSaia PJ, Creasman WT. *Clinical Gynecologic Oncology.* 6th ed. St. Louis: Mosby; 2002:259–288.
5. Kinkel K, Lu Y, Mehdizade A, Pelte MF, Hricak H. Indeterminate ovarian mass at US: incremental value of second imaging test for characterization—meta-analysis and Bayesian analysis. *Radiology.* 2005;236:85–94.
6. Landis SH, Murray T, Bolden S, Wingo PA. Cancer statistics, 1998. *Cancer J Clin.* 1998;48:6–29.
7. Juretzka MM, Crawford CL, Lee C, et al. Laparoscopic findings during adnexal surgery in women with a history of nongynecologic malignancy. *Gynecol Oncol.* 2006;101:327–330.
8. Ascher SM, Cooper C, Scoutt L, Imaoka I, Hricak H. Diagnostic imaging techniques in gynecologic oncology. In: Hoskins WJ, Perez CA, Young RC, Barakat RR, Markman M, Randall ME, eds. *Principles and Practice of Gynecologic Oncology.* 4th ed. Philadelphia: Lippincott Williams & Wilkins; 2005:223–266.
9. DePriest PD, Varner E, Powell J, et al. The efficacy of a sonographic morphology index in identifying ovarian cancer: a multi-institutional investigation. *Gynecol Oncol.* 1994;55:174–178.
10. Gallup DG, Talledo E Management of the adnexal mass in the 1990s. *South Med J.* 1997;90:972–981. Review.
11. Bast RC Jr, Klug TL, St John E, et al. A radioimmunoassay using a monoclonal antibody to monitor the course of epithelial ovarian cancer. *N Engl J Med.* 1983;309:883–887.
12. Myers ER, Bastian LA, Havrilesky LJ, et al. *Management of Adnexal Mass.* Evidence Report/Technology Assessment no.130. AHRQ pub. no. 06-E004. Rockville, MD: Agency for Healthcare Research and Quality; February 2006.
13. Høgdall EV, Christensen L, Kjaer SK, et al. Protein expression levels of carcinoembryonic antigen (CEA) in Danish ovarian cancer patients: from the Danish MALOVA ovarian cancer study. *Pathology.* 2008;40:487–492.
14. Hoffman, MS. Overview of the evaluation and management of adnexal masses. In: Barbieri RL, Falk SJ, Mann WJ, Goff B, eds. *UpToDate.* Available at: *http://www.uptodate.com.* Accessed August 13, 2008.
15. Padilla LA, Radosevich DM, Milad MP. Limitations of the pelvic examination for evaluation of the female pelvic organs. *Int J Gynaecol Obstet.* 2005;88:84–88.
16. DePriest PD, van Nagell Jr JR, Gallion HH, et al. Ovarian cancer screening in asymptomatic postmenopausal women. *Gynecol Oncol.* 1993;51:205–209.
17. Modesitt SC, Pavlik EJ, Ueland FR, DePriest PD, Kryscio RJ, van Nagell JR Jr. Risk of malignancy in unilocular ovarian cystic tumors less than 10 centimeters in diameter. *Obstet Gynecol.* 2003;102:594–599.
18. Junor EJ, Hole DJ, McNulty L, Mason M, Young J. Specialist gynaecologists and survival outcome in ovarian cancer: a Scottish national study of 1866 patients. *Br J Obstet Gynaecol.* 1999;106:1130–1136.
19. Ghezzi F, Cromi A, Bergamini V, et al. Should adnexal mass size influence surgical approach? A series of 186 laparoscopically managed large adnexal masses. *BJOG.* 2008;115:1020–1027.
20. Eltabbakh GH, Charbonneau AM, Eltabbakh NG. Laparoscopic surgery for large benign ovarian cysts. *Gynecol Oncol.* 2008;108:72–76.
21. Paulsen T, Kaern J, Trope C. Improved Three-Year Disease-Free Survival for Patients with FIGO Stage I Ovarian Cancer without Capsule Rupture:

A Population-Based Study. Abstract no. 254. Society of Gynecologic Oncologists 39th annual meeting, Tampa, March 2008.

22. Gol M, Baloglu A, Yigit, et al. Accuracy of frozen section diagnosis in ovarian tumors: is there a change in the course of time? *Int J Gynecol Cancer.* 2003;13:593–597.

23. Rose PG, Rubin SC, Nelson BE, et al. Accuracy of frozen section (intraoperative consultation) diagnosis of ovarian tumors. *Am J Obstet Gynecol.* 1994;171:823–826.

24. Twaalfhoven FC, Peters AA, Trimbos JB, et al. The accuracy of frozen section diagnosis of ovarian tumors. *Gynecol Oncol.* 1991;41:189–192.

25. Ozols RF, Rubin SC, Thomas GM, Robboy SJ. Epithelial ovarian cancer. In: Hoskins WJ, Perez CA, Young RC, Barakat RR, Markman M, Randall ME, eds. *Principles and Practice of Gynecologic Oncology.* 4th ed. Philadelphia: Lippincott Williams & Wilkins; 2005:895–987.

26. ACOG/ Society of Gynecologic Oncologists Committee Opinion no. 280: The Role of the Generalist Obstetrician-Gynecologist in the Early Detection of Ovarian Cancer. December 2002.

27. Society of Gynecologic Oncologists Practice Guidelines. Referral guide: when to refer to gynecologic oncologists. *Gynecol Oncol.* 2000;78, S1–S13.

CHAPTER 9

Ovarian Tumors of Low Malignant Potential

Rabbie K. Hanna, MD
Department of Obstetrics and Gynecology, University of North Carolina at Chapel Hill, NC, USA

John T. Soper, MD, FACOG
Department of Obstetrics and Gynecology, University of North Carolina School of Medicine, Chapel Hill, NC, USA

Pathology Notes: Chad Livasy, MD
Associate Professor, Department of Pathology and Laboratory Medicine, University of North Carolina School of Medicine, Chapel Hill, NC, USA

Background

Ovarian tumors of low malignant potential (LMP), or "borderline" ovarian cancer, was mistaken for true epithelial ovarian cancer for many decades. However, it was realized that some women diagnosed with "ovarian cancer" had an indolent course and their disease was different from women with invasive epithelial ovarian cancer. The pathologic differences distinguishing invasive epithelial ovarian carcinomas from ovarian LMP were recognized by FIGO and WHO in the 1970s.[1] Patients affected by these tumors are usually younger than women who develop epithelial ovarian cancer, with an average age at diagnosis of 40 to 44 years (10–15 years younger than those with ovarian cancer). Overall, these patients have an earlier stage at presentation, lower recurrence rates, longer survival, and late recurrences compared to invasive ovarian cancer. Thus, the overall prognosis of these tumors is excellent (Table 9.1).[2] Ovarian tumors of low malignant potential represent approximately 15% of all primary epithelial ovarian cancers.

Histologic subtypes

Epithelial LMP tumors are defined histologically by the presence of a complex architecture in addition to nuclear atypia and mitotic activity but, most importantly, lack invasion of the underlying stroma, which distinguishes LMP tumors from ovarian carcinoma. Ovarian tumors of low malignant potential are generally classified according to their epithelial characteristics as serous (50%), mucinous (46%), and mixed, endometroid, clear cell, or Brenner tumors (3.9%). Serous LMP tumors, the most common histologic type, are bilateral in 30% of patients and can be associated with extra-ovarian implants in up to 35% of cases. Extra-ovarian disease follows the typical spread pattern of epithelial ovarian carcinoma, with the potential for both peritoneal and retroperitoneal/lymphatic spread. These implants are further classified into invasive and noninvasive, depending on whether there is invasion into the underlying stroma.

Gynecological Cancer Management: Identification, Diagnosis and Treatment, Edited by Daniel L. Clarke-Pearson and John T. Soper. Published 2010 by Blackwell Publishing, ISBN: 978-1-4051-9079-4.

Table 9.1 Survival of patients with ovarian tumors of low malignant potential

Stage	No. patients	5-year survival (%)	10-year survival (%)
Stage I	2310	99	97
Stage II	158	98	90
Stage III	228	96	88
Stage IV	87	77	67

From Trimble CL, Kosary C, Trimble EL. Long-term survival and patterns of care in women with ovarian tumors of low malignant potential. *Gynecol Oncol.* 12002;86:34–37.

Mucinous tumors are classified as either intestinal (85%) or endocervical (15%) subtypes depending on the nature of the epithelial lining. Diffuse non-invasive peritoneal implants that produce abundant mucus, or pseudomyxoma peritonei, are identified in 10% of these tumors. Often pseudomyxoma peritonei results from metastasis from an appendiceal or other gastrointestinal primary site. Thus evaluation of the peritoneal cavity, gastrointestinal tract, gallbladder, and performance of appendectomy is of utmost importance when operating on patients with mucinous LMP.[3]

Pathology notes

Serous tumors of low malignant potential

The borderline category of ovarian neoplasms is an ongoing challenging and controversial area in gynecologic pathology. Approximately 15% of ovarian serous neoplasms fall into the borderline (low malignant potential) category. The vast majority of these tumors behave in a benign fashion, particularly for patients with stage I lesions. Patients with stage I LMP tumors have a disease-free survival rate of 98% and a disease-specific survival rate of 99.5%. The potentially malignant behavior appears to be essentially confined to the patients with advanced stage (approximately 30% of patients with serous LMP tumors). Pathologic evaluation of tumor architecture and characterization of extra-ovarian implants plays an essential role in identifying patients at high risk for malignant behavior.

There are two histologic patterns of serous LMP tumors, the typical type and the micropapillary/cribriform type. The micropapillary pattern is important to recognize as it has been shown to be associated with more aggressive clinical behavior, ovarian surface involvement, bilaterality, and peritoneal implants[4–7]. The micropapillae in these tumors have cores containing minimal to absent connective tissue and are lined by cells showing a high nuclear/cytoplasmic ratio (Plate 9.1). The papillae should be at least 5 times as long as wide and the micropapillary pattern should measure at least 5 mm in one dimension on at least one slide for diagnosis. Adequate sampling of ovarian tumors by the pathologist is an essential part of correctly identifying these neoplasms, and it is recommend that at least 1 section/centimeter of maximum tumor diameter be studied. Micropapillary serous tumors should be clearly identified as such in pathology reports.

Approximately 20% to 30% of serous LMP tumors will be found to have peritoneal implants at the time of initial surgery. These implants are classified by the pathologist as noninvasive, non-invasive desmoplastic, or invasive based on histologic clues. Accurate classification of implants can be particularly difficult, especially for those lacking underlying normal tissue in the biopsy (therefore, the gynecologic surgeon is encouraged to excise peritoneal implants rather than take a biopsy of lesions). Tumor invasion of underlying tissue is the most important adverse prognostic feature, and these tumors behave as well-differentiated

Pathology notes (*continued*)

serous carcinomas. In the absence of underlying normal tissue, histologic patterns showing micropapillary architecture or solid nests of cells surrounded by a cleft are associated with a poor prognosis. Patients with noninvasive peritoneal implants associated with typical serous LMP tumors have a very good prognosis. Correct pathologic classification of implants is very important in predicting the long-term prognosis for patients.

A minority of serous LMP tumors may show small foci of stromal invasion in the ovary. These tumors have been designated as "serous LMP tumors with microinvasion." The size criteria used in the literature to define microinvasion has been variable, ranging from 3 to 5 mm in the maximum linear dimension or up to 10 mm². Most studies have shown a similar good prognosis for these tumors as serous LMP tumors lacking this finding.

Typical serous LMP tumors with an absence of an exophytic surface component have been shown to have a very low risk of peritoneal involvement by tumor. On the contrary, serous LMP tumors with a micropapillary component or ovarian surface involvement show a high risk for peritoneal disease. Documentation of ovarian surface involvement by typical or micropapillary serous LMP is clinically important and should be noted in the pathology report.

Regional lymph node involvement at presentation has been reported in 21% to 25% of patients with serous LMP tumor. The origin of lymph node involvement by serous LMP tumor is unexplained. Possibilities include both true embolic disease versus de novo origin from preexisting nodal endosalpingiosis. Microscopic regional lymph node involvement at presentation does not appear to be associated with adverse prognosis.

Mucinous tumors of low malignant potential

Mucinous borderline (low malignant potential) tumors are typically unilateral (> 95%), large (often >15 cm), multilocular cystic neoplasms with a smooth ovarian surface. Histologically, it is a noninvasive mucinous tumor with varying degrees of epithelial proliferation often associated with mild to moderate nuclear atypia, intestinal differentiation, and scattered mitotic figures. The survival for stage I mucinous LMP tumor of the ovary is essentially 100%. The real challenge in evaluating ovarian mucinous LMP neoplasms is confirming that they are indeed ovarian primaries and not metastatic mucinous neoplasms. The pathologist relies on patient clinical history, ovary gross and microscopic findings, and immunohistochemistry to properly classify these neoplasms. Metastatic tumors that may mimic a primary ovarian mucinous LMP tumor include appendix, pancreas, endocervix, and occasionally colorectal carcinomas. These metastatic tumors may show histologic features very similar to primary ovarian mucinous LMP tumors. An adnexal mass may be the first presenting symptom for these patients, who then fall under the care of a gynecologist.

Much helpful information can be obtained simply from the gross appearance of the ovaries. Tumors showing bilateral ovarian involvement, a nodular growth pattern, surface involvement by tumor, and extra-ovarian disease are at high suspicion for metastasis to the ovary from another primary site. Ovarian mucinous tumors associated with pseudomyxoma peritonei (PMP) are definitionally metastatic and of probable appendiceal origin (Fig. 9.1), with the very rare exception being GI mucinous neoplasms arising within ovarian teratomas.[8, 9] Histologic clues to metastasis include signet-ring cell forms (GI or breast metastasis), nodular distribution of tumor, ovarian surface involvement, extensive pseudomyxoma ovarii, and zones of "dirty necrosis" with surrounding garland pattern of epithelium (colorectal metastasis). Pathology reports of mucinous LMP tumors should document the presence or absence of ovarian surface involvement.

Pathology notes (*continued*)

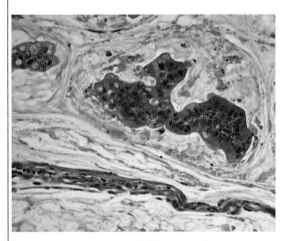

Figure 9.1 Metastatic well-differentiated mucinous adenocarcinoma with a metastasis in the omentum. This patient presented with bilateral adnexal masses. Intraoperative frozen section examination of the ovaries at the time of surgery revealed LMP. The appendix was removed and confirmed to be the primary site for this mucinous neoplasm.

The metastatic tumor most likely to simulate a primary ovarian mucinous tumor of LMP is an appendiceal mucinous tumor. Histologic evaluation of the appendix is required to definitively evaluate for the presence or absence of an appendiceal primary, as these tumors may be quite small. Based on frozen section that suggests an ovarian mucinous neoplasm, the gynecologic surgeon is encouraged to perform an appendectomy to evaluate for an occult appendiceal primary.

Immunohistochemistry can be very helpful in determining the origin of mucinous neoplasms involving the ovary. Cytokeratin 7 and cytokeratin 20 immunostains can help resolve problematic cases; however, the correct diagnosis requires integration of several factors, including patient clinical history. If a patient has any history of prior malignancy, it is important to let your pathologist know. Multiple other tumor types, including lung and breast, have been known to metastasize to the ovary.

It should be noted that frozen section evaluation of mucinous neoplasms has certain limitations. It is practical to examine only 1 or 2 sections at the time of intraoperative frozen section. Mucinous tumors can be very heterogeneous, such that sampling errors are likely to occur. Permanent sections are typically submitted at a rate of 1 section/cm of maximum tumor dimension. For a 16-cm tumor with 16 histologic sections, diagnostic features of LMP may only be found on 2 sections. As a result, a frozen section diagnosis of mucinous cystadenoma may occasionally be followed by a final diagnosis of mucinous LMP. Clues to metastasis (eg, bilateral disease, small tumor size, extra-ovarian disease) should be evaluated at frozen section such that potential primary sites can be evaluated intraoperatively.

Lastly, rare primary mucinous LMP tumors may be associated with microinvasion, often defined by invasive foci <3 to 5 mm in the greatest dimension or <10 mm^2. Another variant finding is the presence of focal high-grade intraepithelial carcinoma without associated stromal invasion. Mucinous LMP tumors showing microinvasion or intraepithelial carcinoma still have an excellent prognosis, with overall survival of approximately 95%.

Endometrioid tumors of low malignant potential

Endometrioid LMP tumors are rare, and experience with these tumors is limited in the literature. Based on current understanding, endometrioid borderline tumors are considered to be essentially benign and do not have a low malignant potential; however, the studies to date are not large and lack long-term follow-up. The most problematic area for the pathologist in the classification of these tumors is the separation of borderline tumors from well-differentiated endometrioid adenocarcinomas.

Surgical staging and management

The staging assigned to this category of ovarian tumors uses the FIGO staging for ovarian carcinoma. Survival is related to stage and presence or absence of invasive implants. In general, surgical removal of the primary lesion and resection (debulking) of implants is the cornerstone of treatment. LMP tumor implants are not chemosensitive, unless they contain invasive elements. Complete debulking of gross extra-ovarian noninvasive implants will decrease morbidity resulting from the slow growth of these lesions, and will assure that the patient has been adequately evaluated for invasive disease. Sutton and associates reported that in a group of 32 women with stage III optimally debulked LMP tumors that were treated with >6 cycles of cisplatin and cyclphosphamide ± doxorubicin, only one patient died of disease during the study duration, with a median follow-up of 31 months. This was despite a relatively low complete response rate; only 6 of 15 patients who underwent a second-look laparotomy had a completely negative reassessment.[10]

Although LMP tumors that appear to be early stage have microscopic noninvasive metastases involving peritoneal surfaces and retroperitoneal lymph nodes with approximately the same frequency as ovarian carcinomas, the clinical importance of comprehensive surgical staging has not been established. In general, surgical staging with lymph node dissection is performed when there is a significant probability that the primary lesion is a true ovarian carcinoma.

Patients with invasive extra-ovarian implants, however, have a prognosis that is affected by tumor differentiation and the amount of residual disease, similar to advanced invasive ovarian carcinoma. If invasive extra-ovarian implants are documented, chemotherapy with a platin/taxane combination is recommended, similar to the treatment of ovarian carcinoma.

Clinical Scenario 1

A 36-year-old woman presents with vague lower abdominal pain. Examination reveals an 11-cm left adnexal mass.

What is the clinical presentation of patients with LMP tumors, and how should this patient be evaluated?

Most patients with LMP tumors present with a unilateral adnexal mass. They may be asymptomatic or have pelvic/abdominal pressure, abdominal distention, or pelvic pain. Acute pelvic pain may represent ovarian torsion. Given that many women with LMP tumors are of reproductive age, immediate surgical exploration and ovarian cystectomy in the setting of severe acute pain associated with an adnexal mass will offer the best chance of preserving ovarian tissue. The symptoms caused by LMP tumors cannot be distinguished from those of epithelial ovarian cancer. Therefore, further investigation and surgery will usually be necessary for a persistent adnexal mass.

Further evaluation should include a pelvic ultrasound examination to better characterize the architecture of the mass. Despite their limitations in premenopausal women, CA-125 and CEA would be reasonable laboratory tests to obtain.

An ultrasound examination confirms an 11-cm cystic left adnexal mass most likely originating from the left ovary with findings of multiple septations and solid components in some of its cystic structures.

What are the sonographic findings that might suggest an ovarian LMP tumor?

There are no sonographic findings that are characteristic of ovarian LMP tumors. Common sonographic findings include a cyst within the ovary of small to medium size with mural nodularity or intraluminal excrescences, increased vascular flow in the nodules, and preserved surrounding ovarian parenchyma. LMP tumors may have low-level echoes within the cystic components of the mass, reminiscent of typical endometriomas. Evidence of peritoneal dissemination and peritoneal fluid (ascites) may be more suggestive of epithelial ovarian cancer, but may also be found in LMP tumors. Finally, some LMP tumors may present as simple cysts. While not initially concerning, serial follow-up sonograms often show temporal evolution with more features suspicious for malignancy in later scans.[11]

Are there any tumor markers that aid in the diagnosis of LMP?

CA-125 levels are elevated in 92% of patients with advanced-stage serous LMPs, but in only 25% of women with stage I serous LMPs.[12] Serial CA-125 values tend to progressively elevate over time in patients with ovarian carcinomas and LMP tumors. Serum CEA levels may be elevated in mucinous LMP tumors and in gastrointestinal malignancies (see below for a more detailed discussion of the association of mucinous ovarian tumors and gastrointestinal malignancies). Although CA-125 and CEA levels are not diagnostic of LMP, an elevated level of one of these markers should raise suspicion and may suggest that the clinician seek consultation with a gynecologic oncologist.

Clinical Scenario 2

After removal of a 9-cm ovarian mass that had no surface nodules or excrescences, frozen section is obtained. The pathologist reports a possible serous borderline tumor of the left ovarian complex cyst that was removed.

How accurate is a frozen section for these tumors?

Most of the information concerning the accuracy of intraoperative frozen section biopsies for LMP tumors is based on retrospective studies. Frozen section results should be interpreted with caution because some lesions are upgraded to ovarian cancers on final pathology (for a more detailed discussion, see the "Pathology Notes" earlier in this chapter). One large study has reported a sensitivity and positive predictive value (PPV) of 71.1% and 84.3%, respectively. Overdiagnosis was found in 6.6% (21/317) and true ovarian cancer was under-diagnosed in 30.6% (97/317).[13] Frozen section is less accurate in large tumors and mucinous lesions because small foci of invasion might be missed since only 1 or 2 sections of the tumor are able to be evaluated during the frozen section evaluation.

Following removal of the involved ovary (reported as LMP on frozen section), what surgical procedures should be performed?

When the diagnosis of an ovarian LMP tumor is suspected from a frozen section biopsy, particularly if there is any suspicion of an invasive lesion, comprehensive surgical staging should be performed. In regard to the affected ovary itself, a unilateral oophorectomy should be performed. If preservation of fertility is not required, total abdominal hysterectomy with bilateral salpingo-oophorectomy is the treatment of choice. Staging for possible ovarian cancer includes exploration of the entire abdominal cavity with peritoneal washings, infracolic omentectomy, and random peritoneal biopsies. If possible, all gross lesions should be resected. Evaluation of the lymph nodes includes selective bilateral pelvic and para-aortic lymphadenectomies, removing para-aortic lymph nodes to the level of the insertion ovarian veins into the vena cava and left renal vein. Women with mucinous lesions should undergo appendectomy because some will have a clinically occult appendiceal primary malignancy that is metastatic to the ovary.

In women who desire child-bearing, the contralateral ovary and uterus should be left in place and care should be taken to avoid trauma that might result in adhesions and tubal occlusion. Careful inspection and palpation of the contralateral ovary is necessary because of the risk of bilaterality, and if there is a suspicious mass or lesion, an ovarian cystectomy or wedge biopsy may be performed. Wedge or random biopsies of a normal contralateral ovary in the absence of lesions, however, are not recommended because of the risk of adhesions that might compromise fertility. In women who have fertility-sparing staging surgery, ipsilateral selective pelvic and para-aortic lymphadenectomy is usually performed to limit adhesions involving the contralateral adnexum.

It is crucial to perform a comprehensive staging procedure if an invasive lesion is suspected, be it via laparotomy or laparoscopy, because the final stage of the disease will be the basis of discussing treatment, prognosis, and survival rates with the patient if an invasive ovarian carcinoma is diagnosed on final pathology. If complete comprehensive staging cannot be performed at initial surgery, it is preferable to manually and visually explore the abdominal cavity and await final pathology results.

Clinical Scenario 3

A 34-year-old nulligravida undergoes laparoscopic ovarian cystectomy. An isolated 5-cm right ovarian cyst is dissected away from the ovarian stroma intact and placed in an endoscopic pouch, where it is drained prior to removal. Despite ultrasound and gross visual impression of a simple cyst (Fig. 9.2), final pathology results indicate that this is a serous LMP tumor. The patient wishes optimal preservation of fertility.

What are the options for management in this patient?

As initially mentioned, thorough surgical staging is important if the diagnosis of invasive ovarian cancer is suspected. In this patient, the diagnosis of LMP has been histologically established and invasive ovarian carcinoma excluded. The role of comprehensive surgical staging for patients with LMP apparently confined to a single ovary has not been established, and adhesions produced by a staging procedure in this patient might have an adverse effect on fertility. In general, fertility preservation in patients with LMP tumors can be achieved with multiple operative options including a unilateral cystectomy or unilateral adnexectomy for unilateral lesions and a bilateral cystectomy or unilateral adnexectomy and contralateral cystectomy for bilateral lesions.[14, 15] Preservation of functional ovarian tissue (cystectomy) does increase the risk of recurrence when compared to radical surgery

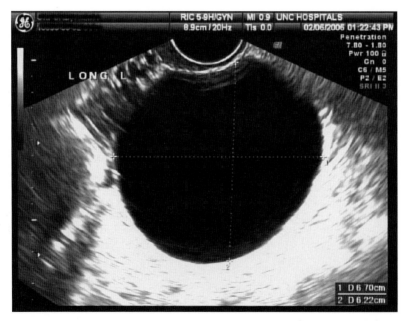

Figure 9.2 Clinical Scenario 3. Ultrasound of ovarian cyst. (Image compliments of Alice Chuang, MD, Department of Obstetrics and Gynecology, University of North Carolina.)

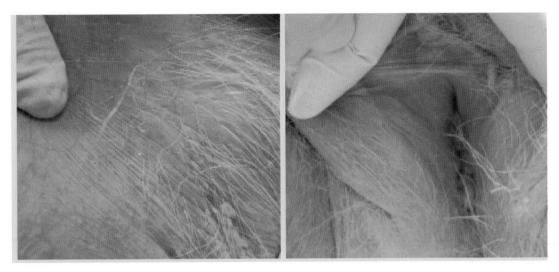

Plate 1.1 Long-standing lichen sclerosis (interlabial view, right) and pre-biopsy close-up view of site B in Plate 1-2.

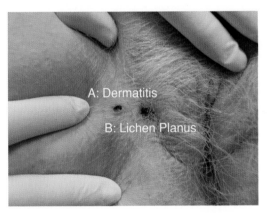

A: Dermatitis

B: Lichen Planus

Plate 1.2 Superimposed contact dermatitis on the background of lichen planus. The dark areas are biopsy sites and silver nitrate applied for hemostasis.

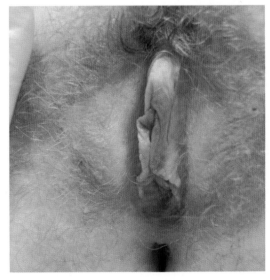

Plate 1.3 Redness and scaling of labia majora indicative of contact dermatitis.

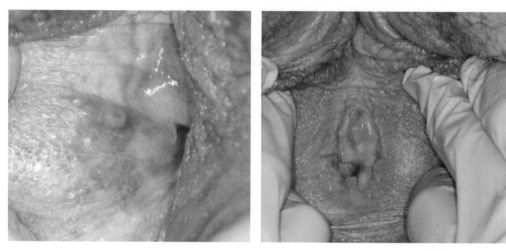

Plate 1.4 Lacy lesions of vulvar lichen planus.

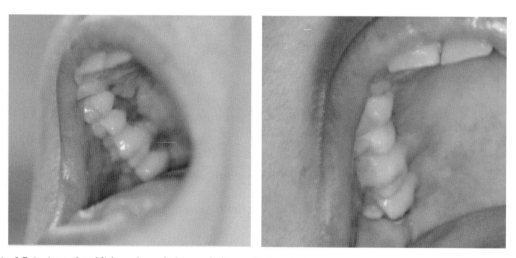

Plate 1.5 Lesions of oral lichen planus before and after methotrexate treatment.

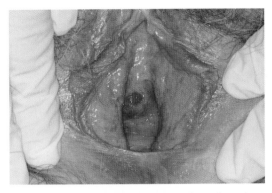

Plate 1.6 Glossy "wet" labia minora with patchy redness and irregular margins of heart's line with loss of keratinized epithelium in inner labial folds.

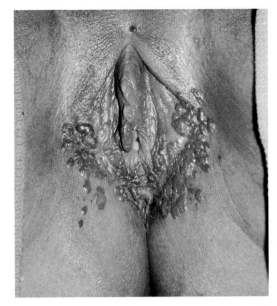

Plate 2.1 Photo of extensive hyperpigmented lesions of the vulva and perianal regions. Biopsy consistent with VIN III.

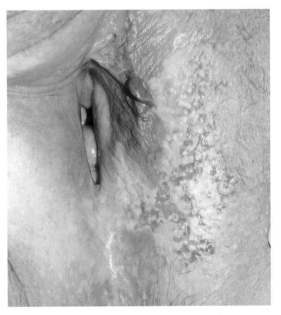

Plate 2.2 Lesion on left vulva. Biopsy: Paget disease.

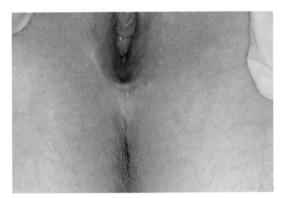

Plate 2.3 Raised irregular lesion of the perineum in a background of atrophy (LSA).

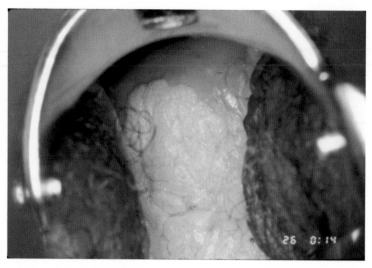

Plate 3.1 Colposcopy of anterior vagina after application of acetic acid. The thick white epithelium of VAIN III is readily apparent.

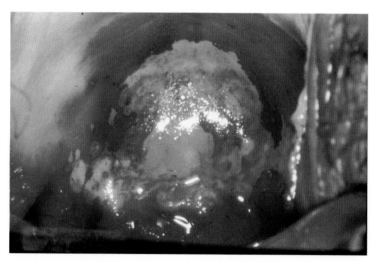

Plate 3.2 After application of Lugol solution, the VAIN II lesion is readily identified as "nonstaining" as opposed to the areas of dark brown indicating uptake in glycogenated squamous epithelium.

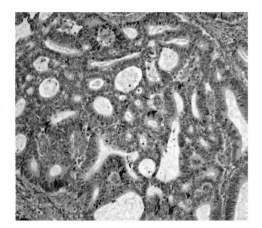

Plate 4.1 Cribriform pattern of invasive endocervical adenocarcinoma. This field shows numerous confluent punched-out glandular spaces over a broad area indicative of stromal invasion. This case was associated with metastasis to one of the patient's ovaries. Both tumors showed diffuse strong immunoreactivity for p16.

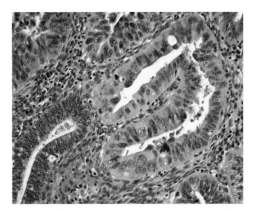

Plate 5.1 Endometrial intraepithelial carcinoma (EIC). This polypectomy specimen contains multiple glands lined by cells with high-grade malignant cytology in contrast to the one benign atrophic gland in the bottom left corner. The degree of cytologic atypia is beyond what is observed in EIN/atypical hyperplasia. The tumor cells demonstrated diffuse strong immunoreactivity for p53, supporting the diagnosis.

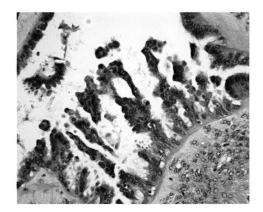

Plate 9.1 Serous borderline tumor with micropapillary features. The tall micropapillae lack stroma within their core and are lined by cuboidal cells with high nuclear/cytoplasmic ratios. There is no evidence of stromal invasion in this high-power field.

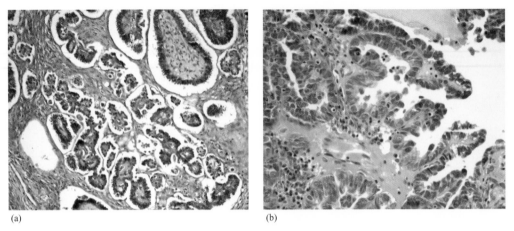

(a)   (b)

Plate 10.1 **(a)** Example of low-grade serous carcinoma with micropapillary architecture, pink cytoplasm, uniform oval nuclei, and rare mitoses. In contrast, **(b)** shows a high-grade serous carcinoma with large pleomorphic nuclei with distinct nucleoli. Mitotic figures were readily identified in other areas of the slide.

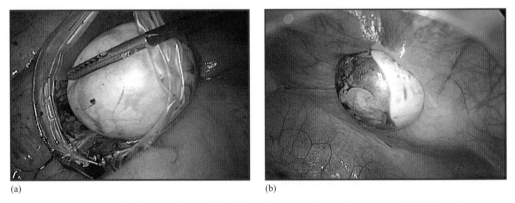

(a)   (b)

Plate 10.2 Specimen retrieval with an endoscopic bag during laparoscopic oophorectomy. **(a)** Placing the ovary involved with a cystic neoplasm into the endoscopic bag. **(b)** The cyst can be aspirated within the bag to facilitate removal through a laparoscopic port site without intraperitoneal spill or contamination of the subcutaneous tissue.

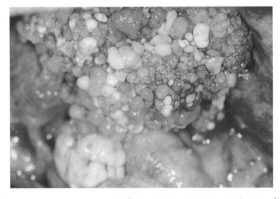

Plate 10.3 Photograph of surface excrescences on a papillary serous ovarian carcinoma diagnosed by laparoscopy.

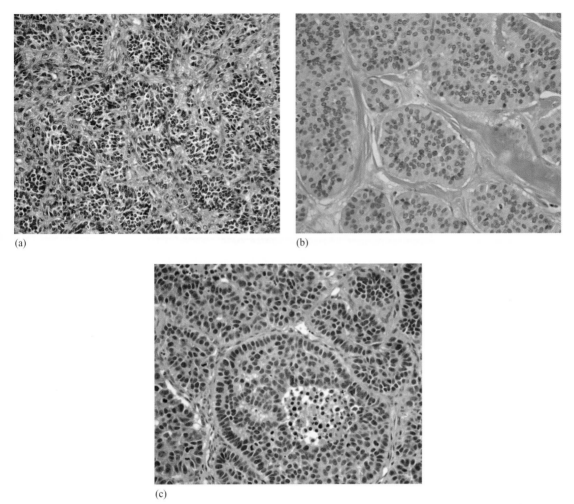

(a)

(b)

(c)

Plate 11.1 Adult granulosa cell tumor and its mimics. **(a)** Adult granulosa cell tumor with a nested growth pattern. Mitotic figures were difficult to find in this case (< 1 mitotic figure/10 high-power fields). **(b)** Ovarian carcinoid tumor with a nested pattern. Immunohistochemistry for neuroendocrine markers were strongly positive and inhibin stain was negative. **(c)** High-grade small-cell carcinoma with a nested pattern. The mitotic count for this cases was markedly elevated (35 mitoses/10 high-power fields). Multiple foci of geographic necrosis were noted and the tumor cells were strongly positive for neuroendocrine markers and negative for inhibin expression.

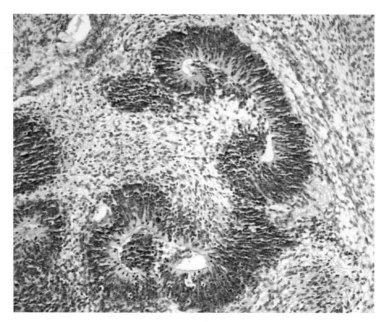

Plate 12.1 Immature teratoma. Primitive neuroepithelial rosettes as shown here have distinctive histology and are the most reliable histologic finding to define the presence of immature elements in teratoma.

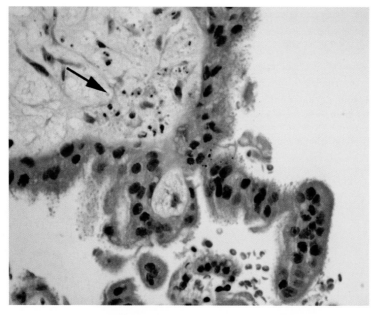

Plate 14.1 Early complete mole. The identification of abundant karyorrhexis debris (*arrow*) within villi showing edema and diffuse trophoblastic proliferation are very supportive for the diagnosis of early complete mole.

(oophorectomy). Both Zanetta and associates[16] and Rao and colleagues[15] had similar recurrence rates—19% and 16% versus 5% and 4%, respectively, for patients undergoing fertility-sparing surgeries compared to surgical treatment that included hysterectomy with removal of both adnexae. The risk of recurrence increases when fertility-sparing surgeries are performed on bilateral or multifocal lesions.[17] If recurrence does occur, surgical resection alone is usually curative. Favorable features that are associated with decreased risk of recurrence are small, grossly unilateral lesions, and intact removal of the cyst.

What surveillance would be recommended after cystectomy for LMP?

Transvaginal ultrasound is the most effective diagnostic technique for the follow-up of young patients treated conservatively for early borderline tumors. This has been studied retrospectively by Zanetta and associates[17] in addition to physical examinations and CA-125 measurements. They recommended ultrasound evaluations every 3 months for the first 2 years and every 6 months thereafter. CA-125 levels were measured every 6 months for serous tumors. There have not been any prospective studies to confirm this schedule of surveillance. Other radiologic modalities, such as CT or MRI scans, should be used if there is a high clinical suspicion of recurrence outside of the pelvis.

This patient has chronic anovulation and was considering ovarian stimulation with clomiphene prior to ovarian cystectomy. What are the risks associated with ovarian stimulation and LMP tumors?

There are no prospective clinical trials that show any association between the recurrence of ovarian borderline tumors and the subsequent use of "fertility drugs." Several retrospective studies have attempted to evaluate the effect of fertility medications on the ovary and subsequent development of ovarian cancer. The interpretation of such an association is complicated by the fact the

infertility itself may elevate ovarian cancer risk.[18] In a case control study, Ness and coworkers[18] found that among nulligravida women, fertility drug use was significantly associated with LMP serous tumors (OR = 2.43, 95% CI: 1.01, 5.88) but not with invasive serous adenocarcinoma (OR = 1.11, 95% CI: 0.51, 2.42) or with borderline or invasive mucinous tumors, endometrioid, clear cell, undifferentiated, or other histologic types of ovarian tumors. This association was not observed in gravid women who were subfertile.

Clinical Scenario 4

A 28-year-old G1P1 presents for a postoperative visit after unilateral salpingo-oophorectomy and comprehensive staging of a serous borderline tumor of the left ovary. She is stage IA and desires preservation of fertility. She is concerned about the potential that surgery may have diminished her chances of subsequently conceiving.

What is her ability to conceive following this procedure?

Similar to patients who undergo adnexectomy for benign lesions, fertility is maintained in the majority of patients who undergo conservative surgery for LMP tumors of the ovary. Twelve of the 25 patients reported by Morris and colleagues[1] conceived 24 pregnancies without complications after conservative treatment for LMP. Another investigator[19] reported a 48% pregnancy rate in women who underwent a conservative staging operation for patients with ovarian LMP tumors. Depending on initial stage of disease, patients are at an increased risk for late LMP tumor recurrence, and should undergo close follow-up with physical examination, ultrasound evaluation of the preserved ovary, and tumor marker surveillance until child-bearing is complete. After completion of child-bearing, completion surgery with hysterectomy and removal of all remaining ovarian tissue is recommended, because of an increased risk for developing a second ovarian LMP or invasive lesion in the remaining ovary.

What is the role of genetic testing in the evaluation of this patient?

A genetic predisposition for invasive ovarian cancer has been established in patients who carry a high-risk BRCA-1 or BRCA-2 mutation. This is especially prevalent among women of Ashkenazi Jewish ancestry. This association, however, does not include borderline tumors of the ovary. Gotlieb and associates[20] studied a total of 1269 women diagnosed with ovarian tumors over a 5-year period in Israel. A total of 233 (18.3%) were identified to have ovarian LMP tumors and 256 (20.2%) had stage I or II invasive ovarian cancers. One hundred seventeen borderline tumors and 161 early-stage invasive tumors were analyzed for the presence of the 185delAG, 5382insC BRCA1, and 6174delT BRCA2 Jewish founder mutations. They found that the prevalence of Jewish founder mutations involving BRCA1 and BRCA2 was only 4.3% of patients with borderline tumors as compared to 24.2% of patients with early-stage ovarian cancer.[20] Based on these and other studies, we do not recommend genetic testing unless invasive ovarian cancer or other high-risk features are present in the family history.

What is her risk of recurrence after unilateral salpingo-oophorectomy?

Recurrences of serous borderline tumors occur at a median of 5 to 7 years after initial surgery. The rate of recurrence is dependent on the initial surgical procedure, with patients who underwent fertility-sparing surgery having a risk of recurrence approaching 19% compared to 4.6% of those who underwent surgery that included bilateral salpingo-oophorectomy.[11] Patients treated with conservative surgery for LMP ovarian tumors should be encouraged to undergo completion TAH/USO after they no longer wish childbearing. Zanetta and coworkers[16] reported that the rate of recurrence with progression into invasive lesions was only 2%. Among 7 patients with invasive recurrences, 5 were of the serous subtype and the other 2 of mucinous subtypes. Six of these 7 patients had initial fertility-sparing surgery.[16]

Clinical Scenario 5

A 54-year-old woman is explored for an 8-cm right adnexal mass. At the time of hysterectomy and bilateral salpingoophorectomy, she has tumor rupture. Several 1 to 2-cm pelvic implants are removed and a 3-cm omental implant is removed with omentectomy. Elective appendectomy is performed. There is no retroperitoneal lymphadenopathy and all grossly visible implants have been removed. Final pathology reveals a unilateral mucinous LMP with noninvasive extra-ovarian implants. The appendix is histologically normal. Cytology prior to tumor rupture was negative.

What adjuvant treatment is required for this patient?

Patients with early-stage LMP tumors that have been completely resected do not benefit from adjuvant chemotherapy.[21] Long-term follow-up every 3 months for the first 2 years, and then every 6 months until at least 5 years after surgery, would include clinical examinations, CA-125 levels, and vaginal sonographic examinations or CT scans.[17] Recurrent lesions should be approached with an attempt at complete surgical debulking with special emphasis on close pathologic examination to rule out recurrence as malignant lesions or LMP with invasive implants.

Patients who have advanced-stage LMP tumors present more challenging decision-making. Sutton and associates[10] documented that advanced LMP lesions with optimally debulked residual disease rarely responded to platin-based chemotherapy as determined by second-look laparotomy, yet had a very low mortality caused by ovarian cancer. In patients with noninvasive implants and complete surgical debulking, no further treatment is required, but close clinical follow-up is recommended. Adjuvant chemotherapy may be considered in patients with noninvasive implants, but this is controversial. Although adjuvant chemotherapy is most often recommended for patients with invasive metastatic implants, there are no randomized clinical trials that have established efficacy. Some retrospective studies have documented an improved survival in patients with invasive implants from LMP tumors treated with chemotherapy, but there have not been any prospective studies to confirm these findings.

Clinical Scenario 6

A 43-year-old woman is explored for bilateral 7-cm complex masses with solid components and increased free fluid on preoperative ultrasound. CA-125 value was 59 U/mL. At the time of TAH/BSO, she has bilateral mucinous LMP tumors confirmed by frozen section. There is 300 mL free gelatinous ascites with "egg white" consistency and a few firm implants involving the omentum that are removed with omentectomy.

What additional surgical procedures should be performed?

When a mucinous ovarian tumor is found, the abdomen should be carefully explored for evidence of a GI primary lesion. Most cases of pseudomyxoma peritonei are associated with a primary malignancy of the appendix. Because the appendiceal primary may be very small, appendectomy should be performed in all cases of suspected pseudomyxoma or mucinous LMP tumors of the ovary. An attempt should be made to debulk all solid metastatic implants, and all of the mucinous ascites should be evacuated.

What is the management of pseudomyxoma peritonei?

Principles of management include appendectomy with complete debulking of peritoneal implants and evacuation of all of the mucinous ascites. Unfortunately, the majority of patients will relapse after surgical debulking, but in the absence of treatment, it may be years before patients become symptomatic from recurrent disease. In the past, management included close clinical and radiographic follow-up, with carefully sequenced surgical debulking when patients developed clinically significant progression. A small GOG study suggested a benefit using intraperitoneal (IP) 5-fluorouracil in a few patients with pseudomyxoma.[22] Currently, other investigators are studying aggressive surgical debulking combined with intraoperative IP chemotherapy with hyperthermia.[23] It is currently recommended that patients with this relatively rare malignancy be referred to centers that specialize in the management of pseudomyxoma peritonei.

References

1. Morris RT, Gershenson DM, Silva EG, Follen M, Morris M, Wharton JT. Outcome and reproductive function after conservative surgery for borderline ovarian tumors. *Obstet Gynecol*. l2000;95:541–547.

2. Trimble CL, Kosary C, Trimble EL. Long-term survival and patterns of care in women with ovarian tumors of low malignant potential. *Gynecol Oncol*. l2002;86:34–37.

3. Cadron I, Leunen K, Van Gorp T, Amant F, Neven P, Vergote I. Management of borderline ovarian neoplasms. *J Clin Oncol*. l2007;25:2928–2937.

4. Burks RT, Sherman ME, Kurman RJ. Micropapillary serous carcinoma of the ovary: a distinctive low-grade carcinoma related to serous borderline tumor. *Am J Surg Pathol*. 1996;20:1319–1330.

5. Seidman JD, Kurman RJ. Subclassification of serous borderline tumors of ovary into benign and malignant type: a clinicopathologic study of 65 advanced stage cases. *Am J Surg Pathol*. 1996;20;1331–1345.

6. Burks RT, Kurman RJ. Case review: micropapillary serous carcinoma of the ovary. *Pathol Case Rev*. 1997;2:154–159.

7. Eichorn JH, Bell DA, Young RH, et al. Ovarian serous borderline tumors with micropapillary and cribriform patterns: a study of 40 cases and comparison with 44 cases without these patterns. *Am J Surg Pathol*. 1999;23:397–409.

8. Ronnett BM, Kurman RJ, Zahn CM, et al. The morphologic spectrum of ovarian metastases from appendiceal adenocarcinomas. A clinocopathologic and immunohistochemical analysis of tumor often misinterpreted as primary ovarian tumors or metastatic tumors from other gastrointestinal sites. *Am J Surg Pathol.* 1997;21:1144–1155.

9. Ronnett BM, Shmookler BM, Diener-West M, et al. Immunohistochemical evidence supporting the appendiceal origin of pseudomyxoma peritonei in women. *Int J Gynecol Pathol.* 1997;16:1–9.

10. Sutton GP, Bundy BN, Omura GA, Yordan EL, Beecham JB, Bonfiglio T. Stage III ovarian tumors of low malignant potential treated with cisplatin combination therapy (a Gynecologic Oncology Group study). *Gynecol Oncol.* l1991;41:230–233.

11. Alfuhaid TR, Rosen BP, Wilson SR. Low-malignant-potential tumor of the ovary: sonographic features with clinicopathologic correlation in 41 patients. *Ultrasound Q.* l2003;9:13–26.

12. Rice LW, Berkowitz RS, Mark SD, Yavner DL, Lage JM. Epithelial ovarian tumors of borderline malignancy. *Gynecol Oncol.* l1990;39:195–198.

13. Tempfer CB, Polterauer S, Bentz EK, Reinthaller A, Hefler LA. Accuracy of intraoperative frozen section analysis in borderline tumors of the ovary: a retrospective analysis of 96 cases and review of the literature. *Gynecol Oncol.* l2007;107:248–252.

14. Chan JK, Lin YG, Loizzi V, Ghobriel M, DiSaia PJ, Berman ML. Borderline ovarian tumors in reproductive-age women. Fertility-sparing surgery and outcome. *J Reprod Med.* l2003;48:756–760.

15. Rao GG, Skinner EN, Gehrig PA, Duska LR, Miller DS, Schorge JO. Fertility-sparing surgery for ovarian low malignant potential tumors. *Gynecol Oncol.* l2005;98:263–266.

16. Zanetta G, Rota S, Chiari S, Bonazzi C, Bratina G, Mangioni C. Behavior of borderline tumors with particular interest to persistence, recurrence, and progression to invasive carcinoma: a prospective study. *J Clin Oncol.* l2001;19:2658–2664.

17. Zanetta G, Rota S, Lissoni A, Meni A, Brancatelli G, Buda A. Ultrasound, physical examination, and CA 125 measurement for the detection of recurrence after conservative surgery for early borderline ovarian tumors. *Gynecol Oncol.* l2001;81:63–66.

18. Ness RB, Cramer DW, Goodman MT, et al. Infertility, fertility drugs, and ovarian cancer: a pooled analysis of case-control studies. *Am J Epidemiol.* l2002;155:217–224.

19. Swanton A, Bankhead CR, Kehoe S. Pregnancy rates after conservative treatment for borderline ovarian tumours: a systematic review. *Eur J Obstet Gynecol Reprod Biol.* l2007;135:3–7.

20. Gotlieb WH, Chetrit A, Menczer J, et al. Demographic and genetic characteristics of patients with borderline ovarian tumors as compared to early stage invasive ovarian cancer. *Gynecol Oncol.* l2005;97:780–783.

21. Barnhill DR, Kurman RJ, Brady MF, et al. Preliminary analysis of the behavior of stage I ovarian serous tumors of low malignant potential: a Gynecologic Oncology Group study. *J Clin Oncol.* l1995;13:2752–2756.

22. Look KY, Stehman FB, Moore DH, Sutton GP. Intraperitoneal 5-fluorouracil for pseudomyxoma peritoneii. *Int J Gynecol Cancer.* l1995;5:361–365.

23. Lutton NJ, Moran BJ. Clinical results of cytoreduction and HIPEC in pseudomyxoma peritonei. *Cancer Treat Res.* 12007;134:319–328.

CHAPTER 10

Early Epithelial Ovarian Cancer

Alberto Mendivil, MD
Department of Obstetrics and Gynecology, University of North Carolina School of Medicine, Chapel Hill, NC, USA

Wesley C. Fowler, Jr., MD, FACOG, FACS
Department of Obstetrics and Gynecology, University of North Carolina School of Medicine, Chapel Hill, NC, USA

Pathology Notes: Chad Livasy, MD
Associate Professor, Department of Pathology and Laboratory Medicine, University of North Carolina School of Medicine, Chapel Hill, NC, USA

Background

Epithelial ovarian cancer (EOC) is the second most common gynecologic malignancy, with approximately 21,650 cases diagnosed annually in the United States and an estimated 15,520 deaths. It is the most common cause of death among women with gynecologic malignancies and the fifth most common cancer in American women.[1] A woman's lifetime risk for ovarian cancer is 1.4%, with the peak incidence in the 6th and 7th decades of life. Family history of breast or ovarian cancer can increase the lifetime risk to 15% to 60%. A strong family history refers to women having two or more first-degree relatives diagnosed with breast and/or ovarian cancer. Patients with familial gastrointestinal cancers diagnosed before the age of 45, and those with a personal history of breast cancer, also carry a greater risk. Autosomal dominant inheritance is noted in hereditary site-specific ovarian cancer, Lynch II syndrome, and hereditary breast/ovarian cancer. DNA mismatch repair genes MSH2 and MLH1 when mutated are found in the Lynch II syndrome. Mutations in BRCA1 and BRCA 2 are often found in patient with breast and ovarian cancer which can account for as much as 90% of cancers in women with familial ovarian cancer histories.[2] (See Chapter 7).

The majority of women with ovarian cancer initially are diagnosed in advanced stage (stage III or IV) due to the lack of screening tests and nonspecific symptoms. The overall survival of these women is approximately 30%. Factors that have an impact on prognosis include initial stage, volume of residual disease at the completion of the initial surgical procedure, grade of tumor, patient performance status, response to platin-containing chemotherapy regimens, and age.[3]

Patients with early-stage (stage I and II) ovarian cancer have a much more favorable prognosis. Critical to an optimal outcome for these women is correct comprehensive surgical staging and treatment with appropriate adjuvant chemotherapy. (Table 10.1).[4,5]

A single layer of peritoneal mesothelium that is derived from the ceolomic layer during embryogenesis surrounds the ovary. The totipotential nature of this epithelial layer can lead to malignant transformation and can differentiate to any cell type found in the Müllerian tract, including fallopian tube, uterus, cervix, and ovarian stroma. It

Gynecological Cancer Management: Identification, Diagnosis and Treatment, Edited by Daniel L. Clarke-Pearson and John T. Soper. Published 2010 by Blackwell Publishing, ISBN: 978-1-4051-9079-4.

Table 10.1 The 1986 FIGO staging system of ovarian malignancies

FIGO stage	Description (based on surgical and pathologic findings)
I	Disease limited to the ovaries
Ia	Disease limited to one ovary, no ascites, no surface involvement, capsule intact
Ib	Disease limited to both ovaries, no ascites, no surface involvement, capsule intact
Ic	Either stage Ia or Ib with ascites containing malignant cells or positive peritoneal cytology, capsule ruptured, or surface involvement
II	Disease involving one or both ovaries with pelvic extension
IIa	Extension or metastases to the fallopian tube or uterus
IIb	Disease spread to other pelvic organs\including the pelvic sidewall
IIc	Either stage IIa or stage IIb with ascites containing malignant cells or positive peritoneal cytology, capsule ruptured, or surface involvement
III	Peritoneal implants outside pelvis and/or positive retroperitoneal or inguinal lymph nodes
IIIa	Grossly limited to the true pelvis, negative nodes, microscopic seeding of abdominal peritoneum
IIIb	Implants of abdominal peritoneum 2 cm or less; nodes negative
IIIc	Abdominal implants greater than 2 cm and/or positive retroperitoneal or inguinal nodes
IV	Distant metastases; positive pleural effusion, parenchymal liver or spleen metastases

From Changes in definitions of clinical staging for carcinoma of the cervix and ovary: International Federation of Gynecology and Obstetrics. *Am J Obstet Gynecol.* 1987;156:263–264.

Table 10.2 Histology and cellular subtype of epithelial ovarian neoplasms[7]

Histologic/cellular type	Example
Serous/endosalpingeal	
Benign	Cystadenoma
Borderline	Surface papillary tumor
Malignant	Cystadenocarcinoma
Mucinous/endocervical	
Benign	Cystadenoma
Borderline	Cystic tumor
Malignant	Cystadenocarcinoma
Endometrioid/endometrial	
Benign	Cystadenoma/ adenofibroma
Borderline	Cystic tumor
Malignant	Cystadenocarcinoma
Clear cell/Müllerian	
Benign	Cystadenoma/ adenofibroma
Borderline	Cystic tumor
Malignant	Adenocarcinoma
Transitional cell/transitional	
Benign	Brenner
Borderline	Proliferating Brenner type
Malignant	Malignant Brenner/ non-Brenner transitional cell
Squamous cell/squamous	
Mixed epithelial/mixed	
Undifferentiated/anaplastic	

From Kaku T, Ogawa S, Kawano Y, et al. Histological classification of ovarian cancer. *Med Electron Microsc.* 2003;36:9–17.

is thought that ovarian cancers develop from the surface epithelium or post-ovulatory exposure to sex-steroid hormones or other cellular chemicals. Theories to account for EOC include incessant ovulation, gonadotropin stimulation, hormonal stimulation, and inflammation.[6] Any part of the ovary can undergo rapid, uncontrolled proliferation and may subsequently undergo malignant transformation. Table 10.2 outlines the various epithelial ovarian neoplastic cell types and histologies.[7]

Pathology notes

Survival for stage I ovarian cancer is > 90%. Accurate staging is an essential part of predicting prognosis and guiding therapy. Pathology reports from all staged ovarian cancers should include the AJCC pathologic stage in the report. Accurate pathologic staging includes gross inspection of the ovary at the time of frozen section to evaluate for capsule rupture or the presence of tumor on the ovarian surface. Detailed gross inspection of omentum is also extremely important as metastases may be small, consisting only of microscopic disease. The omentum can be serially sectioned into thin slices for inspection and then palpated for firm regions. Any abnormalities need to be submitted for histologic evaluation. Cytology results of peritoneal washings or ascites should be incorporated into the final AJCC pathologic stage.

Early-stage ovarian cancers are closely tied to the epithelial type of the carcinoma. The prevalence of stage I ovarian cancer by histologic type is as follows: serous (4%), clear cell (36%), endometrioid (53%), mucinous (83%), and Brenner (100%).[8] Although the vast majority of ovarian carcinomas are serous carcinomas, most stage I ovarian cancers show mucinous, endometrioid, or clear cell histology. Serous carcinomas tend to be relatively smaller and bilateral with rapid spread to pelvic and abdominal cavities. The lead time from grossly detectable disease to extraovarian spread is brief for serous carcinomas. Grading of serous carcinomas is particularly relevant to lower-stage cases. Based on clinical outcome data and molecular genetic alterations observed in serous ovarian carcinoma, serous carcinoma can be divided into the usual high-grade serous carcinoma (p53 mutations) and the much rarer low-grade serous carcinoma (KRAS, BRAF mutations). The low-grade serous carcinomas are frequently associated with serous tumors of low malignant potential and show a survival advantage over high-grade serous carcinoma. The distinction between low- and high-grade serous carcinoma can be made on routine histology (Plate 10.1) with high interobserver agreement.[9]

The majority of primary mucinous adenocarcinomas of the ovary are large (mean size 18 cm), unilateral, and well differentiated. Areas resembling a mucinous borderline tumor or cystadenoma are commonly found within the tumor. Ovarian mucinous adenocarcinomas can further be divided into those with a confluent glandular pattern (90% survival) and those with an infiltrative pattern (survival < 50%). For any mucinous adenocarcinoma involving the ovary, it is imperative that metastasis be excluded. Gross features raising concern for metastasis include bilaterality and relatively small tumor size. Histologic clues to metastasis include signet-ring cell forms (GI or breast metastasis), nodular distribution of tumor, ovarian surface involvement, extensive pseudomyxoma ovarii, and zones of "dirty necrosis" with surrounding garland pattern of epithelium (colorectal metastasis).

Tumors with endometrioid histology are commonly stage I. While there is no uniform consensus on the grading of these tumors, the WHO recommends the FIGO system as used in the endometrium. Ovarian endometrioid adenocarcinoma may occur in conjunction with endometrial endometrioid adenocarcinoma and it can be difficult to determine if the tumors represent synchronous primaries or endometrial primary with ovarian metastasis. Well-differentiated, noninvasive/superficially invasive tumors are unlikely to metastasize to the ovary. Poorly differentiated, deeply invasive carcinomas with lymphovascular space invasion are much more likely to metastasize to the ovary. Ovarian endometrioid adenocarcinomas seen in association with endometriosis or adenofibroma favor an independent ovarian primary. Bilateral ovarian endometrioid adenocaricnomas with small size (<5 cm), with invasive growth pattern and mulinodularity, favor metastasis from the corresponding endometrial adenocarcinoma. In practice it may not always be possible to determine whether the tumors are independent or endometrial carcinoma with metastasis to ovary.

Pathology notes (*continued*)

The prognosis of clear cell carcinoma has not been shown to correlate with grade; therefore clear cell carcinoma is typically not graded. For the pathologist, it is important to distinguish clear cell carcinoma from its mimics including dysgerminoma, steroid cell tumor, metastatic renal clear cell carcinoma, and metastatic GI carcinoma.

Kurman and colleagues have proposed a model for ovarian carcinogenesis. In their discussion, they divide tumors into two groups similar to uterine cancer and designated type I and type II. Type I tumors present in early stage are typically low grade and more biologically indolent. Examples of these type I tumors are low-grade micropapillary lesions with serous, mucinous, endometrioid, and clear cell histology. Type II tumors present in advanced stage, are high grade, and are aggressive. This category of tumors would include high-grade serous carcinoma, clear cell, and carcinosarcoma of the ovary.[10, 11] There are some tumor types that may have characteristics of both categories such as neuroendocrine carcinoma of the ovary. These tumors may often present in the early stage but are very aggressive and refractory to conventional combination chemotherapy. Low and high-grade serous carcinomas typically arise through different genetic pathways. Low-grade serous carcinomas, for example, arise through alteration oncogenes (RAS), whereas high-grade carcinomas may arise via mutations in the tumor-suppressor genes (p53 system, BRCA1/2).[12]

Clinical Scenario 1

A 35-year-old para 0010 is being considered for laparoscopic oophorectomy for a 7-cm cyst (Fig. 10.1).

What clinical features can be used preoperatively to distinguish benign from malignant adnexal masses?

In the United States, women have a 5% to 10% chance of developing an ovarian neoplasm. Of these patients, 1% to 2% will have a malignant neoplasm. Approximately 300,000 women are hospitalized every year for management of an ovarian neoplasm. About 1 in 10 women will have surgery for an adnexal mass in their lifetime. The incidence of malignant adnexal tumors varies according to age. Patients less than 45 years old who have an adnexal mass will have a malignancy in 6% to 10% of cases, 33% to 50% in patients over 45 years of age, and 50% of cases in patients less than 10 years of age.[13]

In patients with adnexal masses, there are many features and physical findings than may predict either a benign or malignant etiology. A thorough history and physical examination may provide clues to assist in distinguishing benign and malignant adnexal masses. In patients with early EOC, physical exam findings may differ from patients with advanced EOC. Patients may describe pain, bloating, early satiety, intermittent nausea and/or vomiting, (and if the mass is large), pelvic pain and/or pressure, or difficulty with defecation, particularly if the mass is fixed in the posterior cul-de-sac. Patients may describe low-grade fevers or malaise. Often, patients may not experience any symptoms at all. The presence of a fixed, solid, irregular pelvic mass palpated on physical examination may be suspicious of an ovarian malignant neoplasm. However, patients with leiomyomas, tubo-ovarian abscesses, or severe endometriosis may have symptomatic fixed lesions palpated on examination that are completely benign. A malignancy can also be present in the absence of a pelvic mass especially if a patient has abdominal ascites or a palpable upper abdominal mass. There are limitations to the physical examination, especially among women who are obese. Adnexal masses larger

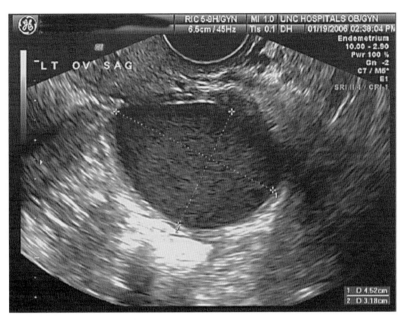

Figure 10.1 Smooth-walled ovarian cyst with internal echos (4.5 × 3.2 cm). (Image compliments of Alice Chaung, MD, Department of Obstetrics and Gynecology, University of North Carolina.)

than 5 cm can easily go undetected in these obese patients. Palpable lymphadenopathy is not a reliable finding, especially in patients with early EOC.

Tumor markers can be useful tools preoperatively in distinguishing benign from malignant neoplasms. CA-125 is a glycoprotein with a high molecular weight found in the epithelium of the embryonic colon.[14] It is the most common biomarker used in ovarian cancer. CA-125 is elevated in over 80% of all women with ovarian cancer. It carries a sensitivity of 50% in stage I and 80% in stage II EOC with a positive predictive value (PPV) of 10%. CA-125 combined with targeted ultrasonography increases the PPV to 20%.[15] Other medical conditions can elevate CA-125, which affects its utility, particularly in premenopausal women. CA-125 can be elevated in pregnancy, infection, leiomyomas, endometriosis, other malignancies, and any other type of disruption to the peritoneal cavity. The presence of pleural or peritoneal fluid or disease involvement of a serosal surface can also elevate the CA-125 serum level.[14] Furthermore, CA-125 can be ele-

vated in 1% of healthy women and may fluctuate during the menstrual cycle. If one must follow CA-125 in a menstruating woman, it is useful to obtain the test at approximately the same time early in the cycle, such as day 3. It is useful to have CA-125 evaluated by the same laboratory whenever possible.

CA-125 has historically not been a good screening test for ovarian cancer. The sensitivity data are based on large studies done in the late 1980 and 1990s. The sensitivity of the CA-125 serum test for detecting women with ovarian cancer is 67% to 80%. The specificity ranges between 98% and 99%. However, because of the low prevalence of the disease in the population, the PPV is only 26%.[16,17] The Prostate, Lung, Colorectal, and Ovarian Cancer Screening (PLCO) trial is evaluating the utility of CA-125 and transvaginal ultrasound as screening tools for ovarian cancer. In this study, which started enrollment in 1993 and ended in 2003, over 28,000 women were screened. A PPV of only 1% and 3.7% were found for transvaginal ultrasound and CA-125, respectively. The

PPV value was far less than what was previously reported in the literature for CA-125, and the authors concluded that this might have been due to the multicenter nature of the trial. The interim conclusions further noted that most cancers were diagnosed in late stages, too many surgical procedures were performed to find one cancer, and only about 5% of surgical procedures found ovarian cancer.[17]

Other tumor markers have also been used as screening tools for ovarian cancer with some improvement in sensitivity but a decrease in specificity. These include CEA, OVX1, M-CSF, CA-125II, CA 72-4, CA 15-3, lipid-associated sialic acid (LASA), HE4, mesothelin, osteopontin, kallikrein(s), and soluble EGF receptor.[15, 18] Zhang and colleagues studied 498 serum samples and used a modeling tool to test the use of four serum markers (CA125II, CA 72-4, CA 15-3, M-CSF) to screen women for ovarian cancer. Using these four markers, they calculated sensitivity of 71% for detecting women with EOC. Since ovarian cancer has a prevalence of 1 in 2500 in the United States, a good screening test would need to have a sensitivity of 75% and a specificity of 99.7%.[19]

A new test that has come to the market for epithelial ovarian cancer screening is called OvaSure, released through LabCorp. The test employs six molecular markers to screen women for ovarian cancer (Leptin, prolactin, insulin-like growth factor II, osteopontin, macrophage inhibitory factor, and CA-125). It was initially studied in serum samples of 365 healthy controls and 160 patients with ovarian cancer. In control patients, the specificity was 99.67%. In the patients with ovarian cancer, the serum panel identified all stage III and IV disease and 89% of stage I/II disease.[20] On July 2, 2008, the Society of Gynecologic Oncologists (SGO) released a statement regarding the use of OvaSure:

The SGO recognizes the need for accurate early detection biomarkers for ovarian cancer. For this reason, SGO reviewed the literature regarding OvaSure, a serum-based diagnostic test for ovarian cancer. After reviewing OvaSure's materials, it is our opinion that additional research is needed to validate the test's effectiveness before offering it to women outside of the context of a research study conducted with appropriate informed consent under the auspices of an institutional review board. SGO is committed to actively following and contributing to this vitally important research. As physicians who care only for women with gynecologic cancers, our hope is that these cancers can either be prevented or detected early. Because no currently available test has been shown to reliably detect ovarian cancer in its earliest and most curable stages, we will await the results of further clinical validation of OvaSure with great interest.

The use of radiologic imaging with transvaginal ultrasound (TVU) is another important tool that has been studied for screening women for EOC. Historically, however, transabdominal (TAU) ultrasound by itself has not improved detection rates. A European prospective study of over 5000 women using TAU for ovarian cancer screening found a detection rate of 100%, but the PPV was only 2.3%, and the specificity was 97.7%.[21] Fishman and colleagues performed a large multicenter trial of TVUs in over 4500 women who were at high risk for developing EOC. The authors found that ultrasound alone was of limited value as an independent modality for detecting early-stage ovarian cancer.[22] Using ultrasound in combination with serum markers is another potential way of screening women at high risk for developing EOC. Previously, it was noted that the PPV for EOC using CA-125 screening alone was 4.6%. When combining CA-125 and TVU, the PPV increased to 40%. Using combined-modality screening was highly sensitive for detecting advanced-stage disease.[23] In the end, the goal of screening should be to decrease ovarian cancer–specific mortality. In order to achieve this goal, screening tests must have both a high sensitivity for early disease and specificity beyond the results achieved by current technology.

Other imaging modalities can be used to detect adnexal masses. Computed tomography (CT) scans can evaluate the abdominal cavity and assess for the presence of enlarged pelvic and para-aortic lymph nodes. It is useful if there is a known cancer but not very informative for screening. Magnetic resonance imaging (MRI) is somewhat better in describing masses than CT scans. It is similar to CT in providing information about the abdomen and pelvis although at a greater cost compared to CT. Positron emission tomography (PET) scans may be useful in the diagnosis of tumor recurrences, but the role for PET scans in the initial evaluation of a woman with an adnexal mass has not been established. Finally, there are significant costs associated with CT, MRI, and PET scans compared to transvaginal sonography.

What gross features can be used to distinguish benign from malignant ovarian tumors at the time of laparoscopy?

Using a laparoscopic approach to women with adnexal masses can be a feasible method and is widely accepted for diagnosing and subsequently treating EOC. The risk of encountering an ovarian malignancy in a simple cyst in premenopausal women is less than 1%. In postmenopausal patients the same lesion will be malignant in up to 3% of cases. Furthermore, a complex mass with the some or all the characteristics listed in Table 10.3 may increase the rate of unsuspected malignancy to greater than

Table 10.3 Ultrasound findings of adnexal masses that may indicate a malignancy[22]

Ultrasound Characteristics For The Ovary
Cystic mass with thick septation
Internal papillae
Solid components
Neovascularity
Low-resistant blood flow
Bilateral masses
Ascites
Matted bowel
Irregular borders

From Leng JH, Lang JH, Zhang JJ, et al. Role of laparoscopy in the diagnosis and treatment of adnexal masses. *Chin Med J (Engl)*. 2006;119:202–206.

13%.[24, 25] There are visual cues that the surgeon should be familiar with to raise the suspicion of malignancy. During the initial survey, a thorough evaluation of the pelvis and upper abdomen should be performed including the surface of the contralateral ovary, the uterine serosa, the appendix (if applicable), the bowel serosa, liver surface, diaphragm, and omentum. Two findings on the ovary that may raise suspicions for a malignancy are papillary projections on the outer surface of the ovary (Fig. 10.2) or protruding into the cystic cavity and a solid-appearing texture.[24] Gross tumor implants need to be biopsied and sent for frozen section. Free fluid in the pelvis should be collected and sent to pathology. If no fluid is seen, 50 to 100 mL of an isotonic saline solution should be used to wash the pelvis and aspirate for cytologic evaluation. Leng and colleagues studied over 2000 patients with benign-appearing adnexal masses by ultrasound and normal CA-125 serum levels. Forty-one patients had intracystic vegetations and 6 of these patients had invasive carcinoma (15%). While this number appears high, the rate of malignancy in the total studied population was only 0.3%.[24] Another study of 667 patients with adnexal masses having benign characteristics found a 5.7 % rate of unexpected intracystic vegetations, with 14% of those cases showing borderline tumors. There were no cases of invasive carcinoma.[26] Laparoscopic evaluation of adnexal masses can be performed in patients with lesions that have benign ultrasound characteristics and a normal CA-125 value with a less than 1% rate of invasive carcinoma.

Clinical Scenario 2

A 29-year-old woman presents with an adnexal mass and an abnormal ultrasound of the ovary (Fig. 10.2). Despite the abnormal ultrasound, given the patient's age, the mass was felt unlikely to be ovarian cancer. However, during laparoscopic salpingo-oophorectomy papillary serous

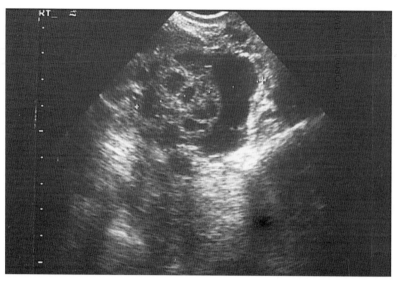

Figure 10.2 Serous carcinoma of the ovary. Note the papillary excrescences, thick septations, and internal echogenic material (nodularity). (Image compliments of Alice Chuang, MD, Department of Obstetrics and Gynecology, University of North Carolina.)

ovarian cancer is diagnosed by frozen section. No extra-ovarian lesions are noted.

What is appropriate staging for presumed early ovarian cancer?

Surgical staging is vital in assessing a patient with early EOC. Appropriate surgical staging is diagnostic, therapeutic, and prognostic. Ovarian cancer has been historically staged via laparotomy. Recently, series have evaluated the use of laparoscopy to stage early EOC. While it is not expected that the general gynecologist has the skill or training to perform a full staging procedure via laparoscopy for early EOC, it is important rather to be able to recognize key anatomic disruptions or deviations and to be able to communicate them to a consultant either intraoperatively or postoperatively. These anatomic deviations include lymphadenopathy, gross tumor implants (including approximate size and location), involvement of contralateral ovary, and abnormalities of intestinal structures (ie, potential for primary site of disease).

Appropriate staging for EOC, particularly for apparent early EOC, is critical because it may affect postoperative management. For example, patients with fully staged IA or IB grade I carcinomas typically do not require additional therapy. However, any patient with stage IC grade I lesions, advanced-stage disease, or any stage disease with high-grade histology such as grade III lesion, clear cell, carcinosarcoma, or neuroendocrine, requires postoperative combination chemotherapy. The importance of staging can be illustrated by published reports showing inadequate initial staging of patients sent to tertiary care centers. Young and colleagues evaluated 100 patients with a diagnosis of "early EOC" (stage IA-IIB). After restaging, 31% of patients were "up-staged" based on positive para-aortic lymph node metastases, unsuspected disease in the pelvic peritoneum, ascites fluid, or disease on the diaphragm.[27]

If carcinoma is encountered during laparoscopy it is important to thoroughly evaluate the abdomen and pelvis both visually and with tissue sampling. This can be performed by the initial primary surgeon or with an appropriate consultant trained to perform a thorough lymphadenectomy. Aspiration of peritoneal ascetic fluid or pelvic washings (isotonic saline solution) should be sent for cytologic evaluation; this includes fluid collected from the peri-hepatic region. The entire affected ovary and tube should be removed. If fertility is not desired, the contralateral ovary and uterus should also be removed. Biopsies of the peritoneum should be taken from the following locations: anterior and posterior cul-de-sac, bilateral abdominal paracolic gutters, intestinal mesentery, and omentum. Any grossly abnormal tissue should be removed, including scar tissue. Suspicious pelvic and/or para-aortic lymph nodes should be removed. If no enlarged or suspicious lymph nodes are seen, a thorough pelvic lymphadenectomy and para-aortic lymphadenectomy to the level of the gonadal vessels should be employed to assess for microscopic stage IIIC disease. Lymph node metastases even in apparent stage I disease may be detected in up to 14% of patients.[28]

Laparoscopy can be used successfully to stage early EOC in highly selected individuals. It is important to note that laparoscopic staging is a fairly new concept and should be performed by trained advanced laparoscopists with the ability to perform a thorough exploration and lymph node dissection. The standard laparoscopic staging involves a full infrarenal para-aortic and pelvic lymphadenectomy, removal of the remaining adnexa, and total laparoscopic or laparoscopic-assisted vaginal hysterectomy when appropriate. A study by LeBlanc and colleagues evaluated 28 patients referred for completion staging. All but one was successfully staged via laparoscopy. Twenty-one percent of patients were upstaged for positive peritoneal implants or positive para-aortic lymph node metastases.[29] Outcomes from laparoscopy and laparotomy are similar in terms of accuracy and adequacy of staging. Patients who underwent laparoscopy had shorter hospital stays compared to laparotomy.[30]

A concern in staging early EOC via laparoscopy is the possibility of port-site metastases. The reported rate ranged from 1% to 2.3%.[31, 32] Interestingly, Huang and colleagues reported on 6 cases of port-site metastases from 31 patients who underwent laparoscopic staging for EOC over an 8-year period.[33] This rate (19%) appears to be an exception rather than the rule.

Is fertility-sparing surgery an appropriate option for a patient with presumed early-stage epithelial ovarian cancer?

With women delaying child-bearing with increased frequency, the potential for fertility-sparing management of malignant adnexal masses will also increase in frequency. There is greater availability of options for preservation of fertility for women with gynecologic malignancies. In early EOC, fertility-sparing surgery can be used with favorable outcomes. For fertility-sparing procedures to be effective, the patient first must be willing to retain her fertility and be aware of the risks. Factors that may affect a woman's options include age, tumor grade, success of initial comprehensive staging, family history, and known causes of infertility, if applicable. The patient must be fully aware of her condition to make an informed decision. Finally, the treatment should never compromise the possibility of a cure.

The peak age of EOC is in the 6th and 7th decades of life, with a lifetime risk of 1.4%. The risk is greater if the patient is BRCA 1/2 positive, or has multiple first-degree family members with either breast or ovarian cancer. Over 70% of patients present with advanced-stage disease. Stage I disease is found in 25% of patients, who typically have a greater than 90% 5-year survival. Patients with stage IA or IB disease can defer platinum-based chemotherapy and elect to undergo intensive surveillance with every 3 months CA-125 serum level, pelvic exam, and transvaginal ultrasound at 3 to 6-month intervals. Patients with stage IA disease with high-grade histologies should receive platinum-based chemotherapy. Schilder reported on 52 patients who underwent fertility-sparing staging for early EOC (stage IA-IC) who achieved 31 pregnancies in 17 patients. Unfortunately, there were also 3 recurrences in the same group; 10-year survival for this cohort was 93%.[34]

Hereditary ovarian cancer syndromes constitute about 10% of EOC cases. Patients with a history of breast cancer or BRCA gene mutation or multiple first-degree relatives with breast or ovarian may be at greater risk for developing EOC. Those with BRCA 1 mutations have a 40% to 50% risk of developing ovarian cancer in their lifetime, while there is a 15% to 25% increased risk for patients with BRCA 2 mutations.[35]

Fertility-sparing surgery for EOC involves complete evaluation of the entire pelvis, upper abdomen, and tissue sampling. It consists of unilateral salpingo-ophorectomy, with or without biopsy of the contralateral ovary, bilateral pelvic and para-aortic lymph node dissection, peritoneal biopsies, pelvic washings, and infracolic omentectomy. These can be safely done via laparoscopy if appropriate.

What if this patient's wishes are not known at the time of surgery?

When taking a patient to surgery for an adnexal mass, preoperative risk should be assessed based on ultrasound findings, CA-125 level if available, and family history. If the patient has a significant preoperative risk for malignancy, the patient should be consented for the possibility of full surgical staging as appropriate (including complete hysterectomy and bilateral salpingo-ophorectomy). If future fertility is desired, fertility-sparing surgical staging should be performed. A more unsettling scenario is when the patient has a low preoperative risk but a malignancy is encountered and the patient's desire to retain fertility is not known. The surgeon has two options: terminate the surgery and return at a later date for completion of staging, or speak to a family member, if available, and discuss the options for immediate staging versus completion surgery at a later date. In either case, a surgeon with the appropriate training to properly stage the patient's malignancy should perform the surgery. Regardless of the surgical decision, the safety of the patient should always be the surgeon's number one priority.

Several important factors are necessary for a patient to qualify for fertility-sparing surgery. The tumor must be unilateral, free of adhesions, well encapsulated, and with no presence of ascites or evidence of extra-ovarian spread. The entire abdomen and pelvis must be thoroughly evaluated along with the opposite ovary. Occult tumor involvement in the contralateral ovary occurs in 7% to 10% of cases.[36] If the contralateral is normal in size, shape, and consistency, a biopsy is not necessary; however, wedge biopsy may be safely performed.

Patients have successfully achieved viable pregnancies after fertility sparing-surgery for early EOC. Once child-bearing is complete, the uterus and remaining ovary should be removed. The risk of recurrence is low, especially with well-differentiated tumor in true stage I disease. Zanetta and associates reported on 99 patients with stage I disease, and 5 out of 53 (9%) patients managed conservatively recurred; 3 patients recurred in the contralateral ovary (3.5%).[37] A study from Italy showed a recurrence rate of 11.8% after conservative surgery and involved the preserved ovary in 7% of cases.[38]

What are the consequences of tumor rupture in a patient with presumed early-stage epithelial ovarian cancer?

The concept of intraoperative rupture and its effect on prognosis has historically been controversial. However, intraoperative rupture does change postoperative management. Patients with stage IA or IB low-grade tumors require no additional therapy, whereas stage IC patients (via intraoperative rupture or otherwise) require adjuvant combination chemotherapy. Early studies regarding intraoperative rupture showed no difference in survival. Other studies have shown a worse prognosis for iatrogenic stage IC disease (overall survival of 93% for stage IA versus 73% for IC-ruptured).[39] Mizuno and colleagues also showed a worse prognosis for patients with iatrogenic stage IC disease versus stage IA. More importantly, rupture occurring some time prior to surgery may lead to seeding the peritoneal cavity and thus lead to worse outcomes.[40] It is important to contain the tumor in a bag during laparoscopic surgery for an adnexal mass and avoid uncontrolled rupture when at all possible (Plate 10.2).

If comprehensive staging cannot be performed, what is/are the appropriate surgical procedure(s)?

When confronted with a malignant mass during laparoscopic surgery, one may follow these simple recommendations. First, survey the entire abdomen and pelvis, noting any evidence of tumor implants as well as the character of the contralateral ovary, and ensure that this information is reflected in the operative report. Second, collect pelvic washings, as these may be helpful in counseling the patient after surgery about the need for further surgery and/or subsequent chemotherapy. Third, it is best to resist the temptation to proceed with lymph node sampling or further removal of pelvic organs if one is not an accomplished laparoscopic surgeon, as this may lead to an increase in pelvic adhesions and disruption of retroperitoneal surgical planes and landmarks. Such disruptions make minimally invasive surgery more technically challenging less likely to complete. Finally, it is not necessary to convert the case to a laparotomy from laparoscopy due to the findings of a malignancy. Avoiding laparotomy in this circumstance will help eliminate delay for future surgery.

What is the survival of early-stage epithelial ovarian cancer patients?

Survival for early EOC is excellent compared to advanced-stage disease. Five-year survival for stage IA and IB disease is 89% and 65%, respectfully. In contrast, 5-year survival for stage IIIC disease is 29%.[41] Patients with stage IA and IB well-differentiated lesions do not benefit significantly from adjuvant chemotherapy and are treated with surgery alone.[42] In patients with stage IA disease with a high-risk histology such as grade III tumor or clear cell, adjuvant treatment is required and usually consists of combination chemotherapy with carboplatin and paclitaxel for given every 21 days for six cycles.

Clinical Scenario 3

Frozen section of an ovarian cyst removed via laparoscopy in a 35-year-old woman has returned compatible with a poorly differentiated ovarian adenocarcinoma. Further laparoscopic evaluation reveals gross tumor implants on the omentum and diaphragms (Plate 10.3).

What is the appropriate surgical procedure for this apparently advanced ovarian cancer?

Over 70% of patients with EOC present with advanced-stage disease. Five-year survival for these patients decreases as the stage advances: 43% for stage IIIA, 41% for stage IIIB, 29% for stage IIIC, and 13% for stage IV.[43] The cornerstone of treatment whenever possible is initial cytoreductive surgery (ie, surgical debulking). Consultation with a gynecologic oncologist experienced in managing patients with advanced EOC is critical for improved patient outcomes. The extent of cytoreductive surgery (optimal versus suboptimal tumor debulking) affects survival. Optimal cytoreduction is defined as removing all tumor implants greater than 1 cm in diameter, while suboptimal cytoreductive surgery results in remaining tumor implants that are greater than 1 cm in diameter. Advanced EOC encountered during laparoscopy or initial laparotomy often requires the use of advanced surgical techniques such as bowel resection or radical hysterectomy. In general, the goal of surgery in women with advanced EOC is to establish a diagnosis through pathologic evaluation of tissue, assess the extent of disease (stage), and removed any visible sign of tumor if possible (optimal cytoreduction).

While many patients with early EOC can be staged via laparoscopy or laparotomy, patients with advanced disease most often require laparotomy. The surgery is typically performed via vertical skin incision. This type of incision provides the best method of exposure to the upper abdomen that may be required for surgery involving the liver, diaphragm, or spleen. The first step in the operation is to get a sense of the extent of disease and obtain enough tissue to send for frozen section and make a diagnosis. Can the patient be optimally cytoreduced? This question may often dictate the radical nature of the operation. For example, if the patient has extensive upper abdominal disease, such as parenchymal liver metastases or diaphragmatic disease, a rectosigmoid resection may not be indicated for cytoreduction unless the patient has symptoms of obstruction. These patients may benefit equally from simple hysterectomy and bilateral salpingo-oophorectomy. The omentum should be removed (infracolic or total), especially if it is infiltrated by tumor, as removal of the omentum will add to the tumor debulking and decrease postoperative ascites formation. The pelvic and para-aortic lymph nodes should be assessed and removed if they are enlarged or if there is no evidence of gross disease > 2 cm outside the pelvis (less than stage IIIC disease).

The ultimate goal of cytoreductive surgery in advanced ovarian cancer is to remove all visible signs of tumor. Multiple studies have evaluated optimal and suboptimal cytoreduction and consistently shown that optimal cytoreduction to at least less than 1 cm residual disease positively impacts survival.[44,45] Conversely patient with suboptimal residual disease had a worse 5-year survival. Patients with a large initial tumor burden fared worse than patients with small initial volume disease even if both categories of patients were reduced to < 1 cm disease remaining.[46] Optimal cytoreductive surgery may include extensive resection of disease in the upper abdomen including partial hepatectomy, distal pancreatectomy, diaphragmatic stripping or resection, and splenectomy. While these procedures add to operative time, they are not associated with increased rates of complications.[47]

What is the role of pelvic and para-aortic lymphadenectomy in patients with obvious stage III disease?

The goal of cytoreductive surgery in advanced-stage EOC is resection of all tumor implants to less than 1 cm for maximal survival benefit. Systemic lymphadenectomy versus resection of bulky lymph nodes in the pelvic and para-aortic region has been studied in stage III disease. While median progression-free survival was better in patients who underwent systemic lymphadenectomy, there was no difference in overall survival. Patients in the systemic lymphadenectomy group had longer operating times and greater rates of blood transfusions.[48] In general, our practice in advanced (stage IIIC or IV) disease is to remove any bulky pelvic or para-aortic lymph nodes that would result in optimally debulking the patient.

What is the difference in survival of early and late epithelial ovarian cancer?

Survival in EOC is largely dependent on the amount of initial tumor volume and histologic subtype. Patients with stage IA-IB grade I disease require no additional therapy after comprehensive surgical staging. Those with grade III histologies and disease stage greater than IC require adjuvant combination chemotherapy typically with carboplatin and paclitaxel given every 3 weeks for 6 cycles. Five-year survival in early-stage disease ranges from 89% for stage IA to 68% for stage IB. In advanced-stage disease, 5-year survival is worse for stage IIIC (29%) and stage IV (13%) disease.[43]

First-line chemotherapy for EOC is comprised of two agents, carboplatin and paclitaxel. The drugs are typically delivered via an indwelling central venous access catheter (port-a-cath). Our practice is to give the first cycle of chemotherapy as an inpatient to assess for chemotherapy-related hypersensitivity reactions. The remaining 5 cycles are given every 21 days as an outpatient. Carboplatin is dosed by area under the curve (AUC = 6) and paclitaxel is given at 175 mg/m^2. The main side effects of carboplatin are fatigue, neutropenia, and anemia. The main side effects of paclitaxel are alopecia, peripheral neuropathy, neutropenia, and anemia.[49] Chemotherapy may also be delivered via intraperitoneal (IP) port-a-cath. A large randomized study through the Gynecologic Oncology Group showed a progression-free survival advantage of 5 months for patients who underwent initial IP chemotherapy versus traditional IV chemotherapy.[50]

References

1. Jemal A, Siegel R, Ward E, et al. Cancer statistics, 2008. *CA Cancer J Clin.* 2008;58:71–96.
2. Wong AS, Auersperg N. Ovarian surface epithelium: family history and early events in ovarian cancer. *Reprod Biol Endocrinol.* 2003;1:70.
3. Amos CI, Shaw GL, Tucker MA, Hartge P. Age at onset for familial epithelial ovarian cancer. *JAMA.* 1992;268:1896–1899.
4. Vergote I, Trimbos BJ. Treatment of patients with early epithelial ovarian cancer. *Curr Opin Oncol.* 2003;15:452–455.
5. Changes in definitions of clinical staging for carcinoma of the cervix and ovary: International Federation of Gynecology and Obstetrics. *Am J Obstet Gynecol.* 1987;156:263–264.
6. Landen CN, Jr., Birrer MJ, Sood AK. Early events in the pathogenesis of epithelial ovarian cancer. *J Clin Oncol.* 2008;26:995–1005.
7. Kaku T, Ogawa S, Kawano Y, et al. Histological classification of ovarian cancer. *Med Electron Microsc.* 2003;36:9–17.
8. Seidman JD, Horkayne-Szakaly I, Haib M, et al. The histologic type and stage distribution of ovarian carcinomas of surface epithelial origin. *Int J Gynecol Pathol.* 2004;23:41–44.
9. Malpica A, Deavers MT, Tornos C, et al. Interobserver and intraobserver variability of a two-tier system for grading ovarian serous carcinoma. *Am J Surg Pathol.* 2007;31:1168–1174.
10. Kurman RJ, Visvanathan K, Roden R, Wu TC, Shih Ie M. Early detection and treatment of ovarian cancer: shifting from early stage to minimal volume of disease based on a new model of carcinogenesis. *Am J Obstet Gynecol.* 2008;198:351–356.
11. Shih Ie M, Kurman RJ. Ovarian tumorigenesis: a proposed model based on morphological and molecular genetic analysis. *Am J Pathol.* 2004;164:1511–1518.
12. Bell DA. Origins and molecular pathology of ovarian cancer. *Mod Pathol.* 2005;18(suppl):S19–S32.
13. Koonings PP, Campbell K, Mishell DR Jr., Grimes DA. Relative frequency of primary ovarian neoplasms: a 10-year review. *Obstet Gynecol.* 1989;74:921–926.
14. Rapkiewicz AV, Espina V, Petricoin EF III, Liotta LA. Biomarkers of ovarian tumours. *Eur J Cancer.* 2004;40:2604–2612.
15. Murta EF, Nomelini RS. Early diagnosis and predictors of malignancy of adnexal masses. *Curr Opin Obstet Gynecol.* 2006;18:14–19.
16. Woolas RP, Xu FJ, Jacobs IJ, et al. Elevation of multiple serum markers in patients with stage I ovarian cancer. *J Natl Cancer Inst.* 1993;85:1748–1751.
17. Jacobs I, Davies AP, Bridges J, et al. Prevalence screening for ovarian cancer in postmenopausal women by CA 125 measurement and ultrasonography. *BMJ.* 1993;306:1030–1034.
18. Bast RC, Jr., Badgwell D, Lu Z, et al. New tumor markers: CA125 and beyond. *Int J Gynecol Cancer.* 2005;15(suppl):274–281.
19. Zhang Z, Yu Y, Xu F, et al. Combining multiple serum tumor markers improves detection of stage I epithelial ovarian cancer. *Gynecol Oncol.* 2007;107:526–531.
20. Visintin I, Feng Z, Longton G, et al. Diagnostic markers for early detection of ovarian cancer. *Clin Cancer Res.* 2008;14:1065–1072.
21. Campbell S, Bhan V, Royston P, Whitehead MI, Collins WP. Transabdominal ultrasound screening for early ovarian cancer. *BMJ.* 1989;299:1363–1367.
22. Fishman DA, Cohen L, Blank SV, et al. The role of ultrasound evaluation in the detection of early-stage epithelial ovarian cancer. *Am J Obstet Gynecol.* 2005;192:1214-1222; discussion 1221–1222.
23. Olivier RI, Lubsen-Brandsma MA, Verhoef S, van Beurden M. CA125 and transvaginal ultrasound monitoring in high-risk women cannot prevent the diagnosis of advanced ovarian cancer. *Gynecol Oncol.* 2006;100:20–26.
24. Leng JH, Lang JH, Zhang JJ, et al. Role of laparoscopy in the diagnosis and treatment of adnexal masses. *Chin Med J (Engl).* 2006;119:202–206.
25. Muzii L, Angioli R, Zullo M, Panici PB. The unexpected ovarian malignancy found during operative laparoscopy: incidence, management, and implications for prognosis. *J Minim Invasive Gynecol.* 2005;12:81–89; quiz 90–91.

26. Marana R, Muzii L, Ferrari S, Catalano GF, Zannoni G, Marana E. Management of adnexal cystic masses with unexpected intracystic vegetations detected during laparoscopy. *J Minim Invasive Gynecol.* 2005;12:502–507.

27. Young RC, Decker DG, Wharton JT, et al. Staging laparotomy in early ovarian cancer. *JAMA.* 1983;250:3072–3076.

28. Benedetti-Panici P, Greggi S, Maneschi F, et al. Anatomical and pathological study of retroperitoneal nodes in epithelial ovarian cancer. *Gynecol Oncol.* 1993;51:150–154.

29. Leblanc E, Querleu D, Narducci F, et al. Surgical staging of early invasive epithelial ovarian tumors. *Semin Surg Oncol.* 2000;19:36–41.

30. Park JY, Kim DY, Suh DS, et al. Comparison of laparoscopy and laparotomy in surgical staging of early-stage ovarian and fallopian tubal cancer. *Ann Surg Oncol.* 2008;15:2012–2019.

31. Childers JM, Aqua KA, Surwit EA, Hallum AV, Hatch KD. Abdominal-wall tumor implantation after laparoscopy for malignant conditions. *Obstet Gynecol.* 1994;84:765–769.

32. Nagarsheth NP, Rahaman J, Cohen CJ, Gretz H, Nezhat F. The incidence of port-site metastases in gynecologic cancers. *JSLS.* 2004;8:133–139.

33. Huang KG, Wang CJ, Chang TC, et al. Management of port-site metastasis after laparoscopic surgery for ovarian cancer. *Am J Obstet Gynecol.* 2003;189:16–21.

34. Schilder JM, Thompson AM, DePriest PD, et al. Outcome of reproductive age women with stage IA or IC invasive epithelial ovarian cancer treated with fertility-sparing therapy. *Gynecol Oncol.* 2002;87:1–7.

35. Khoury-Collado F, Bombard AT. Hereditary breast and ovarian cancer: what the primary care physician should know. *Obstet Gynecol Surv.* 2004;59:537–542.

36. Benjamin I, Morgan MA, Rubin SC. Occult bilateral involvement in stage I epithelial ovarian cancer. *Gynecol Oncol.* 1999;72:288–291.

37. Zanetta G, Chiari S, Rota S, et al. Conservative surgery for stage I ovarian carcinoma in women of childbearing age. *Br J Obstet Gynaecol.* 1997;104:1030–1035.

38. Colombo N, Parma G, Lapresa MT, Maggi F, Piantanida P, Maggioni A. Role of conservative surgery in ovarian cancer: the European experience. *Int J Gynecol Cancer.* 2005; 15(suppl):206–211.

39. Sainz de la Cuesta R, Goff BA, Fuller AF, Jr., Nikrui N, Eichhorn JH, Rice LW. Prognostic importance of intraoperative rupture of malignant ovarian epithelial neoplasms. *Obstet Gynecol.* 1994;84:1–7.

40. Mizuno M, Kikkawa F, Shibata K, et al. Long-term prognosis of stage I ovarian carcinoma. Prognostic importance of intraoperative rupture. *Oncology.* 2003;65:29–36.

41. Heintz AP, Odicino F, Maisonneuve P, et al. Carcinoma of the ovary. FIGO 6th annual report on the results of treatment in gynecological cancer. *Int J Gynaecol Obstet.* 2006;95(suppl):S161–S192.

42. Young RC, Walton LA, Ellenberg SS, et al. Adjuvant therapy in stage I and stage II epithelial ovarian cancer. Results of two prospective randomized trials. *N Engl J Med.* 1990;322:1021–1027.

43. Heintz AP, Odicino F, Maisonneuve P, et al. Carcinoma of the fallopian tube. FIGO 6th annual report on the results of treatment in gynecological cancer. *Int J Gynaecol Obstet.* 2006;95(suppl):S145–S160.

44. Chi DS, Eisenhauer EL, Lang J, et al. What is the optimal goal of primary cytoreductive surgery for bulky stage IIIC epithelial ovarian carcinoma (EOC)? *Gynecol Oncol.* 2006;103:559–564.

45. Bristow RE, Montz FJ, Lagasse LD, Leuchter RS, Karlan BY. Survival impact of surgical cytoreduction in stage IV epithelial ovarian cancer. *Gynecol Oncol.* 1999;72:278–287.

46. Hoskins WJ, Bundy BN, Thigpen JT, Omura GA. The influence of cytoreductive surgery on recurrence-free interval and survival in small-volume stage III epithelial ovarian cancer: a Gynecologic Oncology Group study. *Gynecol Oncol.* 1992;47:159–166.

47. Eisenhauer EL, Abu-Rustum NR, Sonoda Y, et al. The addition of extensive upper abdominal surgery to achieve optimal cytoreduction improves survival in patients with stages IIIC-IV epithelial ovarian cancer. *Gynecol Oncol.* 2006;103:1083–1090.

48. Panici PB, Maggioni A, Hacker N, et al. Systematic aortic and pelvic lymphadenectomy versus resection of bulky nodes only in optimally debulked advanced ovarian cancer: a randomized clinical trial. *J Natl Cancer Inst.* 2005;97:560–566.

49. Sun CC, Ramirez PT, Bodurka DC. Quality of life for patients with epithelial ovarian cancer. *Nat Clin Pract Oncol.* 2007;4:18–29.

50. Armstrong DK, Bundy B, Wenzel L, et al. Intraperitoneal cisplatin and paclitaxel in ovarian cancer. *N Engl J Med.* 2006;354:34–43.

CHAPTER 11
Ovarian Sex Cord–Stromal Tumors

Emma Rossi, MD
Department of Obstetrics and Gynecology, University of North Carolina School of Medicine, Chapel Hill, NC, USA

John T. Soper, MD, FACOG
Department of Obstetrics and Gynecology, University of North Carolina School of Medicine, Chapel Hill, NC, USA

Pathology Notes: Chad Livasy, MD
Associate Professor, Department of Pathology and Laboratory Medicine, University of North Carolina School of Medicine, Chapel Hill, NC, USA

Background

Sex cord–stromal tumors (SCSTs) are relatively uncommon ovarian neoplasms that arise from cells making up the nongerm cell and nonepithelial tissue of the ovary. Sex cords of the ovary originate from the coelomic epithelium that covers the primitive gonad. During embryologic development, this epithelium proliferates and then grows down into the mesenchyme of the ovary in cords of cells. These sex cords later incorporate the primordial germ cells that migrate from the wall of the yolk sac. The cells of the sex cords (granulosa cells and Sertoli cells) together with the stromal cells (theca cells, Leydig cells, and fibroblasts) make up the matrix of the ovary. While the sex cord cells dominate normal ovarian hormonal production, stromal cells also contribute.

Sex cord–stromal tumors comprise only 7% of malignant ovarian neoplasms, but are responsible for 90% of functional ovarian neoplasms.[1] These tumors are typically associated with steroid hormone production, and functional sex cord–stromal tumors can be categorized into either estrogenic or androgenic tumors. Table 11.1 outlines the typical hormonal profiles of the different types of SCSTs. However, there is variability within the group, and the endocrinologic function of these tumors cannot be rigidly predicted by their dominant cell type. A physician should always consider SCSTs when evaluating conditions of sex hormone excess, and these effects are variable depending on the age of the patient, ranging from precocious puberty, virilization, or postmenopausal bleeding. The hormonal production of SCSTs can result in pathology beyond that of the tumor itself, and physicians must be aware of these patients' increased breast and endometrial cancer risk, particularly in the setting of hyperestrogenism.

Sex cord–stromal tumors can be separated into the subcategories of granulosa–stromal or Sertoli–stromal cell tumors. The former include granulosa cell tumors, thecomas, and fibromas; and the latter include Sertoli cell tumors, Sertoli–Leydig cell tumors, and Leydig cell tumors. These two subcategories comprise the majority of sex cord–stromal tumors. In addition, gynandroblastomas are rare SCSTs that are benign, containing a minimum of 10% of both Sertoli–Leydig and

Gynecological Cancer Management: Identification, Diagnosis and Treatment, Edited by Daniel L. Clarke-Pearson and John T. Soper. Published 2010 by Blackwell Publishing, ISBN: 978-1-4051-9079-4.

Table 11.1 Hormonal profiles of sex cord–stromal tumors

Tumor type	Hormonal profile
Granulosa-cell tumor	Estrogenic
Thecoma	Estrogenic
Fibroma	Hormonally inert
Sertoli-cell tumor	Estrogenic
Sertoli–Leydig cell tumor	Androgenic
Sex cord tumor with annular tubules	Estrogenic
Gynandroblastoma	Androgenic or estrogenic (most commonly androgenic)
Leydig cell tumor	Androgenic
Stromal luteoma	Estrogenic

granulosa cell elements.[2] Sex cord tumor with annular tubules (SCTAT) is a rare SCST that is frequently associated with Peutz–Jeghers syndrome.[3] SCTAT tumors contain cells that are characteristic of both Sertoli and granulosa cells.

Granulosa–stromal cell tumors

Granulosa–stromal cell tumors comprise 70% of sex cord–stromal tumors. The most common tumor in this group is the fibroma, which is a benign, unilateral, solid tumor typically found in a postmenopausal population. When associated with ascites and pleural effusions, ovarian fibromas are part of a condition known as Meigs' syndrome.[4]

Granulosa cell tumors have malignant potential. They are subcategorized into adult and juvenile types, with the former comprising 95% of cases reported.[5] These tumors tend to be large, unilateral, and predominantly solid. Thecomatous components (granulosa–thecomas) result in areas of yellow coloration. Histologically the characteristic findings include cells arranged in rosettes called Call–Exner bodies,[6] and cells containing pale cytoplasm with "coffee bean"–shaped grooved nuclei. These histologic findings are frequently found in the adult variety of granulosa cell tumors, but rarely observed in the juvenile subtype. Pure thecomas are highly hormonally active but benign solid tumors, which feature luteinized cells.

Pathology notes

Adult granulosa cell tumor

Granulosa cell tumors are uncommon neoplasms comprising 1% to 2% of all ovarian neoplasms. The discussion here will focus on adult granulosa cell tumors. Adult granulosa cell tumors are low-grade malignant neoplasms with approximately 93% of cases presenting as stage I. The most relevant factors related to pathologic diagnosis of adult granulosa cell tumors are exclusion of other more or less aggressive neoplasms with similar histology and the documentation of potentially important prognostic factors. Tumors with morphology similar to adult granulosa cell tumors include cellular fibroma/thecoma, stromal sarcomas, carcinoid tumor, small-cell carcinoma, and poorly differentiated endometrioid adenocarcinoma (Plate 11.1). Special stains including inhibin, synaptophysin (neuroendocrine marker), cytokeratin, and reticulin are often helpful in the classification of ovarian neoplasms consisting of monomorphic small blue cells. Distinction from carcinomas, particularly the highly aggressive small-cell carcinoma, is of utmost clinical importance. Small-cell carcinomas are typically unilateral and comprised of a relative monomorphic population of epithelioid cells with high nuclear/cytoplasmic ratios, similar to granulosa cell tumors. An elevated mitotic count is the first clue that a tumor may represent a carcinoma with unusual histology rather than a granulosa cell tumor and indicates the need for special stains.

Pathology notes (*continued*)

Stage is the most important prognostic factor for adult granulosa cell tumors. As most granulosa cell tumors present at stage I, there has been a lot of interest in evaluating prognostic factors to predict which patients are at higher risk of recurrence. Most of the reported studies have a limited number of cases due to the rarity of adult granulosa cell tumors. The results in the literature have been conflicting for several of the prognostic factors evaluated in stage I patients.[7] Capsular rupture appears convincing as an adverse prognostic indicator associated with higher risk for developing recurrent disease. Large tumors (>15 cm) have been reported to have a lower 5-year survival when compared to small tumors (<5 cm). Mitotic index has been evaluated in several studies, with variable results. A study using clearly specified and reproducible methodology found no correlation between tumor recurrence and mitotic count or Ki-67 staining index.[8] Additionally, there was no difference in proliferation between stage I and higher-stage tumors.

Pathology reports for adult granulosa cell tumors should include tumor type, tumor size, and intactness of the ovarian capsule. Reporting of mitotic count is reasonable to include, as the prognostic significance of an elevated mitotic count is not yet completely resolved. Tumors with > 10 mitoses/10 high-power fields deserve consideration as carcinomas or sarcomas mimicking a granulosa cell tumor and may indicate the need for special stains to confirm the diagnosis.

Sertoli–stromal cell tumors

Sertoli–stromal cell tumors include Sertoli, Leydig, and Sertoli–Leydig cell tumors and are sex cord–stromal tumors that mimic the sex cord cells found in the male testis. They are a rare group of tumors, making up 0.5% of all ovarian neoplasms.[9] Up to 82% of these tumors are hormonally active.[10] They are named according to their cellular components, with the most common form of this tumor type being the mixed Sertoli–Leydig form. Pure Sertoli cell tumors tend to be somewhat larger than the pure Leydig cell tumors (4–7 cm compared with 1–3 cm).[10] This may reflect diagnosis of the Leydig cell tumors at an earlier point in their development because of their greater production of male hormones. Pure Sertoli cell tumors may secrete either estrogen or renin, leading to hypertension and hypokalemia[10, 11] in approximately 50% of cases. Sertoli–Leydig or pure Leydig cell tumors are highly androgenic, and in women are usually discovered in the evaluation of hirsuitism or virilization.[12] These tumors are almost always unilateral and clinically confined to the ovary at the time of diagnosis.[9] They almost always contain at least one solid component on imaging, with 70% being purely solid.[10] As a group, they are considered to have very low malignant potential.

Pathology notes

Ovarian sex cord–stromal neoplasms

Sex cord–stromal tumors of the ovaries are a diverse group of neoplasms comprising approximately 10% of all ovarian tumors. Most sex–cord stromal neoplasms show either benign (eg, fibroma, thecoma) or low-grade malignant (eg, granulosa cell tumor, steroid cell tumor, Sertoli–Leydig tumor) biological behavior. Adult granulosa cell tumor has been discussed previously and will not be further discussed here. The diversity of histology observed in this group of

Pathology notes (*continued*)

tumors presents several challenges for the pathologist, especially for the uncommon sex cord–stromal tumors. The pathologist's chief task is to segregate the true sex cord–stromal tumors from other tumor types that show similar histopathologic features. Special stains are often required to make this distinction. Pathology reports from these tumors should include tumor type, tumor size, grade/differentiation (if applicable), and statement clarifying likely biological behavior for borderline and low-grade malignant neoplasms.

Almost 90% of ovarian sex cord–stromal neoplasms fall into the fibroma/thecoma group and are clearly benign. The diagnosis and management of the usual fibroma/thecoma is straightforward. Predicting the biological behavior of the small subset of tumors in this group that shows increased mitotic activity is problematic. Most cellular fibromas showing increased mitotic activity (>3 mitotic figures/10 high-power fields) without associated cytologic atypia demonstrate benign biological behavior.[13] Tumors associated with marked adhesions show a higher risk of recurrence. Tumors showing both increased mitotic rate and cytologic atypia are classified as fibrosarcoma. Cellular fibromatous tumors showing cytologic atypia and a low mitotic index fall into the uncertain malignant potential group, but these tumors are exceedingly rare.

The Sertoli–Leydig cell tumors show tremendous variation in histologic appearance. The tumors are classified into well, moderately, and poorly differentiated tumors based on the histologic pattern. The main challenge for the pathologist in these cases is to exclude other tumors, especially carcinomas, mimicking a Sertoli–Leydig cell tumor. A classic example includes some endometrioid adenocarcinomas that form small tubules resembling a Sertoli–Leydig cell tumor (Plate 11.1).

Steroid cell tumors are rare tumors comprising <1% of all sex cord–stromal neoplasms. The WHO currently recognizes three groups of steroid-producing tumors, including (1) stromal luteoma, (2) Leydig cell tumor, and (3) steroid cell tumor, NOS. The diagnosis of Leydig cell tumor is defined by the identification of crystalloids of Reinke. Tumors that cannot be classified as stromal luteoma or Leydig cell tumor fall into the steroid cell tumor, NOS group. In contrast to the benign behavior of stromal luteoma and Leydig cell tumor, steroid cell tumors (NOS) show uncertain malignant potential. Studies have shown that up to 34% of these tumors behave in a malignant fashion.[14] Gross and histologic features more frequently associated with aggressive clinical behavior include high mitotic index (> 2/10 high-power fields), large tumor size (>7 cm), geographic tumor necrosis, and moderate to severe nuclear atypia. Pitfalls in the diagnosis of steroid cell tumor include pregnancy luteoma and metastatic renal cell carcinoma.

Clinical Scenario 1

A 15-year-old girl (para 0) presents with acute abdominal pain, hemoperitoneum, and a 12-cm complex mass on ultrasound. Spontaneous rupture of a largely solid unilateral ovarian mass is found at laparotomy, with no apparent metastases. Frozen section reveals "poorly differentiated ovarian malignancy."

What are appropriate tumor markers to consider?

The most commonly found ovarian cysts in adolescent populations are functional cysts. However, the most commonly found solid ovarian tumors in the juvenile population are germ cell tumors and sex cord–stromal tumors.[15] Many germ cell tumor types are associated with elevations in a variety of serum tumor markers.

Alpha-fetoprotein is frequently elevated in endodermal sinus tumors, mixed germ cell tumors, and immature teratomas. Lactate dehydrogenase (LDH) is frequently elevated in dysgerminomas. Human chorionic gonadotropin (hCG) is often elevated in ovarian choriocarcinoma and in mixed germ cell tumors. CA-125 is a sensitive but nonspecific marker for epithelial ovarian cancer, but can also be elevated in other malignancies or in a number of benign conditions in a premenopausal population such as endometriosis, intraperitoneal infection or inflammation, and ascites.[16]

Juvenile granulosa cell tumor should also be considered in this 15-year-old patient, and can be associated with elevations in serum inhibin levels. Inhibin is an ovarian glycoprotein hormone that is produced by the granulosa cells of the ovary and acts at the pituitary to inhibit FSH secretion. It consists of an alpha unit and two beta subunits. Inhibin levels have been found to be elevated in most granulosa cell tumors and 100% of thecomas.[17] It is also found to be elevated in a number of other benign and malignant tumors of the ovary, such as mucinous cystadenocarcinoma. While both alpha and beta units can be elevated, it is inhibin B which is the predominant form in GCTs.[18] A normal inhibin value does not exclude this pathology, because juvenile granulosa cell tumors are less commonly associated with an elevated inhibin level compared to adult granulosa cell tumors.[19] Additionally, inhibin levels are difficult to interpret in a premenopausal female, because this is a hormone produced by normal granulosa cells of the ovary, and inhibin secreted by a tumor may not elevate inhibin levels above normal range. Estrogen levels might well be within normal range for a menstruating woman. Serum specimens for all tumor markers mentioned above should be obtained either preoperatively or within a few hours of surgery, because many are cleared rapidly and may become undetectable within a few days after removal of the tumor.

Müllerian inhibitory substance (MIS) is an emerging potential tumor marker for GCTs. Like inhibin, MIS is also produced by granulosa cells of the ovary.[20] MIS has been found to be elevated in a significant number of GCTs preoperatively, reducing in values after treatment, and reemerging with elevated levels more than 11 months before clinically detectable recurrence.[21] However, MIS is not as yet available clinically as a tumor marker because investigation into its clinical applications is not yet complete.

What is appropriate intraoperative management for this patient?

When an adnexal mass is removed, immediate pathologic evaluation with frozen section should be requested.[22] Accuracy of frozen section evaluation is thought to range between 91% and 97% for gynecologic pathologies.[23, 24] The ovarian tumor types that present the greatest numbers of misdiagnoses or challenges at the time of frozen section are mucinous tumors and metastatic ovarian malignances.[25] However, frozen section evaluation of sex cord–stromal tumors can also present diagnostic difficulties. In particular, it may be difficult for the pathologist to appreciate the differences in mitotic activity that distinguish fibromas from fibrosarcomas, and the histologic morphology of granulosa cell tumors on frozen section may be confused for cellular fibromas, transitional cell carcinoma, undifferentiated carcinomas, or yolk sac tumor.[26]

While at least 75% of premenopausal patients with complex adnexal masses undergoing surgery will have benign pathology,[23] all patients undergoing surgery for adnexal masses should receive preoperative counseling about the surgical staging options should the pathology reveal malignancy. When there is no evidence of gross metastatic disease, and clinically the tumor appears to be confined to the ovary, it is appropriate to perform fertility-sparing surgery in a patient who has not yet completed child-bearing.[27] In fertility-sparing surgery, the uterus and contralateral ovary are not removed. However, surgical staging should include peritoneal cytology, omentectomy, performing biopsies of the peritoneum, sampling pelvic and para-aortic lymph nodes, collecting cytology of the diaphragm, and performing a thorough exploration of the abdomen. Of course, any suspicious lesions should be excised. If there is any question of the diagnosis or if comprehensive surgical staging cannot be performed and a unilateral ovarian tumor is encountered, it is preferable to simply obtain washings, remove the affected adnexum, manually and visually explore the upper abdomen, and await permanent histology to determine whether further surgery is needed.

At the time of surgery, close inspection of the contralateral ovary should take place, because 2% to 8% of sex cord–stromal tumors are bilateral,[28–30] but a normal-appearing contralateral ovary should not be biopsied, because this is more likely to produce adhesions or result in complications from bleeding than to yield a diagnosis of an occult bilateral lesion. Five-year survival is equivalent (97% versus 98%, $p = 0.061$) between premenopausal women with low grade sex cord–stromal tumors who received fertility-sparing sugery and those who were fully staged.[27] Patients who have undergone fertility-sparing surgery should consider hysterectomy and contralateral oophorectomy once child-bearing is completed.[27]

What is the prognosis of juvenile granulosa cell tumor?

Stage of disease is the most important prognostic factor for juvenile granulosa cell tumor (JGCT).[31] Ninety percent of JGCTs are stage IA or IB with a 97% 3.5-year survival rate. Isosexual precocious puberty is associated with favorable prognosis, although it is unclear as to whether this is secondary to symptoms prompting earlier diagnosis. While early-stage JGCT is associated with good prognosis, advanced JGCT is associated with aggressive and rapidly progressive disease. In this way JGCT differs from the adult form of the tumor, which behaves more indolently and is associated with a longer time to recurrence.[32] Therefore, the period of intense postoperative surveillance for a patient with stage I juvenile granulosa cell tumor can be reduced given that recurrence is anticipated to occur earlier in the course of disease.

Clinical Scenario 2

A 7-year-old girl presents with telarche, vaginal spotting, and on ultrasound has a 5-cm right adnexal solid mass.

What is the differential diagnosis in this patient?

This child is presenting with signs of isosexual precocity. Precocious puberty can be divided into two classifications: gonadotrophin releasing hormone (GnRH)-dependent precocious puberty, and GnRH-independent precocity. GnRH-dependent precocity is "true" precocious puberty, and involves early activation of the hypothalamic–pituitary–gonadal axis. GnRH-independent precocious puberty results in sexual maturation due to extrapituitary secretion, exposure to human chorionic gonadotropin (hCG), or sex steroid secretion independent of the hypothalamic–pituitary–gonadal axis. In girls, GnRH-dependent processes predominate, the majority of which have an idiopathic etiology.[33] Nonidiopathic causes include central nervous system (CNS) tumors,[34] CNS irradiation,[35] previous excess androgen exposure,[36] and primary hypothyroidism.[37] The latter is felt to be a result of thyropin (TSH) directly activating FSH receptors secondary to hormonal structural similarities.[38]

GnRH-independent isosexual precocity results from unregulated secretion of excess sex hormones from either the gonads or the adrenal glands, or from exogenous sources. Examples of these pathologies include granulosa, Sertoli, or theca cell tumors of the ovaries, exogenous estrogens, or adrenal pathologies such as congenital adrenal hyperplasia or androgen-secreting tumors. McCune–Albright syndrome (MAS) is a genetic disease that is a rare cause of GnRH-independent precocious puberty and is also characterized by café-au-lait skin pigmentation and fibrous dysplasia of the bone.[39] Because this patient has an adnexal mass, a sex cord–stromal tumor would be the most likely diagnosis, but other causes must be excluded.

What is an appropriate evaluation before surgery?

The question of what age constitutes pathologic or precocious sexual development is a controversial one. There is a wide range of normal age of onset of pubertal development. Factors such as gender, race, and genetics all influence age of puberty.[40] Taking these factors into account, evaluation for an underlying pathologic cause of precocity should be reserved for Caucasian girls with breast or pubic hair development before the age of 7, and African-American girls before the age of 6.[41]

It is important to perform a thorough history and physical examination to help determine the underlying etiology of isosexual precocity. Particular focus should be made to enquiring about symptoms of central nervous system disorders including a history of CNS disease, trauma, headaches, or seizures. The patient should be asked about a history of exogenous estrogen exposure or abdominal pain. The pattern of sexual characteristic development should be established. Girls who report a normal sequence and pace of pubertal development are more likely to have a GnRH-dependent etiology for their presentation, whereas girls whose pubertal characteristics have developed at an abnormal pace or order are more likely to have a peripheral or GnRH-independent pathology.[42]

On physical examination, fundoscopy should be performed as well as evaluation of visual fields. Breast and hair development should be observed and objectified using Tanner and Ferriman–Gallway stages. Plain radiographs of the wrist should be obtained to evaluate for bone age. Finally, in order to differentiate between central precocity and GnRH-independent precocity, a GnRH stimulation test should be performed. Basal luteinizing hormone (LH) levels are assessed, and then drawn again after administering GnRH. GnRH-independent precocity (such as from ovarian GCT) is associated with stable inhibin levels at baseline and after GnRH administration, and this result should prompt the physician to perform abdominal and pelvic imaging (such as with ultrasound and CT scan).

Serum levels of estradiol, cortisol, DHEAS, and 17-hydroxyprogesterone should be obtained. If levels of inhibin increase from baseline with the GnRH stimulation test, imaging of the brain (with MRI or CT scan) should follow to evaluate for a central cause of precocity, although 90% of central precocity is idiopathic and not associated with measurable central nervous system disease.

Clinical Scenario 3

A 34-year-old nulligravida presents with a solid 9-cm adnexal mass and menorrhagia. She desires to preserve fertility, if possible. At surgery, a bosselated 9-cm solid tumor replacing the left ovary is removed intact and is classified as "mixed granulosa and theca cell tumor" on frozen section. No apparent metastases or ascites are noted; the uterus and contralateral adnexal structures appear normal.

What is the significance of granulosa cells or other histologic features in a mixed granulosa–thecal cell tumor?

In adult-form GCTs, the granulosa cells appear round, pale with little cytoplasm, and contain a classically grooved nucleus (coffee bean). They arrange themselves in rosettes called "Call–Exener bodies." Seventy percent of adult-form granulosa cell tumors contain a mixture of granulosa cells and theca cells that are lipid laden (luteinized) ovarian stromal cells. It is the androstenedione produced by these theca cells that is converted into estradiol by the granulosa cells, and therefore it is the theca cell component of the granulosa–theca cell tumor that in turn produces many of the clinical manifestations of these tumors such as sexual precocity in children, abnormal uterine bleeding in premenopausal women, and postmenopausal bleeding in an older population.

Thecomas are benign tumors that contain theca cells and fibrous tissue, and are typically very hormonally active. They may contain granulosa cell components, and pathology separately categorizes tumors as either granulosa–theca cell or granulosa cell tumors depending on the relative proportion of granulosa cell composition. A granulosa cell tumor contains less than 25% theca cells. A theca cell tumor contains less than 25% granulosa cells, and a granulosa–theca cell tumor contains greater than 25% of each cell type. Theca cell tumors (TCTs) are virtually all benign, while GCTs are malignant but exhibit less malignant activity than most ovarian carcinomas.[1] Because of the difference in prognosis associated with each tumor subtype, it is very important that an accurate histologic diagnosis is obtained. A frozen section finding of greater than 25% granulosa cells within a theca cell tumor suggests a malignant tumor and the surgery should proceed accordingly.

What is appropriate surgical management of this patient?

Surgery for ovarian malignancies serves two important functions: diagnostic staging and therapeutic tumor reduction. In order to accomplish the former, surgery for ovarian malignancies usually includes removal of both ovaries, the uterus, biopsies of pelvic and peri-aortic lymph nodes, biopsies of the omentum, biopsies of the peritoneum, consideration for an appendectomy, and cytology from both peritoneal washings and the diaphragm. Without evaluation of all of these tissues, a physician cannot assign the tumor a surgical stage, and discussions about prognosis and future therapies become more speculative. Ovarian granulosa cell tumors are staged according to the guidelines created by FIGO to stage ovarian malignancies (Table 11.2).

Among sex cord-stromal tumors that have been completely staged, 80% of granulosa–theca cell tumors were stage IA. However, within that same study population, 58% of granulosa cell tumors were stage IA defined at comprehensive staging but only 8% were stage III, and most advanced-stage patients had grossly apparent disease.[1] These findings once again raise the

Table 11.2 FIGO staging of ovarian malignancy

0	No evidence of primary tumor
I	Tumor confined to ovaries
IA	Tumor limited to one ovary, capsule intact No tumor on ovarian surface No malignant cells in the ascites or peritoneal washings
IB	Tumor limited to both ovaries, capsules intact No tumor on ovarian surface No malignant cells in the ascites or peritoneal washings
IC	Tumor limited to one or both ovaries, with any of the following: Capsule ruptured, tumor on ovarian surface, positive malignant cells in the ascites, or positive peritoneal washings
II	Tumor involves one or both ovaries with pelvic extension
IIA	Extension and/or implants in uterus and/or tubes No malignant cells in the ascites or peritoneal washings
IIB	Extension to other pelvic organ No malignant cells in the ascites or peritoneal washings
IIC	IIA/B with positive malignant cells in the ascites or positive peritoneal washings
III	Tumor involves one or both ovaries with microscopically confirmed peritoneal metastasis outside the pelvis and/or regional lymph node metastasis
IIIA	Microscopic peritoneal metastasis beyond the pelvis
IIIB	Macroscopic peritoneal metastasis beyond the pelvis 2 cm or less in greatest dimension
IIIC	Peritoneal metastasis beyond pelvis more than 2 cm in greatest dimension and/or regional lymph node metastasis
IV	Distant metastasis beyond the peritoneal cavity

question for the necessity of complete staging in low-risk tumor populations.

It is acceptable practice to perform fertility-sparing staging in premenopausal women with clinical stage I granulosa–theca cell tumors, as the likelihood of finding distant microscopic disease is extremely small.[27] However, an extensive evaluation of the peritoneal cavity and retroperitoneal structures should take place. When planning surgery to address an adnexal mass, a preoperative discussion should be held with the patient that addresses her desire for future fertility should malignancy be diagnosed. In the patient who is nulliparous and has expressed a desire for future fertility, it would be appropriate to perform staging that does not include hysterectomy and contralateral salpingo-oophorectomy.

If fertility-sparing surgery is performed, it is important to perform sampling of the endometrium as part of the staging procedure, as granulosa cell tumors are associated with an increased risk of endometrial hyperplasia or endometrial cancer, thought to be secondary to their generation of a hyperestrogenic state.[1, 44] One-third of patients with ovarian granulosa cell tumors and menstrual irregularities or postmenopausal bleeding are found to have hyperplasia with atypia and approximately 20% have endometrial adenocarcinoma.[27, 29, 44–46]

What factors influence outcome in patients with granulosa cell tumors?

Stage of disease is the most important prognostic factor when dealing with GCTs.[27] Ninety percent of GCTs are FIGO stage I or confined to the ovary. Stage I tumors have a 5-year survival rate of greater than 90% even among incompletely staged patients,[30] with the 10-year survival rate being 85% to 95%.[45] Conversely, stage III/IV tumors are associated with a 22% to 50% 5-year survival, and 17% to 33% 10-year survival.[45] There are several additional factors that are debated in the literature that might play a role in prognosis such as tumor size, tumor rupture, histologic pattern, nuclear atypical, and mitotic index.

It has been postulated that, independent of stage, tumor size greater than 5 cm is associated with poorer outcomes, such as shorter progression-free survival and 10-year survival in patients with GCT.[28–30] However, these findings have not been consistently reproduced in the

literature,[45, 48, 49] and conversely, there have been recurrences documented in women where the original tumor was microscopic.[50] Tumor rupture is not a consistently demonstrated prognosticator, particularly if the rupture has occurred incidentally at the time of surgery.[51] However, a 26% reduction in 25-year survival was demonstrated in patients with spontaneous rupture of cysts compared with those patients whose GCTs were removed intact.[45] This may reflect a more aggressive underlying pathology for tumors that spontaneously rupture. Other postulated, but not well-substantiated, factors that are associated with poor prognosis in GCTs include histologically diffuse architecture compared with follicular pattern of growth, increased mitotic index, and nuclear atypia.[28, 52, 53] However, the most important and consistent association for prognosis in GCT continues to be stage.

What is appropriate follow-up of patients with granulosa cell tumors treated by surgery?

Adult granulosa cell tumors have an overall good prognosis but with a tendency to late recurrence.[20] The medium time to onset of recurrence is 4 to 6 years.[30] However, recurrence can be as late as 40 years after initial diagnosis.[54] Therefore, lifelong follow-up is necessary. Follow-up visits are recommended at 3-month intervals in the first 2 years, every 6 months in the subsequent 3 years, and then annual but lifelong follow-up thereafter. Visits should include performing a thorough physical examination and drawing serum inhibin levels. Some authors propose performing annual chest radiographs,[20] but the value of this is questionable, and in general, radiographic imaging should be reserved for follow-up of abnormal symptoms, physical examination findings, or elevating serum inhibin levels. The mainstay of treatment of recurrence is early detection of recurrence and secondary surgical resection, because chemotherapy and radiation therapy have limited success in treating this disease, particularly in advanced stages.[55]

Clinical Scenario 4

A 40-year-old woman has progressive symptoms of increased libido, clitoral enlargement, "hoarseness," and hair growth in a beard distribution and over her chest plate, while noticing temporal balding.

What is the appropriate evaluation for this patient?

This patient is demonstrating symptoms consistent with virilization. Virilization in adolescent or adult women involves the acquisition of clitoral enlargement, increased muscle mass, acne, hirsuitism, frontal or crown hair thinning, deepening of the voice, and menstrual disruption with annovulation.[56] The etiology is one of androgen excess, which may be caused by:

- Polycystic ovarian syndrome
- Androgen-producing tumors of the ovary, adrenal glands, or pituitary glands
- Hypothyroidism
- Anabolic steroid exposure
- Congenital adrenal hyperplasia due to 21-hydroxylase deficiency (late onset)

Virilization should not be confused with hirsuitism, which is one of the symptoms of virilization but can occur as an isolated benign condition without other virilizing signs or symptoms. Hirsuitism is defined as excessive terminal hair that appears in a male pattern in women.[57] It can be distinguished from hypertrichosis, which is excessive hair growth in a nonsexual pattern not caused by androgen excess.[58] The etiology of hirsuitism is androgen exposure (both relative amount, and hair follicle sensitivity to the hormone) causing increased development of terminal hairs, which are thicker and more pigmented. It is free testosterone that exerts this effect, and therefore it is associated with conditions that increase total testosterone or androgens, or those that involve a reduction in sex-hormone binding globulin. Benign conditions such as idiopathic hirsuitism and PCOS make up the majority of causes of hirsuitism. However, when the development of hirsuitism is abrupt and short in onset, occurs after the 3rd decade of life, or is associated with symptoms or signs of virilization (such as those seen in this patient), further workup with serology and imaging for underlying pathology should take place.[58]

Evaluation should begin by taking a thorough history, with care to address features such as menstrual history, weight history, medication history, and family history.[59, 60] This information can assist in identifying causes of hirsuitism such as PCOS (with anovulatory cycles and weight gain), exogenous hormone exposure, or familial causes such as adrenal hyperplasia. A physical examination should be performed that identifies the degree and pattern of hair growth and loss. An objective tool developed to measure these changes is the Ferriman–Gallwey score.[61, 62] Scores greater than 8 are considered pathologic in Caucasion and black women, and are concerning for underlying androgen excesses. Physical examination should also include survey of the body habitus, skin (for signs of acne), evaluation for clitoromegaly, and evaluation of laryngeal cartilage development. The abdomen and pelvis should be examined to evaluate for the presence of an adrenal or pelvic mass.

Laboratory testing should be reserved for women with severe hirsuitism of abrupt development, in the 3rd decade of life or later, and for those who exhibit signs of virilization. The cornerstone of laboratory testing for hirsuitism is measurement of serum androgens. Serum total and free testosterone are recommended. However, it is total testosterone (not free) that is more widely available, and more standardized. It includes measurement of both bound (by sex-hormone binding globulin) and free testosterone. Total testosterone may be normal in conditions of low SHBG, such as PCOS, and yet hirsuitism is present because free testosterone is elevated and available to interact with receptors at the hair follicles. Values of total testosterone are rarely greater than 150 ng/dL in benign conditions such as these. A total testosterone value exceeding 150 ng/dL is highly suspicious for an androgen-secreting tumor (such as a Sertoli–Leydig cell tumor of the ovary, or adrenal tumor).[63–66] In order to help differentiate an ovarian versus adrenal source of the increased testosterone level, serum dehydroepiandrosterone sulfate (DHEAS) or dehydroepiandrosterone (DHEA) levels can be drawn. DHEAS or DHEA levels greater than 700 μg/dL are highly suspicious for an adrenal tumor.[63] Additional hormonal evaluation including serum prolactin, basal or stimulated 17-hydroxyprogesterone, and TSH can also be evaluated, particularly if serum androgens are not found to be elevated or if menstrual irregularities are present.[56]

If an androgen-secreting ovarian neoplasm is suspected from the physical examination or laboratory values (total testosterone > 150 ng/dL), a pelvic ultrasound should be performed. Certainly large solid masses in the adnexae would be concerning for a Sertoli–Leydig cell tumor. However, many of these tumors are too small to detect by ultrasound, even if they are able to produce androgen concentrations that can exert a virilizing effect. Sertoli–Leydig–stromal tumors tend to be predominantly solid in ultrasonographic appearance. Leydig tumors are typically smaller (up to 3 cm) than Sertoli cell tumors, which can average 9 cm. Sertoli–Leydig cell tumors are typically of intermediate size.[10] As has been previously mentioned, it is the Leydig cell tumor that is most typically found in an older population (such as that of our patient). Seventy-five percent of Leydig cell tumors are associated with excess androgen production, compared to 50% for Sertoli or Sertoli–Leydig cell tumors.[68] However, these tumors tend to be small, and therefore may evade identification by either pelvic ultrasound or CT scan of the abdomen and pelvis. Therefore a patient who exhibits new-onset virilization, with elevated serum androgen levels and negative imaging, should be offered surgical exploration with possible biopsy of the ovaries.

If a Sertoli–Leydig cell tumor is diagnosed at surgery, what is the appropriate surgical management?

Sertoli–Leydig cell tumors have unknown malignant potential.[12] Tumors are defined as malignant based on the degree of histologic differentiation.[69] Malignant potential is absent in well-differentiated tumors, and as high as 59% in poorly differentiated tumors. Therefore, accurate reporting of frozen section pathology is critically important for the surgeon in making intraoperative decisions. Well-differentiated Sertoli–Leydig cell tumors are confined to stage IA, and therefore, in a premenopausal patient who desires future fertility, a unilateral salpingo-oophorectomy is the recommended surgical management.[12] However, because their malignant potential is unknown, the patient should be recommended to undergo a hysterectomy with contralateral salpingo-oophorectomy after fertility is no longer desired. For the younger patient desiring future fertility whose frozen section pathology reveals a poorly differentiated Sertoli–Leydig cell tumor, the risk for malignant potential is higher (59%), and therefore fertility-sparing surgery with lymph node, omental, and peritoneal sampling should take place, followed by completion hysterectomy with contralateral salpingo-oophorectomy when child-bearing is completed. In older women with a tumor not confined to the ovary, surgical debulking and surgical staging including bilateral salpingo-oophorectomy, hysterectomy, omentectomy, and peritoneal and lymph node sampling is recommended.

What factors influence outcome in patients with Sertoli–Leydig cell tumors?

As with other sex cord–stromal tumors, the prognosis of Sertoli–Leydig cell tumors is most closely associated with tumor stage.[70] Other important prognostic factors are patient age and tumor differentiation. Young age at diagnosis tends to be associated with poor tumor differentiation,[9] and both are associated with worse prognosis. In a combined review of almost 250 cases of Sertoli–Leydig cell tumors, stage IA was found among all well-differentiated tumors, 93% of intermediate-differentiated tumors, and 98% of poorly differentiated tumors. Tumor recurrence occurs in approximately 20% of stage I tumors (of all histologies) and approximately 22% of all stages,[9] and is associated with a 34% risk of mortality.

Unlike its cousin the granulosa cell tumor, most recurrences of Sertoli–Leydig cell tumors occur within the first 36 months after diagnosis.[70] However, they have been reported to have recurred as late as 35 years after diagnosis, and therefore lifelong follow-up is recommended. Initially more intensive surveillance should take place with evaluation every 3 months in the first 2 years, followed by every 6 months until 5 years postoperatively, and annually thereafter. Evaluation should include quantification of serum testosterone levels, thorough physical examination, and imaging of the abdomen and pelvis with CT scanning. Recurrences are most commonly intra-abdominal.

Clinical Scenario 5

A 70-year-old woman presents with right pleural effusion, ascites, and a 10-cm solid adnexal mass. Ca-125 is 125 units/L. Paracentesis yields an acellular transudate.

What is the differential diagnosis in this case?

This clinical scenario is particularly worrisome for an ovarian malignancy. The constellation of signs—pleural effusion, ascites, adnexal mass, and elevated CA-125—are particularly suggestive for an epithelial ovarian malignancy, which is the most common cause of ovarian cancer. Other non-epithelial ovarian malignancies should also be considered. Benign ovarian neoplasms are also a possibility. In a review of 70 patients with an ovarian tumor, 27 of the 38 (71%) patients with malignancy had an elevation in CA-125, whereas only 8 of 32 (25%) patients with a benign tumor had serum elevations in CA-125.[71] Elevations in CA-125 may be found with any condition that causes peritoneal, pleural, or pericardial irritation, including ascites, pleural effusions, infection, or inflammatory conditions (such as arthritis). Therefore,

in this patient, the elevation in CA-125 may be from mesothelial stimulation secondary to the ascites or pleural effusions, and not a function of the ovarian mass.[72] An important consideration in this patient with a modest elevation in CA-125, and acellular acites, is Meigs' syndrome. Meigs' syndrome includes the triad of ascites, pleural effusions, and benign ovarian fibroma.[4] Given the concern for malignancy in a patient of this age, it is important that diagnosis of a benign process such as ovarian fibroma is confirmed by surgical intervention with oophorectomy and exploration of the abdomen.

What is the optimal management of this patient's asymptomatic pleural effusion?

The explanation for the etiology of fluid accumulation within the peritoneal and pleural spaces seen in Meigs' syndrome is controversial. It has been proposed that secretion of substances such as vascular endothelial growth factor (VEGF) causes neovasculature within the fibroma to have increased permeability to proteins that allow for generation of a transudate.[73] This transudate is created at a volume that exceeds peritoneal resorptive capacity, and subsequently exerts an effect across the diaphragm, resulting in sympathetic pleural effusions.[74] Effusions associated with benign fibromas resolve spontaneously after removal of the fibroma.[75] Therefore, expectant management should be followed when observing asymptomatic pleural effusions in the setting of ovarian fibroma. Thoracentesis or a chest tube would be considered preoperatively if it were felt necessary to improve pulmonary function.

Discuss surgical management of a fibroma and features that might suggest a rare scarcoma

Ovarian fibromas are considered benign if they do not contain mitotic activity and have a low cellular density. Cellular fibromas contain increased cellular activity, but fewer than 3 mitoses per 10 high-power fields, and are also considered benign. Surgical management of fibromas can include either a unilateral salpingo-oophorectomy or removal of the tumor alone.[76] Frozen section evaluation should be obtained in order to confirm the benign nature of the lesion. Because the majority of these tumors are benign and require only exision of the tumor, a minimally invasive approach may be considered when planning surgery.

Fibrosarcomas contain 4 or more mitoses per 10 high-power fields, in addition to marked increased cellularity and nuclear atypia. They are aggressive tumors that should be surgically staged.

References

1. Cronje HS, Niemand I, Bam RH, Woodruff JD. Review of the granulose-theca cell tumors from the Emil Novak ovarian tumor registry. *Am J Obstet Gynecol.* 1999;180:323.

2. Fukunaga M, Endo Y, Ushigome S. Gynandroblastoma of the ovary: a case report with an immunohistochemical and ultrastructural study. *Virchows Arch.* 1997;430:77.

3. Westerman AM, Wilson JH. Peutz-Jeghers syndrome: risks of a hereditary condition. *Scand J Gastroenterol Suppl.* 1999;230:64.

4. Meigs JV. Fibroma of the ovary with ascites and hydrothorax; Meigs' syndrome. *Am J Obstet Gynecol.* 1954;67:962.

5. Lack EE, Perez-Atayde AR, Murthy AS, et al. Granulosa theca cell tumors in premenarchal girls: a clinical and pathologic study of ten cases. *Cancer.* 1981;48:1846.

6. Young R, Clement PB, Scully RE. The ovary. In: Sternberg SS, ed. *Diagnostic Surgical Pathology.* New York: Raven; 1989: 1687.

7. Miller K, McCluggage WG. Prognostic factors in ovarian adult granulosa cell tumour. *J Clin Pathol.* 2008;61:881–884.

8. Leuverink EM, Brennan BA, Crook ML, et al. Prognostic value of mitotic counts and Ki-67 immunoreactivity in adult-type granulosa cell tumour of the ovary. *J Clin Pathol.* 2008;61:914–919.

9. Roth LM, Anderson MC. Sertoli Leydig cell tumors—a clinicopathologic study of 34 cases. *Cancer.* 1981;48:187–197.

10. Demidov VN, Lipatenkova J, Vikhareva O, Van Holsbeke C, Timmerman D, Valentin L. Imaging of gynecological disease (2): clinical and ultrasound characteristics of Sertoli cell tumors, Sertoli-Leydig cell tumors and Leydig cell tumors. *Ultrasound Obstet Gynecol.* 2007;31:85–91.

11. Oliva E, Alvarez T, Young RH. Sertoli cell tumors of the ovary: a clinicopathologic and immunohistochemical study of 54 cases. *Am J Surg Pathol.* 2005;29:143.

12. Sachdeva P, Arora R, Dubey C, Sukhija A, Daga M, Singh D. Sertoli-Leydig cell tumor: a rare ovarian neoplasm. Case report and review of literature. *Gynecol Endocrinol.* 2008;24:230–234.

13. Alkushi A, Young RH, Clement PB. Cellular fibromas of the ovary: a study of 62 cases including 24 with ≥4 MFs/10 HPFs. *Mod Pathol.* 2004;17:189A.

14. Hayes MC, Scully RE. Ovarian steroid cell tumors (not otherwise specified). A clinicopathologic analysis of 63 cases. *Am J Surg Pathol.* 1987;11:835–835.

15. Laufer, MR, Goldstein, DP. Benign and malignant ovarian masses. In: Emans JE, Laufer MR, Goldstein DP, eds. *Pediatric and Adolescent Gynecology.* 5th ed. Philadelphia: Lippincott Williams & Wilkins; 2005.

16. Nilof JM, Knapp RC, Schaetzel E, Reynolds C, Bast RC Jr. CA 125 antigen levels in obstetrics and gynecological patients. *Obstet Gynecol.* 1984;64:703–707.

17. Robertson DM, Burger HG, Fuller PJ. Inhibin/activin in ovarian cancer. *Endocr Relat Cancer.* 2004;11:35–49.

18. Petraglia F, Luisi S, Pautier P, et al. Inhibin B is the major form of inhibin/activin family secreted by granulose cell tumors. *J Clin Endocrinol Metab.* 1998;83:1029–1032.

19. Huang JN, Liu YZ, Zhang XM. Clinical analysis of juvenile ovary granulosa cell tumor. *Zhuongha Fu Chan Ki Za Zi.* 2007;42:533–536.

20. Pectasides D, Pectasides A. Granulosa cell tumor of the ovary. *Cancer Treat Rev.* 2008;34:1–12.

21. Rey RA, Lhomme C, Marcillac I, et al. Antimullerian hormone as a serum marker of granulose cell tumors of the ovary: comparative study with serum alpha-inhibin and estradiol. *Am J Obstet Gynecol.* 1996;174:958–965.

22. Scully R, Young RH, Clement PB. Tumors of the ovary and maldeveloped gonads. In: *Atlas of Tumor Pathology.* Washington, DC: AFIP; 1998.

23. Acs G. Intraoperative consultation in gynecologic pathology. *Semin Diagn Pathol.* 2002;19:237–254.

24. Seidman JD, Kurman RJ, Ronnett BM. Primary and metastatic mucinous adenocarcinomas in the ovaries: incidence in routine practice with a new approach to improve intraoperative diagnosis. *Am J Surg Pathol.* 2003;27:985–993.

25. Saglam EA, Usubütün A, Ayhan A, Küçükali T. Mistakes prevent mistakes: experience from intraoperatie consultation with frozen section. *Eur J Obstet Gynecol Reprod Biol.* 2006;125:266–268.

26. Baker P, Oliva E. A practical approach to intraoperative consultation in gynecological pathology. *Gynecol Pathol.* 2008; 27:353–365.

27. Zhang M, Cheung M, Shin J, et al. Prognostic factors responsible for survival in sex cord stromal tumors of the ovary—an analysis of 376 women. *Gynecol Oncol.* 2007;104:396–400.

28. Stenwig JT, Hazekamp JT, Beecham JB. Granulosa cell tumors of the ovary. A clinicopathological study of 118 cases with long-term follow-up. *Gynecol Oncol.* 1979;7:136–152.

29. Fox H, Agrawal K, Langley F. A clinicopathologic study of 92 cases of granulose cell tumor of the ovary with special reference to the factors influencing prognosis. *Cancer.* 1975;35:231–241.

30. Evans AT, Gaffey TA, Malkasian GD, et al. Clinico-pathologic review of 118 granulosa and 82 theca cell tumors. *Obstet Gynecol.* 1980;55:231–238

31. Hirakawa M, Nigai Y, Yagi C, Nashiro T, Inamine M, Aoki Y. Recurrent juvenile granulosa cell tumor of the ovary managed by palliative radiotherapy. *Int J Gynecol Cancer.* 2007.

32. Young RH, Dickerson GR, Scully RE. Juvenile granulosa cell tumors of the ovary: a clinicopathologic review of 125 cases. *Am J Surg Pathol.* 1984;8:575–596.

33. Bridges NA, Christopher JA, Hindmarsh PC, Brook CG. Sexual precocity: Sex incidence and aetiology. *Arch Dis Child.* 1994;70:116.

34. Listernick R, Charrow J, Gutmann DH. Intracranial gliomas in neurofibromatosis type 1. *Am J Med Genet.* 1999;89:38.

35. Ogilvy-Stuart AL, Clayton PE, Shalet SM. Cranial irradiation and early puberty. *J Clin Endocrinol Metab.* 1994;78:1282.

36. Pescovitz OH, Hench K, Green O, et al. Central precocious puberty complicating a virilizing adrenal tumor: treatment with a long-acting LHRH analogg. *J Pediatr.* 1985;106:612.

37. Van Wyk JJ, Grumbach MM. Syndrome of precocious menstruation and galactorrhea in juvenile hypothyroidism: an example of hormonal overlap in pituitary feedback. *J Pediatr.* 1960;57:416.

38. Anasti JN, Flack MR, Frohlich J, et al. A potential novel mechanism for precocious puberty in juvenile hypothyroidism. *J Clin Endocrinol Metab.* 1995;80:276.

39. Weinstein LS, Shenker A, Gejman PV, et al. Activating mutations of the stimulatory G protein in the McCune-Albright syndrome. *N Engl J Med.* 1991;325:1688.

40. Herman-Giddens MD, Slora EJ, Wasserman RC, et al. Secondary sexual characteristics and menses in young girls seen in office practice: a study from the Pediatric Research in Office Settings Network. *Pediatrics.* 1997; 99:505.

41. Kaplowitz PB, Oberfield SE. Reexamination of the age limit for defining when puberty is precocious in girls in the United States: implications for evaluation and treatment. Drug and Therapeutics and Executive Committees of the Lawson Wilkins Pediatric Endocrine Society. *Pediatrics.* 1999;104:936.

42. Heller ME, Dewhurst J, Grant DB. Premature menarche without other evidence of precocious puberty. *Arch Dis Child.* 1979;54:472.

43. Muzii L, Palaia I, Sansone M, et al. Laparoscopic fertility-sparing staging in unexpected early stage ovarian malignancies. *Fertil Steril.* 2009;91:2632–2637.

44. Rabban JT, Gupta D, Zaloudek C, Chen L. Synchronous ovarian granulosa cell tumor and uterine serous carcinoma: a rare association of a high risk endometrial cancer with an estrogenic ovarian tumor. *Gyncecol Oncol.* 2006;103:1164–1168.

45. Bjorkholm E, Silfversward C. Prognostic factors in granulosa cell tumors. *Gynecol Oncol.* 1981;11:261–274.

46. Ohel G, Kaneti H, Schenker JG. Granulosa cell tumors in Israel: a study of 172 cases. *Gynecol Oncol.* 1983;15:278–286.

47. Dockerty MB, Mussey E. Malignant lesions of the uterus associated with estrogen-producing ovarian tumors. *Am J Obstet Gynecol.* 1951;61:147–153.

48. Malmstrom H, Hogberg T, Risberg B, Simonsen E. Granulosa cell tumors of the ovary: prognostic factors and outcome. *Gyncol Oncol.* 1994;52:50–55.

49. Miller BE, Barron BA, Wan JY, Delmore JE, Silva EG, Gershenson DM. Prognostic factors in adult granulosa cell tumor of the ovary. *Cancer* 1997;79(10):1951-5.

50. Miller BE, Barron BA, Dockter ME, Delmore JE, Silva EG, Gershenson DM. Parameters of differentiation and proliferation in adult granulose cell tumors of the ovary. *Cancer Detect Prev.* 2001;25:48–54.

51. Schneider DT, Calaminus G, Wessalowski R, et al. Ovarian sex cord-stromal tumors in children and adolescents. *J Clin Oncol.* 2003;21:2357–2363.

52. Fontanelli R, Stefanon B, Raspagliesi F, et al. Adult granulose cell tumor of the ovary: a clinico pathologic study of 35 cases. *Tumori* 1998;84(1):60-4.

53. Vesco KK, Carney ME. Granulosa cell tumor of the ovary: extensive late recurrence after initial occult microscopic disease. *Obstet Gynecol*. 2002;99:888–891.

54. Crew KD, Cohen MH, Smith DH, et al. Long natural history of recurrent granulose cell tumor of the ovary 23 years after intial diagnosis: a case report and review of the literature. *Gynecol Oncol*. 2005;96:235.

55. Savage P, Constenla D, Fisher C, et al. Granulosa cell tumors of the ovary: demographics, survival and the management of advanced disease. *Clin Oncol*. 1998;10:242–245.

56. Yildiz B. Assessment, diagnosis and treatment of a patient with hirsutism. *Nature Clin Pract*. 2008;4:294–300.

57. Rosenfield RL. Clinical practice: hirsutism. *N Engl J Med*. 2005;353:2578–2588.

58. Martin K, Chang RJ, Ehrmann D, et al. Evaluation and treatment of hirsutism in premenopausal women: an Endocrine Society clinical practice guideline. *J Clin Endocrinol Metab*. 2008;93:1105–1120.

59. McKenna TJ. Screening for sinister causes of hirsutism. *N Engl J Med*. 1994;331:1015.

60. Rittmaster RS. Medical treatment of androgen-dependent hirsutism. *J Clin Endocrinol Metab*. 1995;80:2559.

61. Hatch R, Rosenfield RS, Kim MH, Tredway D. Hirsutism: implications, etiology, and management. *Am J Obstet Gynecol*. 1981;140:815

62. Ferriman D, Gallwey J. Clinical assessment of body hair growth in women. *J Clin Endocrinol Metab*. 1961;21:1440.

63. Meldrum DR, Abraham GE. Peripheral and ovarian venous concentrations of various steroid hormones in virilizing ovarian tumors. *Obstet Gynecol*. 1979;53:36.

64. Friedman CI, Schmidt GE, Kim MH, Powell J. Serum testosterone concentrations in the evaluation of androgen-producing tumors. *Am J Obstet Gynecol*. 1985;153:44.

65. O'Driscoll JB, Mamtora, Higginson J, et al. A prospective study of the prevalence of clear-cut endocrine disorders and polycystic ovaries in 350 patients presenting with hirsutism or androgenic alopecia. *Clin Endocrinol*. 1994;41:231.

66. Derksen J, Nagesser SK, Meinders AE, et al. Identification of virilizing adrenal tumors in hirsute women. *N Engl J Med*. 1994;331:968.

67. Miller KK, Rosner W, Lee H. Measurement of free testosterone in normal women and women with androgen deficiency:comparison of methods. *J Clin Endocrinol Metab*. 2004;89:525.

68. Gheorghisan-Galateanu A, Fica S, Terzea D, Caragheorgheopol A, Horhoianu V. Sertoli-Leydig cell tumor—a rare androgen secreting ovarian tumor in postmentopausal women: case report and review of literature. *J Cell Mol Med*. 2003;7:461–471.

69. Young RH, Scully, RE. Ovarian Sertoli-Leydig cell tumors. A clinico-pathological analysis of 207 cases. *Am J Surg Pathol*. 1985;9:543–569.

70. Metzinger DS, Webb MJ. Surgical management of Sertoli-Leydig cell tumors of the ovary. *CME J Gynecol Oncol*. 2002;7:140–142.

71. Yedema C, Massuger L, Hilgers J, et al. Preoperative discrimination between benign and malignant ovarian tumors using a combination of CA 125 and CA 15.3 serum assays. *Int J Cancer Suppl*. 1988;3:61–67.

72. Abad A, Corzola E, Ruiz F, et al. Meig's syndrome with elevated CA 125: case report and review of the literature. *Eur J Obstet Gynecol*. 1999;82:97–99.

73. Ishiko O, Yoshida H, Sumi T, et al. Vascular endothelial growth factor levels in pleural and peritoneal fluid in Meigs' syndrome. *Eur J Obstet Gynecol Reprod Biol*. 2001;98:129.

74. Samanth KK, Black WC. Benign ovarian stromal tumors associated with free peritoneal fluid. *Am J Obstet Gynecol*. 1970;107:538.

75. Agaba EI, Ekwempo CC, Ugoya SO, Echejo GO. Meigs' syndrome presenting as hemorrhagic pleural effusion. *West Afr J Med*. 2007;26:253.

76. Leung SW, Yuen PM. Ovarian fibroma: a review on the clinical characteristics, diagnostic difficulties and management of 23 cases. *Gynecol Obstet Invest*. 2006;62:1–6.

CHAPTER 12

Germ Cell Tumors of the Ovary

Alberto A. Mendivil, MD
Department of Obstetrics and Gynecology, University of North Carolina School of Medicine, Chapel Hill, NC, USA

Victoria Lin Bae-Jump, MD, PhD
Department of Obstetrics and Gynecology, University of North Carolina School of Medicine, Chapel Hill, NC, USA

Pathology Notes: Chad Livasy, MD
Associate Professor, Department of Pathology and Laboratory Medicine, University of North Carolina School of Medicine, Chapel Hill, NC, USA

Background

Germ cell tumors of the ovary (GCTs) are derived from primitive germ cells of the embryonic gonad and may be either benign or malignant. The benign germ cell tumor (mature teratoma or dermoid) is familiar to all gynecologists and may be managed by ovarian cystectomy in nearly all cases.

This chapter will discuss the malignant germ cell tumors, which are discovered in young women. While these tumors are highly malignant, proper management will usually result in long-term survival as well as preservation of fertility. Success in treating malignant GCTs has resulted from knowledge gained in the treatment of the male (testicular) form of the disease (seminoma and other testicular malignancies), and collaborative clinical trials by groups both inside (Gynecologic Oncology Group) and outside gynecology (Pediatric Oncology Group/Children's Oncology Group).

Ovarian germ cell tumors comprise about 20% to 25% of ovarian neoplasms, but only 3% of these are malignant. The malignant germ cell tumors are relatively rare and very sensitive to chemotherapy, which makes their treatment highly successful. GCTs occur primarily in young women between 10 and 30 years of age (average age 19 years), and represent 70% of ovarian tumors in this age group. Before the late 1980s, treatment consisted of radical surgical resection, followed by prolonged courses of chemotherapy. However, over the past 3 decades, clinical trials have demonstrated excellent outcomes with more conservative surgical and chemotherapy approaches.

GCTs are staged surgically using similar surgical and pathologic criteria as the more common epithelial ovarian cancers according to the International Federation of Gynecology and Obstetrics (FIGO) staging criteria (Chapter 10, Table 10.1).[1] GCTs of the ovary are very similar in histologic subtype to those found in the male testicle. The most common GCT is the benign mature cystic teratoma, which accounts for 25% to 30% of all ovarian tumors. These tumors are typically found in women in the 2nd and 3rd decades of life and rarely in the elderly. Only 10% are bilateral, which makes them amenable to fertility-sparing surgery.

Malignant GCTs, which account for 2% to 3% of ovarian cancers, have several pathologic diagnoses including: dysgerminoma, endodermal sinus

Gynecological Cancer Management: Identification, Diagnosis and Treatment, Edited by Daniel L. Clarke-Pearson and John T. Soper. Published 2010 by Blackwell Publishing, ISBN: 978-1-4051-9079-4.

Table 12.1 Classification of ovarian germ cell tumors

Dysgerminoma
Endodermal sinus tumor
Embryonal carcinoma
Polyembryoma
Non-gestational choriocarcinoma
Teratoma
    Immature
    Mature
    Monodermal or highly specialized
        Struma ovarii
        Carcinoid
Mixed germ cell tumors

From DiSaia PJ, Creasman WT. *Clinical Gynecologic Oncology*. 6th ed. St. Louis: Mosby; 2002.

Table 12.2 Germ cell tumor cell types with associated tumor marker

Cell type	Tumor marker
Dysgerminoma	LDH, hCG[a]
Endodermal sinus tumor	AFP, LDH
	hCG, AFP
Embryonal carcinoma	LDH[a]
Polyembryoma	hCG, AFP
Choriocarcinoma	hCG, LDH[a]
	AFP[a]
Mixed germ cell	LDH[a]
Immature teratoma	AFP[a], LDH[a]

hCG, human chorionic gonadotropin; AFP, alpha-fetoprotein; LDH, lactate dehydrogenase.
[a]Marker may or may not be present.

tumor, immature teratoma, and the mixed primitive germ cell tumor (Table 12.1). Pure embryonal carcinomas, polyembryomas, and nongestational choriocarcinomas are exceedingly rare. Tumor markers are frequently elevated in patients with specific germ cell tumor types, as discussed below (Table 12.2).

Brief description of ovarian GCTs

Dysgerminomas (analogous to male testicular seminoma) are malignant tumors that account for half of ovarian GCTs and 2% of all ovarian malignancies.[2, 3] Approximately 75% of women are diagnosed with stage I disease. Bilateral ovarian disease is more common with dysgerminomas than any of the other malignant GCTs, with involvement of the contralateral ovary occurring in 10% of cases. Patients typically present with acute onset of abdominal pain and a pelvic mass. Grossly, the ovary contains a large, lobulated, solid mass that is cream or tan colored. Central necrosis may be observed. Dysgerminomas can be found in the dysgenetic ovaries of phenotypic females who have a Y chromosome. Women included in this group are those with pure gonadal dysgenesis (46X,Y), mixed gonadal genesis with mosaicism (45X/46X,Y), or complete androgen insensitivity (46X,Y). Given the

increased risk of recurrence and of developing a gonadoblastoma if the dysgenetic ovary is left in situ, a normal karyotype must be confirmed for fertility-sparing surgery.

The tumor marker most frequently elevated in dysgerminomas is lactate dehydrogenase (LDH) (Table 12.2). Occasionally, human chorionic gonadotropin (hCG) can be elevated, and does not necessarily indicate the presence of choriocarcinoma elements.

Endodermal sinus tumors, also called yolk sac tumors, are malignant tumors that account for 20% of ovarian GCTs, representing the second most common tumor type. They are found primarily in young girls and women with a mean age of 18 years of age at presentation.[4] About one-third of patients are pre-menarchal. Grossly, the ovarian mass is yellowish and more friable than those seen with dysgerminomas. These tumors are usually necrotic and contain areas of focal hemorrhage. Patients typically present with the acute onset of abdominal pain and a pelvic mass. Endodermal sinus tumors are known to behave very aggressively, often resulting in rapid growth and extensive intraperitoneal dissemination. The tumor marker commonly elevated in endodermal sinus tumors is alpha-fetoprotein (AFP) (Table 12.2). Serum LDH may also be elevated.

Embryonal carcinomas represent 5% of malignant GCTs. These are one of the most aggressive tumors of the ovary and are typically found in teenagers. The most common presentation of embryonal carcinomas is abdominal pain and a pelvic mass. Clinically, patients also may also present with precocious puberty, abnormal uterine bleeding, hirsutism, or amenorrhea due to the endogenous production of testosterone and estrogen. Serum hCG and AFP are often both elevated (Table 12.2) and can be used to follow patients with embryonal carcinoma. Pregnancy tests may be deceivingly positive since these tumors produce hCG.

Polyembryoma is a rare tumor that is normally found as a component of mixed germ cell tumors. This tumor is very aggressive with extensive local invasion and often distant metastases. The typical patient is pre-pubertal and may show signs of sexual precocity. Patients with these tumors often have elevated levels of hCG and AFP (Table 12.2).

Non-gestational choriocarcinoma in its pure form is extremely rare. Most patients who present with this tumor are younger than 20 years old. Precocious puberty (50% of patients) and irregular vaginal bleeding are common among women with these tumors. Gestational choriocarcinoma associated with pregnancy and non-gestational choriocarcinoma are histologically identical; however, DNA analysis can reliably distinguish between these two entities. If paternal DNA is found within the tumor, this confirms a gestational or placental origin. Ovarian choriocarcinomas, similarly to their gestational counterparts, have a tendency for early hematogenous metastases to such sites as the lung, liver, brain, bone, and vagina. Unfortunately, in contrast to gestational choriocarcinomas, pure ovarian choriocarcinomas respond poorly to chemotherapy and are most often fatal. hCG is a well-known tumor marker for all choriocarcinomas (Table 12.2).

Teratomas present in mature (benign) and immature (malignant) forms. *Mature cystic teratomas (dermoid cysts)* are common, benign, and contain the three germ cell layers: ectoderm (hair, skin, teeth), mesoderm, and endoderm. They account for 95% of all teratomas and have a characteristic appearance on ultrasound. Dermoid cysts are surgically managed by ovarian cystectomy or unilateral salpingo-oophorectomy. These lesions can be bilateral in 10% to 15% of cases. Malignant transformation of dermoid cysts is rare, occurring in less than 2% of cases. The most common cell type in patients with malignant transformation of a dermoid cyst is squamous cell carcinoma.

Immature teratoma is the third most common type of malignant GCT but comprises less than 1% of ovarian teratomas. It consists of all three germ cell layers (ectoderm, mesoderm, and endoderm) and contains immature or embryonal structures (Plate 12.1). These tumors are found classically before the age of 20. They are graded according to the quantity of immature neural tissue seen on histopathologic evaluation, where grade 0 lesions are well differentiated with rare foci of immature neural tissue and grade 3 lesions have large amounts of immature neural tissue, embryonal tissue, atypical cells, and mitotic figures. Tumor grade is an important indicator of the risk of extra-ovarian spread and overall prognosis. Immature teratomas have lost the ability to secrete hormones, and thus there are no characteristic tumors markers. However, AFP and LDH may be elevated in rare cases (Table 12.2).

Mixed germ cell tumors contain at least two malignant germ cell components. Dysgerminoma is the most common malignant GCT found in mixed germ cell tumors (69–80%) and is usually associated with an endodermal sinus tumor. If a dysgerminomatous element is found, the contralateral ovary is involved 10% of the time.

Patients with stage IA dysgerminomas and stage IAG1 unruptured immature teratomas do not require additional therapy. For all others, as well as those with advanced-stage disease, multimodality therapy is required, consisting of fertility-sparing surgery and platinum-based chemotherapy. Advanced stage GCTs is not as ominous a prognostic factor as it is epithelial ovarian cancer. Advanced cases of malignant GCTs are typically very chemosensitive and should be considered potentially curable.

Pathology notes

The most commonly encountered germ cell tumor is the benign mature cystic teratoma (MCT), which is the most common benign tumor in reproductive-age women. Approximately 15% of MCTs are bilateral. Pathologic evaluation of MCT is typically straightforward. The pathologist needs to exclude any immature elements, particularly for younger patients with more solid masses. Immature elements are rare in patients over 30 years of age. Intraoperative diagnosis of MCT can usually be made by gross examination alone when the classic cystic appearance is seen in association with hair and keratinous debris. Frozen section evaluation is appropriate for teratomas showing areas of solid growth. A definitive diagnosis of immature elements on frozen section should be cautioned unless the pathologist sees clear formation of primitive neuroepithelial rosettes (Plate 12.1). A frozen section diagnosis of immature teratoma based solely on immature mesenchymal elements is unreliable, as benign mesenchymal elements or cerebellum formation may lead to an incorrect diagnosis. The pathologist also needs to exclude the presence of carcinoma arising in a mature cystic teratoma. Histologic types of malignant degeneration include squamous cell carcinoma, carcinoids, and thyroid carcinomas. Struma ovarii are monodermal teratomas comprised almost exclusively of thyroid tissue. These tumors are expected to show benign biological behavior unless malignant change is observed. Most malignant struma ovarii have pathologic features of papillary thyroid carcinoma. Evidence of thyroid differentiation can be confirmed with immunohistochemical stains for thyroid transcription factor-1 (TTF1) and thyroglobulin for problematic cases. Teratomas may also show carcinoid differentiation with multiple architectural patterns including insular, trabecular, and goblet cell. Immunohistochemical stains for neuroendocrine markers (synaptophysin and chromogranin) are usually required to make the diagnosis.

Immature teratomas occur predominantly in the first 2 decades of life. Tumors containing immature elements or showing atypical gross features including solid tumor growth should be well sampled. Thorough sampling is required to accurately assess the quantity of immature elements for grading purposes. Tumor grade and stage should be reported for all cases containing immature elements. Immature teratomas should be graded based either on a three-tier scheme from 1 to 3,[5] or a two-tier scheme[6] where the terms "low grade" and "high grade" are used. The grades are determined by the volume of immature elements quantified at 40× magnification. Grade 1 (low-grade), stage I tumors contain scant immature elements (<1 per 40× field on a given slide), and most are expected to show indolent clinical behavior. Peritoneal "metastatic" deposits of mature teratomatous elements composed of mature glial tissue are observed in approximately 10% of patients with immature teratoma, and this phenomenon is termed gliomatous peritonei. This change should be considered biologically benign provided the implants are histologically mature.

Other malignant germ cell tumors include dysgerminoma, yolk sac tumor, embryonal carcinoma, and choriocarcinoma. These tumors are all considered high grade and are not further graded or classified. The pathologist's task for these tumors is to correctly classify the tumor, often with the help of special stains such as alpha-fetoprotein and hCG, and determine whether the neoplasm is pure or mixed. For malignant mixed germ cell tumors, each component should be documented in the pathology report along with their relative percentages.

Frozen section evaluation of malignant germ cell neoplasms can be difficult as they are poorly differentiated tumors with subtle defining features. Multiple sections and special stains are typically needed to classify these tumors. Some carcinomas, such as clear cell carcinoma, show histologic features similar to germ cell tumors, and a definite distinction between the two may not always be able to be made at frozen section. In

Pathology notes (*continued*)

young patients where malignant germ cell tumor is high on the differential, communication of any preoperative AFP or hCG results to the patholo- gist during intraoperative consultation is helpful in subtyping a malignant neoplasm as germ cell in origin.

Incidence

In the United States, the age-adjusted incidence for malignant GCTs is about 0.5 per 100,000, which is about 40 times less than epithelial ovarian cancer. The incidence peaks in the early 20s, and these tumors are three times more common in Asian and black women than Caucasian women, for unknown reasons. GCTs account for about 60% of all ovarian tumors; and of these, 3% are malignant.[7]

Etiology/Biology

The biology of ovarian GCT, like testicular can- cer, is thought to originate from defective meiosis leading to the activation of multiple pathways in- volved in gametogenesis and ultimately, resulting in the development of the unique phenotypes seen in GCT. Genetic instability may result from a defec- tive switch from mitosis to meiosis and in essence, renders cells that are able to express functions and structures unique to both states.[8] Surti and col- leagues found that 65% of teratomas are derived from a single germ cell after meiosis I and failure of meiosis II. Approximately 35% of teratomas arise from failure of meiosis I or mitotic division of pre- meiotic germ cells.[9] Karyotypic abnormalities are common and include chromosome abnormalities. The short arm of chromosome 12 (12p) has been implicated in both ovarian and testicular GCT, sug- gesting that this region plays an important role in the neoplastic transformation of these tumors.[10, 11] PTEN is a tumor suppressor gene that is altered in endometrioid adenocarcinoma of the uterus and has been shown to be absent in 86% of embryonal carcinomas and virtually all teratomas.[12, 13]

Risks/Clinical presentation

Clinically, the typical patient with a GCT is young and may present with any of the following: acute abdominal pain (sometimes mistaken for appen- dicitis), abdominal bloating, precocious puberty, abnormal vaginal bleeding (if the tumor is estrogen secreting), or with a positive pregnancy test (if the tumor is hCG producing). When patients with ma- lignant GCTs experience abdominal pain, it may be due to rupture, hemorrhage, or torsion of the ad- nexal mass. Symptoms may arise acutely due to the characteristic rapid growth of these tumors. Torsion and rupture are reported in 5% and 20% of cases, respectively.

GCTs can present in pregnancy or immediately postpartum. Currently, many pregnancy-related cases are first diagnosed during fetal ultrasound evaluation. Persistently elevated AFP, despite sono- graphic absence of neural tube defects, should war- rant evaluation of the adnexa for a possible GCT (yolk-sac tumor, embryonal carcinoma). Surgery may be required for an enlarged adnexal mass di- agnosed during pregnancy, particularly if serum markers are elevated and/or the patient is symp- tomatic. The optimal time for surgery is generally in the mid-second trimester (See Chapter 13 for a more detailed discussion of management of the adenxal mass in pregnancy).

Malignant GCTs tend to enlarge and progress rapidly. The most common symptom is abdominal pain (55–80%). Stage distribution is virtually the opposite from epithelial ovarian cancer. Approximately 60% to 70% of cases are FIGO stage I or II, 20% to 30% are stage III, and stage IV is rare. Bilateral ovarian involvement is typically seen in patients with dysgerminomas (10–15%) or with metastases from advanced disease;

Table 12.3 Comparison of survival according to stage for GCTs and epithelial ovarian cancers

FIGO stage	5-year survival (%) germ cell tumors	5-year survival (%) epithelial ovarian cancers
I	95–100	78
II	85	71
III	79	40
IV	71	13

otherwise, most tumors are unilateral. Benign cystic teratomas are seen in 5% to 10% of cases and involve the contralateral ovary of patients with unilateral malignant GCT. Malignant tumors metastasize through spread to peritoneal surfaces or via lymphatic and hematogenous routes. Dysgerminomas have a predilection to metastasize via the bloodstream and lymphatic channels.[14] Malignant GCTs in general are more likely than epithelial ovarian cancers to metastasize to the lung and liver parenchyma. There are several recognized prognostic factors for malignant GCTs, including stage, histology (dysgerminoma and immature teratoma are relatively favorable histologic types), preoperative serum tumor marker level (hCG, AFP), and residual disease after primary surgery. Age at diagnosis is not a significant prognostic factor. Five-year survival for GCTs is 100% for stage I, 85% for stage II, 79% for stage III, and 71% for stage IV disease.[15,16] Overall survival is much better for GCTs as compared to epithelial ovarian cancers (Table 12.3).

Clinical Scenario 1

A 19-year-old college student presents to the emergency department with the acute onset of abdominal pain, nausea, and vomiting. She also reports worsening vaginal bleeding during her menstrual cycle and feeling bloated. A 15-cm abdominal-pelvic mass is found on clinical examination.

What is the differential diagnosis of this mass?

Acute onset of abdominal pain in a young woman of child-bearing potential can have many different etiologies and should be quickly triaged to avoid further complications that might compromise fertility. These acute symptoms could be attributed to ectopic pregnancy, appendicitis, ovarian torsion or cyst rupture, tubo-ovarian abscess (TOA), or trauma/domestic violence.

The differential diagnosis for a pelvic mass varies by age group (Table 12.4). In adolescent patients, the etiology of a pelvic mass could be the result of an anatomic anomaly such as Müllerian malformations, appendiceal abscesses, and ovarian tumors (ie, teratomas). In premenopausal patients, etiologies include functional cysts and other benign ovarian neoplasms as well as pregnancy-associated masses such as tubal or corneal pregnancies. Inflammatory causes, such as an appendiceal abscess, tubo-ovarian abscesses, or hydrosalpinx, can also produce the same symptoms. Malignant adnexal masses in this age group are often unilateral and can present with symptoms of acute abdominal pain. The incidence of an ovarian malignancy

Table 12.4 Differential diagnosis of pelvic masses in premenopausal women

Ovarian Masses in Young Women
- Follicular cysts
- Hemorrhagic cysts
- Corpus luteum
- Endometrioma
- Theca lutein cysts
- Neoplasms (benign, borderline, malignant)
- Metastatic disease (breast, colon, endometrium)

Extra-Ovarian Masses
- Ectopic pregnancy
- Hydrosalpinx
- Tubo-ovarian abscess
- Paratubal cyst
- Inflammatory bowel disease
- Pedunculated fibroid
- Appendiceal abscess
- Fallopian tube cancer
- Pelvic kidney

in the premenopausal age group is only about 8%. Epithelial ovarian cancer is extremely rare in women under the age of 20. However, malignant masses may have additional findings on imaging such as ascites, bilateral ovarian involvement, and thick internal septations. There may also be findings consistent with hormone overproduction such as hCG in the case of dysgerminomas[17] or elevated levels of estrogen produced by a granulosa cell tumor. Uterine leiomyomas can also present as distinct pelvic masses, especially those that are pedunculated, and these may undergo torsion or infarction and cause significant discomfort.

What should be included in the evaluation of this patient?

Pregnancy, including ectopic pregnancy, should be immediately ruled out as a cause of abdominal pain in a woman of child-bearing age. A thorough medical history is important to help establish a narrowed differential diagnosis. Menstrual history, use of contraceptives (including an IUD), or past history of STIs may suggest a higher probability of tubo-ovarian abscess. A history of infertility or symptoms of endometriosis (dysmenorrhea, dyspareunia, dyschezia) can lead the examiner to consider endometrioma as the cause for the adnexal mass. A family history of malignancies such as breast or ovarian cancer can place a woman at a much increased risk for epithelial ovarian cancer, raising the suspicion for this as the etiology of an ovarian mass (although epithelial ovarian cancer is very unlikely in a 19-year-old).

A chronic or acute history of gastrointestinal symptoms may suggest appendicitis or inflammatory bowel disease. Onset of pain, fever, nausea, vomiting, undulating pain, bloating, early satiety, and bowel or bladder dysfunction can all serve as clues to assist in making a diagnosis.

A unilateral mobile adnexal cyst that is less than 7 cm in diameter is most often benign, particularly in this patient's age group. Rapidly enlarging, fixed, nodular, or bilateral masses are more concerning for malignancy. However, many benign conditions encountered in the younger premenopausal age group, such as endometriosis or pelvic inflammatory disease with tubo-ovarian abscesses, might produce similar physical findings. Germ cell tumors do not have specific physical findings.

Imaging studies can be useful in establishing an operative plan prior to surgery and can be used to better counsel the patient and/or family members. Ultrasound is currently the best, easiest, and least invasive study for evaluating the adnexa and should be used as the first study of choice. Transabdominal combined with transvaginal ultrasound (TVU) has a high sensitivity and specificity for establishing the diagnoses of certain adnexal masses (endometrioma, dermoid cyst) due to their distinctive characteristic features. Other valuable information includes a description of the complexity of the mass—solid and/or cystic, presence of internal septations, ascites, nodularity, or excrescences. Endometriomas often show homogenous echoes, may have thick walls, and can be unilocular or multilocular (Fig. 12.1). Dermoid cysts (benign cystic teratoma) have densities that differ across the mass due to the presence of bone, hair, and sebaceous material (Fig. 12.2). Serous cysts are typically anechoic, smaller, and bilateral while mucinous cysts have internal echogenicity due to the viscous nature of the mucinous fluid, and tend to be larger and unilateral.[18]

While ultrasound is fast, easy, and relatively inexpensive in evaluating adnexal masses, CT and MRI can also be helpful in establishing a diagnosis. The use of CT exposes the patient to ionizing radiation and iodinated intravenous contrast, which may be relatively contraindicated in circumstances where the patient is pregnant, has impaired renal function, or has an allergy to intravenous contrast. There may also be a delay in acquiring the study or the results in a timely fashion. MRI is excellent at differentiating tissue planes and provides detail in three dimensions. MRI can be limited by the time it takes to obtain the study or if the patient is claustrophobic or allergic to the intravenous contrast agent (rare).[19] CT or MRI are typically not indicated in circumstances where the patient

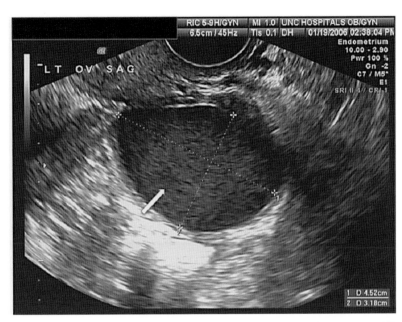

Figure 12.1 Ultrasound image of an endometrioma illustrating the heterogenous echogenic material (*arrow*) representing liquefied coagulated blood; the uniform consistency of the cyst and the clear demarcations are also representative of an endometrioma. (Image compliments of Alice Chuang, MD, Department of Obstetrics and Gynecology, University of North Carolina.)

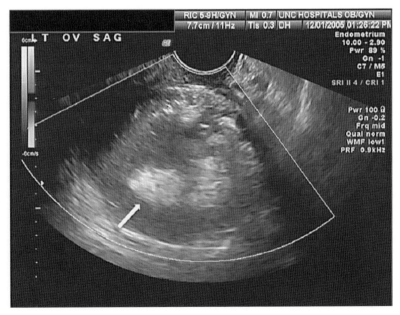

Figure 12.2 Ultrasound of benign cystic teratoma (dermoid cyst). *Arrow* shows an echo-dense area of the cyst representing one of multiple calcified portions of the cyst that may consist of teeth, cartilage, or bone. Dermoid cysts may also contain echo-lucent cystic pockets containing sebum, hair, or serous fluid. (Image compliments of Alice Chuang, MD, Department of Obstetrics and Gynecology, University of North Carolina.)

Table 12.5 Conditions that elevate serum CA-125

Gynecologic	Non-gynecologic	Non-gynecologic cancers
Ovarian cancer	Ascites	Breast cancer
Pelvic inflammatory disease	Mesothelioma	Lung cancer
Uterine fibroids	Lupus	Pancreatic cancer
Uterine cancer	Pleural effusions	Colon cancer
Endometriosis	Liver disease and cirrhosis	
Fallopian tube cancer	Congestive heart failure	
Adenocarcinoma of the cervix	Diverticulitis	
Adenomyosis	Colitis	
Ovarian cysts	Diabetes	
Benign ovarian neoplasms	Pericarditis	
Meig syndrome	Renal disease	
Pregnancy	Sarcoidosis	
Menstruation	Tuberculosis	

is acutely symptomatic from a pelvic mass, because the patient will likely need surgical intervention regardless of the radiographic findings. Postoperatively, CT or MRI imaging may be helpful particularly in cases of ovarian cancer where there is gross residual tumor remaining, and these studies may be used to follow the patient's progress through chemotherapy.

Tumor markers can be useful in suggesting a diagnosis. In this patient's case, a germ cell tumor would be the most likely malignancy and obtaining serum markers for germ cell tumors would be most appropriate (Table 12.2). hCG is useful to exclude pregnancy but can also be elevated in dysgerminomas, embryonal carcinomas, polyembryomas, choriocarcinomas, and mixed germ cell tumors. AFP and LDH can be useful to follow endodermal sinus tumors and other GCTs, but laboratory results of AFP frequently will not be available for several days. In an acute setting, hCG may be available relatively quickly but it is not necessary to delay intervention while awaiting results of other tumor markers, as they will usually not change the initial management of the patient.

CA-125 is another tumor marker frequently used to assess adnexal masses. It is elevated in over 80% of all women with epithelial ovarian cancer. However, other medical conditions may cause CA-125 serum levels to rise, particularly in premenopausal women (Table 12.5). Common gynecologic conditions that can lead to an increase in CA-125 include pregnancy, infection, uterine fibroids, and endometriosis. Any condition that causes disruption or inflammation of the peritoneum may also elevate the serum CA-125. For young premenopausal patients where the risk of epithelial ovarian cancer is extremely low, CA-125 is not very useful in narrowing the differential diagnosis.[20]

Clinical Scenario 2

The patient is an 18-year-old with a pelvic mass that is solid and cystic based on ultrasound findings and measures 15 cm. The mass has a smooth capsule. Intraoperatively, there is 100 mL of ascites and the mass arises from the right adenxae. It is not adherent and there is no other evidence of metastases upon survey of the peritoneal cavity. A cystectomy cannot be performed, so the entire mass (salpingo-oophorectomy) is removed. Frozen section reveals either a germ cell tumor or a granulosa cell tumor. The two diagnoses cannot be confirmed until permanent sections and special stains are used.

What is the proper surgical procedure? Does she need a TAH, BSO? Should the appendix be removed?

Patients with malignant ovarian GCTs or sex cord–stromal tumors (such as granulosa cell tumors) found on frozen section can present a dilemma from the surgeon's point of view. Fortunately, the surgical approach is very similar for all histologic subtypes. The primary message is that ovarian cancers in young women should be managed in a more conservative fashion as compared to older women with epithelial cancers. Most patients with germ cell tumors are young (average age 19 years) and desire to preserve fertility if at all possible. Fortunately, most germ cell tumors are confined to one ovary. Furthermore, given the extreme sensitivity of GCTs to chemotherapy with excellent survival results, we have found that extensive debulking (including a TAH, BSO) is not helpful. Therefore, the surgeon should plan to preserve fertility and avoid hysterectomy and BSO in these cases.

In most cases, a unilateral salpingo-oophorectomy is performed, followed by surgical staging. Staging should include:

- Complete exploration of the peritoneal cavity and palpation of pelvic and paraaortic lymph nodes
- Washings from the peritoneal cavity are submitted for cytologic examination.
- Care should be taken to avoid manipulation and trauma to the contralateral ovary and tube in order to preserve fertility
- Additional staging should include:
  - Omentectomy
  - Pelvic and para-aortic lymphadenectomy
  - Excision of any suspicious lesions

If laparoscopy was used to remove the affected ovary, it is acceptable to proceed with laparoscopic surgical staging if the surgeon is appropriately trained. For advanced-stage disease, laparotomy is still the approach of choice.

Surgical treatment in women who have completed child-bearing traditionally includes total hysterectomy with bilateral salpingo-oophorectomy, bilateral pelvic and para-aortic lymphadenectomy, and biopsies of the pelvic peritoneum including the posterior cul-de-sac, bladder reflection, para-colic gutters and diaphragmatic surface. The omentum should also be removed. In younger women, however, the contralateral ovary and uterus should be preserved if at all possible. Removal of the appendix is not necessary, given the low probability of metastases.

Can fertility-sparing surgery be performed in women with germ cell tumors of the ovary? What are the chances of having a normal pregnancy after being treated with surgery and chemotherapy?

GCTs tumors tend to be unilateral and present at an early stage in about 70% of cases. Fertility-sparing surgical staging is indicated for both malignant GCTs and sex cord–stromal tumors because the ovary is the most common site of disease at diagnosis (95%). Fertility-sparing surgery consists of unilateral salpingo-oophorectomy, pelvic and para-aortic lymph node dissection, peritoneal biopsies (bladder reflection, posterior cul-de-sac, bilateral para-colic gutters, and diaphragmatic surface), and omentectomy. The ipsilateral fallopian tube should be removed because of the intimate vascular and lymphatic connections between the ovary and tube. Survival does not seen to be compromised by using conservative management for patients with early-stage malignant GCTs.

A critical question is whether a patient's fertility is affected by surgery alone. In a study at Charing Cross Hospital, 86% of patients underwent fertility-sparing surgery for primary ovarian disease with the majority (93%) only having unilateral salpingo-oophorectomy. Approximately 54% of these patients had a subsequent successful pregnancy.[21] Another study of 86 patients with malignant GCTs had a fertility-sparing surgery rate of 74%, and 76% of those patients achieved at least one pregnancy. Half of the patients who achieved a pregnancy had received adjuvant chemotherapy, and none of the children born to these patients had any evidence of congenital anomalies.[24]

Fertility-sparing surgery in malignant GCTs does not compromise survival. In a study by Low and Perrin, 74 patients underwent fertility-sparing surgery for malignant GCTs. The average age in their series was 21 years. Approximately 75% were stage I, 4% were stage II, 15% were stage III, and 5% were stage IV. At a follow-up period of 52 months, survival was 98% for early-stage disease (stage I, II) and 94% for patients with advanced disease. Of those patients who underwent chemotherapy, 62% developed amenorrhea but 92% had a normal return to menstrual function at the conclusion of chemotherapy. There were 14 babies born to this cohort of patients who underwent chemotherapy, with no reported congenital anomalies.[25]

For those women who undergo chemotherapy, there is a risk of ovarian dysfunction and failure. Fortunately, the majority of young women who are cancer survivors can anticipate normal menstrual (> 80% of women) and reproductive function. Factors such as older age at the initiation of treatment, greater cumulative drug dose, and longer duration of chemotherapy may contribute to the compromise of ovarian function. The only established method for preservation of child-bearing potential in women at risk for ovarian failure is embryo cryopreservation. This technique should be offered to appropriate candidates before the initiation of chemotherapy. Other experimental techniques with unknown efficacy include cryopreservation of oocytes or ovarian tissue.

Is biopsy of a normal-appearing ovary appropriate or necessary as part of staging?

Staging for malignant GCTs calls for inspection and palpation of gynecologic organs, the peritoneal cavity, and retroperitoneal lymphatic chains. Once the affected ovary is removed and staging is complete, the contralateral ovary should be thoroughly inspected. If the contralateral ovary appears normal, it is best to avoid biopsy or extensive manipulation, including avoiding trauma to the fallopian tube, as this may lead to secondary infertility due to adhesion formation or ovarian failure.[14] Results from reports of fertility-sparing surgery for malignant GCTs have given further credence to keeping the contralateral ovary completely intact. Even if the contralateral ovary contained occult metastatic disease, postoperative chemotherapy will usually result in cure and fertility may be maintained. In cases where there is a small tumor implant on the contralateral ovary, we would advise excision of the implant but preservation of the ovary.

How often is the contralateral ovary involved?

Contralateral involvement of the ovary in malignant GCTs occurs in 10% to 15% of cases. In cases where there is a contralateral lesion, 15% of those tumors are benign cystic teratomas (dermoid cyst). The normal ovary should be smooth and white but may include areas of yellow hue (resolving corpus luteum). Normal ovaries should measure approximately 2 to 3 cm × 2 to 3 cm × 1 to 2 cm in height, length, and width, respectively. Patients with polycystic ovarian syndrome may have ovaries that are double the size of normal.

If the contralateral ovary appears to have a lesion or is enlarged, a wedge biopsy can be safely performed via either laparotomy or laparoscopy. During laparotomy, a fresh #11 scalpel and a pair of smooth forceps can be used to grasp and incise the ovary at the site of the lesion and preferably immediately opposite the hilum. If there is a solid and cystic component to the ovary, it is best to biopsy the solid portion. The size of the biopsy does not need to be large. A portion the size of a small pea is more than sufficient. The specimen should be sent for frozen section for evaluation. Care must be taken in performing biopsies of contralateral ovaries due to the concern of postoperative adhesion formation and impairment of fertility. In most cases, patients with microscopic involvement of the contralateral ovary can be treated successfully with chemotherapy, and the ovary may be preserved.

What tumor markers should be obtained?

Malignant GCTs and sex cord–stromal tumors (such as granulosa cell tumors of the ovary) secrete many different serum tumor markers. When frozen section cannot differentiate between tumor types, markers for both suspected diseases should be obtained as soon as possible (even in the operating room if feasible). For germ cell tumors, AFP, hCG, and LDH may helpful in the follow-up of the patient (Table 12.2). In a young patient, CA-125 will not be useful, as the likelihood of an epithelial ovarian cancer is very small, and this value can be falsely elevated (Table 12.5). Serum total inhibin is a very specific tumor marker for granulosa cell tumors and should be used to follow patients with this disease.[2]

What would be the appropriate management if the frozen section were not obtained and the final pathology returned with a malignant GCT with no evidence of disease on the surface of the ovary?

Data from the Pediatric Oncology Group indicate that restaging is not needed for a patient who was incompletely staged at the initial surgery for malignant GCT. Five-year survival and overall survival are excellent (>90%) for virtually all stages, even among incompletely staged patients.[21, 22] It is important to provide a thorough description of all peritoneal surfaces in the operative report. In addition, it is essential to note if there was pre- or intra-operative rupture of the mass. This information will be valuable for the gynecologic oncologist upon patient referral. If it is unclear as to the presence of metastatic disease, the oncologist may obtain further imaging followed by debulking surgery if necessary. The final surgical stage will dictate expectant management versus the need for postoperative chemotherapy. The most common chemotherapy regimen for

germ cell tumors is a combination of intravenous bleomycin, etoposide and cisplatin given for 3 to 4 cycles.

References

1. DiSaia PJ, Creasman WT. *Clinical Gynecologic Oncology*. 6th ed. St. Louis: Mosby; 2002.
2. Hoskins WJ, Sadie Jenkins Harmon Collection. *Principles and Practice of Gynecologic Oncology*. 4th ed. Philadelphia: Lippincott Williams & Wilkins; 2005.
3. Zalel Y, Piura B, Elchalal U, Czernobilsky B, Antebi S, Dgani R. Diagnosis and management of malignant germ cell ovarian tumors in young females. *Int J Gynaecol Obstet*. 1996;55:1–10.
4. Berek JS, Hacker NF. *Practical Gynecologic Oncology*. 4th ed. Philadelphia: Lippincott Williams & Wilkins; 2005.
5. Norris HJ, Zirkin HJ, Benson WL. Immature (malignant) teratoma of the ovary: a clinical and pathologic study of 58 cases. *Cancer*. 1976;37;2359–2372.
6. O'Conner DM, Norris HJ. The influence of grade on the outcome of stage I ovarian immature (malignant) teratomas and the reproducibility of grading. *Int J Gynecol Pathol*. 1994;13;283–289.
7. Patterson DM, Rustin GJ. Controversies in the management of germ cell tumours of the ovary. *Curr Opin Oncol*. 2006;18:500–506.
8. Adamah DJ, Gokhale PJ, Eastwood DJ, et al. Dysfunction of the mitotic:meiotic switch as a potential cause of neoplastic conversion of primordial germ cells. *Int J Androl*. 2006;29:219–227.
9. Surti U, Hoffner L, Chakravarti A, Ferrell RE. Genetics and biology of human ovarian teratomas. I. Cytogenetic analysis and mechanism of origin. *Am J Hum Genet*. 1990;47:635–643.
10. Houldsworth J, Korkola JE, Bosl GJ, Chaganti RS. Biology and genetics of adult male germ cell tumors. *J Clin Oncol*. 2006;24:5512–5518.
11. Speleman F, De Potter C, Dal Cin P, et al. i(12p) in a malignant ovarian tumor. *Cancer Genet Cytogenet*. 1990;45:49–53.
12. Mutter GL, Lin MC, Fitzgerald JT, et al. Altered PTEN expression as a diagnostic marker for the earliest endometrial precancers. *J Natl Cancer Inst*. 2000;92:924–930.
13. Di Vizio D, Cito L, Boccia A, et al. Loss of the tumor suppressor gene PTEN marks the transition from intratubular germ cell neoplasias (ITGCN) to invasive germ cell tumors. *Oncogene*. 2005;24:1882–1894.

14. Pectasides D, Pectasides E, Kassanos D. Germ cell tumors of the ovary. *Cancer Treat Rev.* 2008;34:427–441.

15. Lai CH, Chang TC, Hsueh S, et al. Outcome and prognostic factors in ovarian germ cell malignancies. *Gynecol Oncol.* 2005;96:784–791.

16. Murugaesu N, Schmid P, Dancey G, et al. Malignant ovarian germ cell tumors: identification of novel prognostic markers and long-term outcome after multimodality treatment. *J Clin Oncol.* 2006;24:4862–4866.

17. Kinkel K, Lu Y, Mehdizade A, Pelte MF, Hricak H. Indeterminate ovarian mass at US: incremental value of second imaging test for characterization—meta-analysis and Bayesian analysis. *Radiology.* 2005;236:85–94.

18. Granberg S, Wikland M. Ultrasound in the diagnosis and treatment of ovarian cystic tumours. *Hum Reprod.* 1991;6:177–185.

19. Murphy KJ, Brunberg JA, Cohan RH. Adverse reactions to gadolinium contrast media: a review of 36 cases. *AJR Am J Roentgenol.* 1996;167:847–849.

20. Murta EF, Nomelini RS. Early diagnosis and predictors of malignancy of adnexal masses. *Curr Opin Obstet Gynecol.* 2006;18:14–19.

21. Billmire D, Vinocur C, Rescorla F, et al. Outcome and staging evaluation in malignant germ cell tumors of the ovary in children and adolescents: an intergroup study. *J Pediatr Surg.* 2004;39:424–429; discussion 429.

22. Rogers PC, Olson TA, Cullen JW, et al. Treatment of children and adolescents with stage II testicular and stages I and II ovarian malignant germ cell tumors: a Pediatric Intergroup Study—Pediatric Oncology Group 9048 and Children's Cancer Group 8891. *J Clin Oncol.* 2004;22:3563–3569.

23. Patterson DM, Murugaesu N, Holden L, Seckl MJ, Rustin GJ. A review of the close surveillance policy for stage I female germ cell tumors of the ovary and other sites. *Int J Gynecol Cancer.* 2008;18:43–50.

24. Tangir J, Zelterman D, Ma W, Schwartz PE. Reproductive function after conservative surgery and chemotherapy for malignant germ cell tumors of the ovary. *Obstet Gynecol.* 2003;101:251–257.

25. Low JJ, Perrin LC, Crandon AJ, Hacker NF. Conservative surgery to preserve ovarian function in patients with malignant ovarian germ cell tumors. A review of 74 cases. *Cancer.* 2000;89:391–398.

26. Schumer ST, Cannistra SA. Granulosa cell tumor of the ovary. *J Clin Oncol.* 2003;21:1180–1189.

27. Ayhan A, Tuncer ZS, Tuncer R, Mercan R, Yuce K. Granulosa cell tumor of the ovary. A clinicopathological evaluation of 60 cases. *Eur J Gynaecol Oncol.* 1994;15:320–324.

CHAPTER 13
Adnexal Masses in Pregnancy

Ursula Balthazar, MD
Department of Obstetrics and Gynecology, University of North Carolina School of Medicine, Chapel Hill, NC, USA

John F. Boggess, MD
Department of Obstetrics and Gynecology, University of North Carolina School of Medicine, Chapel Hill, NC, USA

Background

Adnexal masses have always occurred during pregnancy; however, with the routine use of ultrasound in prenatal care, the finding of an "incidental" adnexal mass in pregnancy has become more common. In 1986, Lavery and colleagues evaluated the presence of adnexal masses in pregnancy detected during ultrasounds on 3918 asymptomatic pregnant patients. During the first trimester, significant adnexal masses were observed in 8.8% of patients, whereas by 16 to 20 weeks, persistent masses were noted in only 1% of patients.[1] Similar series have been performed, which taken together demonstrate that adnexal masses persist into the second trimester in 1% to 2% of pregnant women.[2, 3] Given the relatively high potential that the general obstetrician/gynecologist may encounter an adnexal mass in his or her gravid patients, it is important to address the etiology of these masses as well as appropriate diagnostic measures, management options, and potential complications.

Gynecological Cancer Management: Identification, Diagnosis and Treatment, Edited by Daniel L. Clarke-Pearson and John T. Soper. Published 2010 by Blackwell Publishing, ISBN: 978-1-4051-9079-4.

Etiology

Similar to the non-pregnant state, adnexal masses detected in pregnancy have a variety of potential etiologies, which are generally uterine or ovarian in origin. The differential diagnosis of the adnexal mass in pregnancy is shown in Table 13.1.[2–4]

Because pregnant women are generally in the earlier reproductive age group, the types of tumors found are often different than those tumors found in the later reproductive age group and during menopause. These include functional cysts, endometriosis, benign ovarian neoplasms, borderline (low malignant potential) tumors, and germ cell tumors, rather than malignant epithelial ovarian tumors. Most masses detected in the first trimester are corpus luteal cysts that generally regress spontaneously by the 16th week of pregnancy; this accounts for the significant difference in prevalence of masses diagnosed in the first compared with the second trimester of pregnancy. The relative frequency of all nonfunctional cysts is basically related to the age group of the pregnant patient population rather than the gravid state itself.

Ovarian malignancy is the second most common gynecologic cancer diagnosed during pregnancy after cervical cancer.[5] Between 2% and 10% of adnexal masses in pregnancy are malignant.[3–5] The most common malignant ovarian tumor diagnosed in the pregnant population is the borderline ovarian tumor or tumor of low malignant potential (LMP). This is in contrast to the general population, where approximately 90% of ovarian cancers

Table 13.1 Differential diagnosis of the adnexal mass in pregnancy

Benign masses	Malignant masses
Functional cysts—follicular, corpus luteum	Borderline epithelial tumor (low malignant potential; LMP)
Benign teratomas	Germ cell tumors —dysgerminomas, endodermal sinus tumors, immature teratoma, etc.
Serous cystadenomas	
Mucinous cystadenomas	Epithelial cancers (serous, mucinous, endometroid, etc.)
Paraovarian cysts	Sex cord–stromal tumors —granulosa cell,
Endometriomas	
Luteoma of pregnancy	Sertoli–Leydig cell, gynandroblastoma
Pedunculated leiomyomas	Metastatic tumors to the ovary

Table 13.2 Risk of ovarian malignancy based on sonographic criteria

Risk of ovarian cancer	Sonographic criteria
Low	Unilocular Simple Thin walled Size < 5 cm
Intermediate	Multilocular Complex Thin septations
High	Solid mass Nodules Papillary formations Excrescences Thick septations Size > 5 cm

are invasive epithelial cancers. The younger age of the pregnant patients likely accounts for the higher incidence of the less aggressive borderline tumor, which has a highly favorable prognosis. In a population-based study, ovarian malignancies identified during pregnancy (excluding LMP tumors) were evaluated.[6] Of the 87 invasive ovarian cancers identified during pregnancy, germ cell tumors were most common, accounting for 39.1% of tumors. This is significantly higher than the 15% to 20% incidence of germ cell tumors seen in the non-pregnant population. Dysgerminomas were the most common germ cell tumors identified.[6] Other tumors identified included epithelial tumors, sex cord–stromal tumors, and less common miscellaneous pathology. In general, the overall distribution of ovarian tumors identified in pregnancy is reflective of the younger patient cohort as opposed to intrinsic effects of pregnancy itself.

Diagnostic evaluation

Given overall safety to the fetus and ability to characterize adnexal masses, ultrasound is the most important diagnostic tool used in the evaluation and management of the adnexal mass in the pregnant patient. The same ultrasound parameters for eval-

uation of an ovarian mass in the nongravid patient can be used (Table 13.2). Based on a literature review of studies evaluating ultrasound of ovarian tumors, ultrasound is more able to make an accurate diagnosis of benign tumors rather than malignant tumors.[2] Use of color-flow Doppler has also been suggested to aid in the differentiation of benign and malignant ovarian masses. However, significant overlap exists in blood flow patterns between the two groups, so Doppler does not offer a significant advantage over ultrasound alone.

Because of its known safety in pregnancy, magnetic resonance imaging (MRI) has also been discussed as potentially providing additional diagnostic information in the evaluation of the adnexal mass during pregnancy. Potential benefits of MRI include its ability to develop three-dimensional images, delineate tissue planes, and characterize tissue composition.[2] In a small case series, MRI was able to correctly identify the etiology in 17 out of 17 adnexal masses in pregnancy compared to ultrasound, which only identified 12 out of 17.[7] In general, however, the additional information that MRI provides to the clinical situation is limited by its cost and availability. Most clinical decisions can be made utilizing the information provided by following ultrasound characterization of the adnexal mass alone.

Management: expectant versus surgical

The majority of discussion about the management of the adnexal mass in pregnancy surrounds the decision of expectant versus surgical management. In considering expectant management, the provider must consider the risks to both the mother and the fetus. Adnexal masses identified during pregnancy are associated with a unique set of potential complications to the pregnant patient. Similar to the nongravid state, patients are at risk for torsion, hemorrhage, and rupture. The incidence of torsion for an adnexal mass in pregnancy has been reported to be from 3% to as high as 43%.[5, 8] Studies have also reported the incidence of cyst rupture to be between 9% and 17%. These complications pose a unique threat during pregnancy, where both the mother and the fetus are at risk. Emergency surgery during pregnancy has been linked with adverse fetal events. Hess and associates reported that patients who underwent emergent surgery for management of complications of an adnexal mass during pregnancy had an increased incidence of spontaneous abortion and preterm delivery compared with patients who underwent non-emergent, elective surgical management.[9] While several subsequent case series have shown no difference in perinatal outcome between the elective and emergent laparotomy groups, the patient should be clearly informed of potential risks of observation, emergency surgery, and elective surgery.[6] Another potential benefit for removal of the mass during pregnancy includes preventing obstruction of labor if the mass is located in the posterior cul-de-sac at the time of delivery.[10]

If the decision is made to proceed with surgical removal of the adnexal mass, timing of the procedure is important. Because most masses identified during early pregnancy are corpus lutea or other functional cysts that usually resolve by 16 weeks gestation, elective removal of an adnexal mass is generally recommended if it persists into the second trimester. Delaying surgery until around 16 to 18 weeks prevents unnecessary surgery by allowing resolution of these functional cysts. Additionally, delaying surgery until the second trimester may also decrease the rate of miscarriage from potential disruption of the corpus luteum. Delay also prevents exposure of the fetus to anesthesia during organogenesis, which is typically complete by the end of the first trimester. Additionally, surgery past the early second trimester may require a larger incision to obtain adequate exposure and places the patient at higher risk for premature labor.

While laparoscopy has become the preferred method for evaluating most abnormal ovarian masses in young, nongravid women, adnexal masses in pregnancy have traditionally been removed via laparotomy through a vertical midline incision. Cited concerns for the use of laparoscopy during pregnancy have been related to the enlarged gravid uterus and possible penetrating injury from trocar placement as well as a limited surgical field. Recent case series, however, indicate that laparoscopic removal of adnexal masses in pregnancy is safe and is associated with decreased blood loss, shorter hospital stays, and reduced postoperative pain.[2, 3, 10–12] In two retrospective laparoscopic case series, there were no major intraoperative or postoperative complications reported. Some considerations when performing laparoscopy on the pregnant patient include using an open technique or left upper quadrant entry for initial trocar placement to decrease potential penetrating injury to the gravid uterus. No cervical or uterine instrumentation should be performed. Excessive manipulation of the uterus during the procedure should also be avoided to prevent potential uterine irritability. While laparoscopy appears to be a safe approach in the management of the adnexal mass during pregnancy, the ultimate decision on surgical approach must be based on the skill level and comfort of the provider.

Clinical Scenario 1

A 23-year-old woman presents with an asymptomatic 8.5-cm complex mass with internal echos diagnosed by an obstetric ultrasound at 8 weeks gestation (Fig. 13.1).

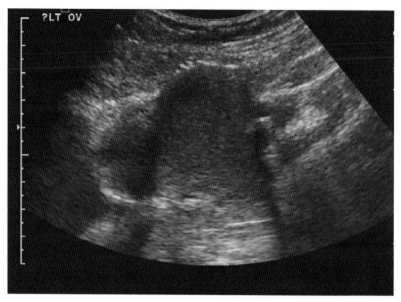

Figure 13.1 Clinical Scenario 1. Ultrasound of cystic mass at 8 weeks gestation. Note diffuse internal echos inside a smooth-walled cyst. (Image compliments of Glenn T. Yamagata, MD, Interventional Radiologist, Greensboro Radiology PA, Greensboro, NC.)

What is the differential diagnosis?

The differential diagnosis of an adnexal mass detected during pregnancy is similar to that of a nongravid reproductive-age female. The most common etiology is a functional cyst either of follicular or corpus luteum origin.[2] The differential diagnosis must also include hemorrhagic cysts, mature cystic teratomas, serous cystadenomas, paraovarian cysts, mucinous cystadenomas, endometriomas, pedunculated leiomyomas, and malignant tumors. There are several other masses unique to pregnancy that, although much less common, should be considered. One example is hyperreactio luteneinalis, which is thought to result from hypersensitivity of the ovary to circulating human chorionic gonadotropin and has a similar appearance to that of a hyperstimulated ovary.[13] Additionally, a luteoma is a rare solid ovarian lesion that occurs in pregnancy and is often associated with maternal hirsuitism or virilization.

What characteristics of adnexal masses in pregnancy are helpful in distinguishing benign from malignant masses?

Ultrasound characteristics are used to help differentiate benign from malignant masses (Table 13.2). Characteristics associated with a benign adnexal mass include simple-appearing, unilocular fluid-filled cysts that are less than 5 cm in diameter. An adnexal mass that persists into the second trimester and is solid, has thick septations, and is greater than 5 cm is likely to be a true neoplasm, benign or malignant, and not likely to resolve with further observation. Some studies that have tried to establish a scoring system to determine the risk of malignancy of an adnexal mass in pregnancy have showed that it is easier to establish the diagnosis of a benign tumor than a malignant one based on ultrasound.[2] In a prospective study on the predictability of ultrasonography, Hermann and

Table 13.3 Effects of pregnancy on gynecologic tumor makers

Tumor marker	Related malignancy	Altered by pregnancy
CA-125	Epithelial ovarian tumors	Yes, increased
CEA	Mucinous ovarian tumors Gastrointestinal malignany	No
AFP	Germ cell tumors Hepatic carcinomas	Yes, increased
Beta-hCG	Germ cell tumors Choriocarcinoma	Yes, increased
LDH	Dysgerminoma	No

colleagues found 95.6% accuracy for nonmalignant masses.[14] Therefore, the likelihood that a mass is malignant cannot be entirely excluded with ultrasound evaluation alone.

How does pregnancy affect frequently used tumor makers?

Tumor markers (eg, CA-125, AFP, hCG, LDH, CEA) are frequently used in the nongravid patient to aid in the diagnosis of adnexal masses, to monitor disease progression, and to monitor response to therapy. The alterations of the most commonly used gynecologic tumor markers caused by pregnancy are shown in Table 13.3.

Because most tumor markers are proteins and antigens associated with cell proliferation and differentiation, they can be altered due to biological functions associated with fetal development and differentiation. Since these many markers may be "falsely positive" in pregnancy, their use is limited.[15] This is especially true for AFP, beta-hCG, and CA-125, which are all elevated during a normal pregnancy. While CA-125 has limited diagnostic use in the differentiation between benign and malignant masses in pregnancy, it can provide a baseline value for future treatment purposes if malignancy is diagnosed.[2, 15] CEA concentrations are not influenced significantly by pregnancy and therefore can be used as a reliable tumor marker in pregnancy. Ad-

ditionally, with the exception of patients with preeclampsia, LDH values change little during pregnancy and therefore can also be used for clinical correlation and monitoring of disease activity.

What are potential complications of an adnexal mass in the first trimester?

The most frequent complication of the adnexal mass in pregnancy is torsion. Retrospective case series have reported the incidence of torsion from 5.4% to 43.8% with the majority occurring during the first trimester.[5] Other potential complications include cyst hemorrhage or rupture. Because the nature of the complications of the adnexal mass during pregnancy can lead to a potential need for emergent surgery for the mother, these complications pose a unique situation where both the mother and the fetus are at risk. Hess and coworkers reported that women who underwent emergent surgery related to complications of an adnexal mass in pregnancy were at greater risk for spontaneous abortion and preterm delivery than patients who underwent elective management.[9] If surgery does occur during the first trimester of pregnancy and there has been potential disruption of a corpus luteal cyst, progesterone support of the pregnancy is indicated.[2] Depending on type of progesterone used, administration is generally two to three times daily vaginally up through 10 weeks gestation.

If the mass persists, what is the optimal gestational age for surgical intervention?

If the decision is made to remove the adnexal mass during pregnancy, it is generally recommended to wait to perform surgery until around 16 to 18 weeks' gestation. Delaying surgery until the second trimester has several potential benefits to the patient. First, most masses diagnosed during early pregnancy are functional cysts and will spontaneously resolve early in the second trimester. Additionally, repeat ultrasound allows for observation of the mass to evaluate for

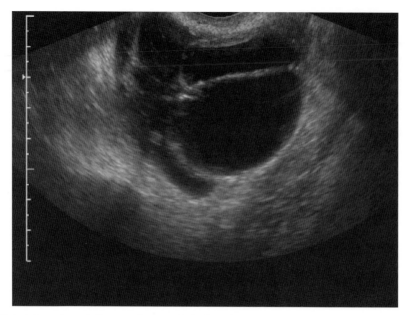

Figure 13.2 Clinical Scenario 1. Follow-up ultrasound of adenxal mass at 14 weeks. Note multiple thin septations. No nodules, solid masses, or free fluid in the cul de sac are noted. (Image compliments of Glenn T. Yamagata, MD, Interventional Radiologist, Greensboro Radiology PA, Greensboro, NC.)

possible enlargement and changes in morphology that may indicate malignancy. As noted above, surgery during the first trimester can potentially disrupt the corpus luteum and thus possibly lead to spontaneous abortion. Also, because the period of organogenesis for the fetus is during the first trimester of pregnancy, it is commonly recommended that all but truly emergent surgery be postponed until later in pregnancy to avoid potential teratogenicity and intrauterine fetal death.

During follow-up scan at 14 weeks gestation, the mass is now 9.5 cm, multicystic with thin septae, and remains asymptomatic (Fig. 13.2).

What are the potential complications of a benign adnexal mass that persists into the second trimester?

The potential complications of torsion, cyst rupture, and hemorrhage all remain the same if the adnexal mass persists into the second trimester. An additional complication is delaying the diagnosis of a potentially malignant mass as observation during pregnancy continues. This is different from the first trimester as the adnexal mass in the second trimester has already proven that it is not resolving spontaneously and therefore less likely to be a benign functional cyst. Furthermore, the consequences of disrupting the corpus luteum have resolved as the pregnancy is now supported fully by the placenta.

What are options for management of this mass?

When discussing the management of the persistent adnexal mass in pregnancy, the risks of expectant management must be weighed against the risks of immediate surgical intervention. The largest benefit of delaying surgery until after delivery of the baby at term would be to avoid the potential adverse effects of surgery and anesthesia on the fetus and the mother. In elective surgery, these risks are very low (2%), whereas Hess and coworkers reported a 40% rate of adverse pregnancy outcomes associated with emergent surgery.[9] More recent studies, however, have shown lower complication rates of emergent surgery during pregnancy.[16] It is difficult to make a single definitive recommendation, as most of the studies investigating adnexal masses in pregnancy are small and retrospective. Therefore, after counseling and thorough evaluation, a patient can be managed expectantly in the appropriate situation, when the risk for malignancy is small. Generally, the indications for expectant management should include ultrasound characteristics strongly consistent with a benign mass, size less than 5 cm, and an asymptomatic mass.

If the patient is not an appropriate candidate for expectant management, then the focus must turn towards a surgical approach. Traditionally, during pregnancy the adnexal mass has been removed through laparotomy via a midline vertical incision. Although laparoscopy has been widely embraced as the gold standard for evaluation of a presumed benign adnexal mass in the nongravid patient, surgeons have been hesitant to perform minimally invasive surgery during pregnancy. The main concerns for laparoscopy during pregnancy involve potential trauma to the gravid uterus as well as a possible negative impact of CO_2 on pregnancy. In recent years, however, there have been several retrospective studies that indicate laparoscopic management of the adnexal mass is safe during pregnancy.[4, 5, 10–12] Laparoscopy also offers significant benefits to the patient including decreased operative blood loss, shorter hospital stay, decreased postoperative pain, and quick recovery.

In general, if laparoscopy is performed for the management of adnexal masses, it should be done by a skilled laparoscopic surgeon comfortable operating on the gravid patient. Fetal heart tones should be checked pre- and postoperatively in the second trimester. Abdominal access should be attained with the open technique or left upper quadrant port placement to decrease the potential for penetrating trauma to the uterus. Port locations should be made based on the anatomy of each patient to allow best access and visualization of the adnexal mass. Additionally, given that pregnancy is a hypercoaguable state, pneumatic compression devices should be utilized throughout the procedure and postoperatively.[17] General inhalation anesthesia should be used for both laparoscopy and laparotomy, as regional anesthesia may be related to a higher risk of preterm labor.[18] If fertility-sparing surgery can be performed, then cystectomy is recommended for this younger reproductive-age population. If the surgery is being performed for concern of malignancy, then oophorectomy should be considered and attempts should be made to avoid intraperitoneal rupture or spill.

Are there measures to prevent premature labor during surgical intervention?

There is no uniform consensus as to whether tocolytics should be used pre- or postoperatively in the management of the adnexal mass during pregnancy to prevent preterm labor. The largest known risk factor for preterm labor in this patient population is the potential need for emergent surgery, which is only preventable by scheduling an elective removal of the mass. Consultation with a maternal–fetal medicine specialist at the institution where the surgery is performed may be considered preoperatively to discuss this issue. In general, though, tocolytics in the second trimester of pregnancy are not routinely used because of the issue of fetal viability.

Other general precautions that might reduce the risk of premature labor include:

- Positioning on the OR table in a right lateral decubitus position to avoid compression of the vena cava and maternal hypotension
- General inhalational anesthesia for both laparoscopy and laparotomy
- Minimizing manipulation of the uterus
- If surgery occurs in third trimester, providing an adequate incision to obtain easy exposure to the mass
- Avoiding air drying of the uterine serosa (apply saline periodically)
- Fetal heart rate monitoring beginning in the postoperative recovery unit

Is there a role for cyst aspiration as management of the adnexal mass?

Given the ability of ultrasound to accurately identify a benign mass, conservative management with needle drainage of the simple cyst offers an additional management option to discuss with the patient who is unable or unwilling to undergo surgical intervention. There are several case reports in the literature of both uncomplicated transabdominal and transvaginal aspiration of ovarian cysts using local anesthesia.[19] Drainage clearly offers the advantage of avoiding surgery and its potential risks to the mother and fetus. It should only be considered when ultrasound characteristics are clearly consistent with a simple cyst. The patient must be aware of risks, which include reaccumulation of the cyst fluid, which has been reported in 30% to 50% of cases, and potential need for surgery later in pregnancy when there are more risks and potential need for laparotomy.[18] There is also the potential risk of rupturing the mass during aspiration, resulting in a chemical peritonitis or spread of a potential malignancy. This technique should be considered in a patient who is not an ideal surgical candidate (eg, obese, anticoagulated, severe pulmonary dysfunction, cardiac disease) who is symptomatic from a simple benign-appearing mass.

If an ovarian malignancy is encountered during the surgery, what is the appropriate management?

If an ovarian malignancy is suspected preoperatively, then surgery should be performed by a gynecologic oncology specialist capable of completing standard surgical staging. This may include oophorecomy, omentectomy, peritoneal washings, and ipsilateral pelvic/para-aortic lymphadenectomy. The same approach to surgical staging in the nongravid patient with an ovarian tumor should be applied to the pregnant patient with the same diagnosis. The level of staging is dependent on the pathology demonstrated at the time of the surgical procedure. In all cases where malignancy is a concern, evaluation by frozen section should be utilized to direct further surgery.[21] Given the desire for future fertility in most pregnant women, the removal or biopsy of a normal-appearing contralateral ovary should not be performed. Further, because of the extreme chemosensitivity of ovarian germ cell malignancies, radical debulking is of little value in these tumors.

The primary types of malignant tumors encountered among adnexal masses diagnosed during pregnancy are similar to their nongravid age equivalents—borderline (LMP) epithelial, germ cell, invasive epithelial, and sex cord–stromal tumors.[3] Given the age of the reproductive patient, the majority of patients with malignancy on frozen section will present with early-stage disease confined to the ovary. For dysgerminoma confined to the ovary (the most common germ cell malignancy) and sex cord–stromal tumors, unilateral salpingo-oophorectomy and peritoneal washings with preservation of the contralateral ovary are generally appropriate.[20] Ovarian tumors of low malignant potential are indolent in nature and in the case of young patients where fertility is a concern, ovarian cystectomy may be performed to preserve the affected ovary. Although this conservative treatment leaves the patient with a 30% risk of recurrence, overall survival is not adversely affected.[20] Surgical resection of the LMP tumor by unilateral salpingo-oophorectomy is also acceptable management for women in their later reproductive years or for women whose tumor is too large to allow for cystectomy. Very few women will present with invasive epithelial ovarian tumors, as this is generally a disease of older women. If the pathology is consistent with an invasive epithelial tumor, then conservative surgery with unilateral salpingo-oophorectomy, peritoneal washings, omentectomy and peritoneal biopsies, and sampling of suspicious pelvic and periaortic nodes should be performed during pregnancy. The complete management plan with total abdominal hysterectomy and contralateral salpingo-oophorectomy may be postponed until after delivery.[3]

The need for adjuvant chemotherapy after a diagnosis of ovarian cancer is dependent on the tumor stage, grade, and histologic type.[2] Potential risks of chemotherapy—including teratogenesis, growth retardation, developmental handicaps, and systemic toxicity—must be considered carefully prior to treatment of the pregnant patient. Deciding upon the most appropriate therapeutic strategy must be case dependent. It is generally not advisable to delay chemotherapy for completion of pregnancy if the risk of cancer progression threatens maternal survival. However, if the tumor is diagnosed in the first trimester, postponement of chemotherapy until the second trimester following the completion of organogenesis is reasonable. In the case of an aggressive tumor such as invasive epithelial cancer, a therapeutic abortion should also be offered to the patient.[20] In general, most experiences with chemotherapy during pregnancy are retrospective and observational, and no studies have evaluated the long-term outcomes of children exposed to intrauterine chemotherapy. Overall, management and treatment of ovarian cancer diagnosed in pregnancy should be coordinated by an interdisciplinary team including a gynecologic oncologist and maternal–fetal medicine specialist.

Clinical Scenario 2

A patient presents at 29 weeks gestation and is found to have a 6-cm asymptomatic adnexal cystic mass on ultrasound.

What are potential complications of a benign mass that persists into the third trimester of pregnancy?

If the clinical and radiologic suspicion is low for malignancy, then a mass first noticed in the third trimester of pregnancy is best managed conservatively with observation until after delivery. The risk of torsion is significantly lower in the third trimester because the large gravid uterus decreases mobility of the adnexa. If surgical management is performed in the third trimester for emergent indications such as torsion, the patient is at increased risk for premature labor, preterm delivery, and poorer pregnancy outcomes compared to the procedures performed in the second trimester.[21] Clearly, if the mass is suspicious for malignancy, then surgical removal is recommended. Given the large size of the gravid uterus in the third trimester, laparotomy via vertical midline incision is the recommended method of surgical intervention. If the surgery is performed and is non-emergent, then there should be a consideration of steroid administration during the third trimester to improve fetal lung maturity. Either dexamethasone or betamethasone can be administered in standard fashion for a scheduled surgery to be performed 48 hours following the initial dose. Emergent surgery should not be delayed for steroid administration.

There is no indication that delivery in the patient with the adnexal mass should be accomplished by elective cesarean section. Regardless of mass size and location, the patient can await spontaneous labor with the plan for vaginal delivery and reevaluation and likely laparoscopic removal of the mass following the postpartum period. If the patient with an adnexal mass does undergo a cesarean delivery for other maternal or fetal indications, then consideration for removal of the mass at the time of delivery is appropriate. Careful inspection of the contralateral ovary should also be performed in the setting of a cesarean section.

References

1. Lavery JP, Koontz WL, Layman L, et al. Sonographic evaluation of the adnexa during early pregnancy. *Surg Gynecol Obstet*. 1986;163:319–323.
2. Leiserowitz G. Managing ovarian masses during pregnancy. *Obstet Gynecol Surv*. 2006;61:463–470.
3. Giuntoli RL, Vang RS, Bristow RE. Evaluation and management of adnexal masses during pregnancy. *Clin Obstet Gynecol*. 2006;49:492–505.
4. Marino T, Craigo SD. Managing adnexal masses in pregnancy. *Contemp Rev Obstet Gynecol*. 2000;45:130–143.

5. Kumari I, Kaur S, Mohan H, Huria A. Adnexal masses in pregnancy: a 5-year review. *Aust NZ J Obstet Gynecol.* 2006;46:52–54.

6. Leiserowitz GD, Xing G, Cress R, et al. Adnexal mass in pregnancy: how often are they malignant? *Gynecol Oncol.* 2006;101:315–321.

7. Kier R, McCarthy SM, Scoutt LM, et al. Pelvic masses in pregnant patients: MR imaging. *Radiology.* 1990;176:709–713.

8. Whitecar P, Turner S, Higby KA. Adnexal masses in pregnancy: a review of 130 cases undergoing surgical management. *Am J Obstet Gynecol.* 1999;181:19–24.

9. Hess CU, Peaceman A, O'Brier WF, et al. Adnexal masses occurring with intrauterine pregnancy: report of 54 patients requiring laparotomy for mature management. *Am J Obstet Gynecol.* 1988;93:585–589.

10. Ribic-Pucelj M, Kobal B, et al. Surgical treatment of adnexal masses in pregnancy. *J Reprod Med.* 2007;52:273–279.

11. Yuen PM, Ng PS, Leung PL, Rogers MS. Outcome in laparoscopic management of persistent adnexal masses during the second trimester of pregnancy. *Surg Endosc.* 2004;18:1354–1357.

12. Mathevet P, Nessah K, Dargent D, Mellier G. Laparoscopic management of adnexal masses in pregnancy: a case series. *Eur J Obstet Gynecol Reprod Biol.* 2003;108:217–222.

13. Chiang G, Levine D. Imaging of adnexal masses in pregnancy. *J Ultrasound Med.* 2004;23:805–819.

14. Herrmann UJ, Gottfried WL, Goldhirsch A. Sonographic patterns of ovarian tumors: prediction of malignancy. *Obstet Gynecol.* 1987;66:777.

15. Sarandkou A, Protonotariou E, Rizos D. Tumor markers in biological fluids associated with pregnancy. *Crit Rev Clin Lab Sci.* 2007;44:151–178.

16. Schmeler KM, Mayo-Smith WW, Peipert JF, et al. Adnexal masses in pregnancy: surgery compared with observation. *Am J Obstet Gynecol.* 2005;105:1098–1103.

17. Guidelines for laparoscopic surgery during pregnancy. *Surg Endosc.* 1998;12:189–190.

18. Hong JY. Adnexal mass surgery and anesthesia during pregnancy: a 10 year retrospective review. *Int J Obstet Anes.* 2006;15:212–216.

19. El-Shawarby SA, Henderson AF, Moss MA. Ovarian cysts during pregnancy: dilemmas in diagnosis and management. *J Obstet Gynecol.* 2005;25:669–675.

20. Sayar H, Lhomme C, Verschraegen CF. Malignant adnexal masses in pregnancy. *Obstet Gynecol Clin North Am.* 2005;32:569–593.

21. Agarwal, N, Parul, Kriplani A, et al. Management and outcome of pregnancies complicated with adnexal masses. *Arch Gynecol Obstet.* 2003;267:148–152.

CHAPTER 14
Gestational Trophoblastic Disease

Rabbie K. Hanna, MD
Department of Obstetrics and Gynecology, University of North Carolina at Chapel Hill, NC, USA

John T. Soper, MD, FACOG
Department of Obstetrics and Gynecology, University of North Carolina School of Medicine, Chapel Hill, NC, USA

Pathology Notes: Chad Livasy, MD
Associate Professor, Department of Pathology and Laboratory Medicine, University of North Carolina School of Medicine, Chapel Hill, NC, USA

Background

The first records of gestational trophoblastic disease (GTD) date to antiquity. The first microscopic description of a hydatidiform mole, and less commonly, a normal pregnancy preceding choriocarcinoma, was by Marchand in 1895, when he described the proliferation of the syncytium and the cytotrophoblasts of the villi in molar pregnancies.[1,2] Hydatidifom moles and malignant gestational trophoblastic neoplasia (GTN) were recognized as relatively uncommon, but potentially devastating diseases occurring in women of reproductive age. Malignant GTN was a rapidly progressing lethal malignancy until Li and associates reported the first complete and sustained remission using chemotherapy in a patient with metastatic choriocarcinoma who was successfully treated with methotrexate.[2] Thus, GTNs were described by Andrew George Ostor (1943–2003) as "God's first cancer and man's first cure."[3]

The normal gestational trophoblast arises from the peripheral cells of the blastocyst in the first few days after conception. Trophoblastic tissue initially grows rapidly into two layers: an inner population of mononucleated cytotrophoblast cells that migrate out and fuse together, forming an outer population of large multinucleated syncytiotrophoblast cells that aggressively invades the endometrium and uterine vasculature generating the placenta.

The development of GTD occurs when the normal regulatory mechanisms controlling the trophoblastic tissue are lost with the subsequent development of partial or complete hydatidiform moles, and other forms of GTD. The World Health Organization (WHO) classified gestational trophoblastic diseases into premalignant GTDs and complete and partial moles, while malignant GTD was referred to as gestational trophoblastic neoplasia (GTN). Histologic criteria for GTN include (1) invasive moles (direct invasion of molar tissue into the myometrium without intervening stroma, with potential for subsequent tumor embolization and hematogenous spread), (2) choriocarcinoma, and (3) placental-site trophoblastic tumors.[1]

Incidence

Estimates for the incidence of various forms of gestational trophoblastic disease vary widely, largely dependent on techniques of case accession. In the

Gynecological Cancer Management: Identification, Diagnosis and Treatment, Edited by Daniel L. Clarke-Pearson and John T. Soper. Published 2010 by Blackwell Publishing, ISBN: 978-1-4051-9079-4.

United States, hydatidiform moles are observed in approximately 1 in 600 therapeutic abortions and 1 in 1000 to 1200 pregnancies.[4] Approximately 20% of patients will be treated for malignant sequelae after evacuation of hydatidiform mole.[4] Gestational choriocarcinoma occurs in approximately 1 in 20,000 to 40,000 pregnancies.[4] Approximately 50% of choriocarcinomas present after term pregnancies, 25% after molar pregnancies, and the remainder after other gestational events. Although much more rare than hydatidiform mole or gestational choriocarcinoma, placental site trophoblastic tumors can develop after any type of pregnancy.[4]

Classification of hydatidiform moles

Complete and partial moles are distinct diseases from a cytologic, pathologic, and clinical standpoint. However, both arise from a nonviable pregnancy, and their management is similar. Table 14.1 compares the clinicopathologic features of complete and partial moles.

Complete hydatiform moles
Complete hydatiform moles are the classic form of molar pregnancy, characterized by the presence of trophoblastic proliferation and hydropic degener-

ation in addition to the absence of histologic evidence of a fetus or fetal vasculature. Complete moles have a normal karyotype of 46,XX in 90% of the cases, usually resulting from an empty ovum fertilized by a single sperm with subsequent reduplication of its haploid set of chromosomes. In approximately 5%, the complete mole has a 46,XY karyotype, which occurs when two sperms (one carrying an X chromosome and the other carrying a Y chromosome) fertilize an empty ovum.[4] This implies that some of the 46,XX karyotype complete moles also result from dispermic fertilization. Fetal development, blood vessels, and fetal red blood cells are not observed in complete moles because the fetus resorbs before the development of the circulatory system.

Partial moles
Most partial moles have a 69,XXX or 69,XXY karyotype derived from a haploid ovum with either reduplication of the paternal haploid set from a single sperm, or less frequently, from dispermic fertilization.[4] Thus one-third of the genetic compliment is derived from the maternal, and two-thirds from the paternal chromosomes. A prominent feature is the presence of various amounts of fetal parts, amnion, and red blood cells.

Table 14.1 Comparison of complete and partial moles

Feature	Complete moles	Partial moles
Karyotype	Most often 46,XX 5% 46,XY All paternal genome	Most often 69,XXX or 69,XXY 2/3 paternal, 1/3 maternal
Pathology		
Fetus	Absent	Sometimes present
Amnion, fetal vessels	Absent	Usually present
Villous edema	Prominent	Variable, focal
Trophoblastic proliferation	Diffuse, slight to severe	Focal, slight to moderate
Clinical presentation		
Diagnosis	Mole	Missed abortion
Uterine size	Large for dates, 53%	Small for dates
Theca lutein cysts	25–35%	Rare
Medical complications	10–25%	Rare
Postmolar GTN	7.8–30%	2.5–7.5%

Pathology notes

The classic histopathologic features of complete mole include generalized villous edema of essentially all villi associated with central cistern formation and enlargement of most of the villi. The villi typically lack vascular formations. The edges of the villi show circumferential hyperplasia of trophoblasts, although the degree of hyperplasia is variable, with loss of the usual trophoblastic polarity. Focal cytologic atypia of trophoblast nuclei is often present. Fetal parts including nucleated RBCs are not identified. For early complete moles (< 12 weeks gestation), the gross and histopathologic features are more subtle. Gross inspection of the villi may not reveal any hydropic change. The degree of hydropic change seen microscopically is also often muted and central cisterns may be absent. Histologic clues to early complete mole include villous edema, identification of trophoblastic hyperplasia, and prominent karyorrhexis of the stromal cells (Plate 14.1). Complete moles are often associated with an exaggerated placental implantation site, and cytologic atypia within the implantation site trophoblasts are typically identified.

In contrast, partial moles show edema and trophoblastic hyperplasia in a subset of the villi; other villi appear small and fibrotic. A mixture of large, edematous chorionic villi and smaller fibrotic villi should raise suspicion of a partial mole. Other supportive features of partial mole include irregular contours with scalloped borders of the large villi associated with trophoblastic inclusions. Irregular patchy trophoblastic hyperplasia is typically seen along the surface of villi. Fetal tissues, while not invariably present, may be seen in partial moles. The implantation site trophoblasts usually show only focal mild atypia.

Hydatidiform mole has historically been recognized as an abnormal placenta characterized by enlarged hydropic chorionic villi with evidence of surrounding trophoblastic proliferation. Due to the earlier clinical detection of possible molar gestations, the classic gross and histologic features are not always seen, or are less prominent. As a result, the recognition and diagnosis of both complete and partial moles has become more difficult. The pathologist's role is to identify hydatidiform moles in dilation and evacuation specimens separating them from their mimics, including hydropic abortus and placental mesenchymal dysplasia. The second role of the pathologist is to clearly distinguish a partial mole from a complete mole.

The recognition of partial moles, particularly early forms, from its mimics is a challenging area for pathologists. A partial mole should always be considered when some villi are dilated and hydropic and others are not. A definitive diagnosis of early partial hydatidiform mole may not always be possible on routine histology. DNA ploidy studies are recommended for problematic cases, as approximately 99% of partial moles show a triploid DNA content with the remaining 1% showing a tetraploid DNA content. When evaluating DNA content, it is important that the pathologist select a test block containing abundant chorionic villi rather than abundant decidua.

The recognition and diagnosis of complete moles is typically more straightforward than with partial moles, but a definitive diagnosis of early complete mole still represents a challenge for the pathologist. In most cases, the diagnosis can be made on routine histology. For particularly problematic cases, immunohistochemistry for p57 can be performed. This stain is positive when a maternal allele is present. Complete moles do not have maternal chromosomes, resulting in complete loss of p57 expression in chorionic villi trophoblasts. Pathologists should ideally select a block that contains both chorionic villi and decidua as the decidua cells serve as positive internal controls.

Placental site nodules (PSNs) are small, circumscribed foci of hyalinized implantation site containing intermediate trophoblasts typically identified in endometrial biopsies/curettings. These are benign lesions that typically occur in women of reproductive age, although pregnancy history

Pathology notes (*continued*)

may be remote, and may be associated with bleeding. PSNs are benign non-neoplastic lesions and are not to be confused with true trophoblastic neoplasms such as placental site trophoblastic tumors (PSTTs). On occasion the pathologist may have difficulty distinguishing a benign exaggerated placental implantation site from a PSTT. Immunohistochemistry for Ki-67 can be particularly helpful for these cases.[5] The Ki-67 index in exaggerated placental implantation sites and placental site nodules is typically near zero (< 5%). In contrast, the Ki-67 index in PSTT is usually 15% or higher.

For frankly malignant trophoblastic tumors, due to the differences in response to therapy, it is important for the pathologist to clearly segregate the tumors into the appropriate diagnostic category distinguishing choriocarcinoma from PSTT or epithelioid trophoblastic tumor. This segregation can usually be achieved with routine histology and immunohistochemical studies for hCG, hPL, and p63.

Clinical features of hydatidiform moles

The availability of accurate and sensitive testing for human chorionic gonadotropin (hCG) and the widespread use of ultrasound have led to earlier diagnosis of molar gestations. Clinical features of molar pregnancies include the following.

1 Elevated hCG values. Average values are significantly higher in complete moles when compared to partial moles, which have a pre-evacuation value of less than 100,000 IU/L in more than 90% of cases.[1]

2 First-trimester vaginal bleeding (89–97%)[4,7] is the most common presentation (mimicking a a threatened spontaneous abortion). Some of these patients may notice the passage of the hydropic vesicles manifested as grape-like tissue. A minority of these patients (5%) develop anemia.[4]

3 Enlarged uterus for gestational age (38–51% in complete moles versus 8–11% in partial moles). Retained blood and chorionic tissues may expand the uterine cavity and contribute to the characteristic ultrasound appearance (Fig. 14.1). The size of the uterus is associated with hCG value.[4,7]

4 Hyperemesis gravidarum (20–6% of complete moles). The presence of an enlarged uterus and/or high values of hCG is associated with an increased frequency of excessive nausea and vomiting.[8]

5 Preeclampsia in the first and early second trimester (12–27% in complete moles versus 4% in partial moles), with the rare occurrence of eclampsia. The presence of early preeclampsia is highly suggestive of a molar pregnancy. It develops in patients with excessive uterine enlargement and high values of hCG.[4]

6 Hyperthyroidism, which occurs almost exclusively in patients with very high hCG values, is due to the cross-reactivity between the hCG and TSH at the TSH receptor level.[4] Thyroid storm may occur at the time of anesthesia induction for molar evacuation if the hyperthyroid status is not well controlled with medications.

7 Theca lutein ovarian cysts (Fig. 14.2) usually are present at the time of presentation, but can develop after molar evacuation. They are also caused by elevated hCG levels.[9] Other signs of ovarian hyperstimulation, such as pleural effusion and ascites, have been documented in rare cases. Theca lutein cysts could be complicated by ovarian torsion or rupture, depending on the size. They tend to resolve after molar evacuation over an interval of 8 weeks to several months, without specific intervention. Patient education about symptoms of torsion is crucial.

8 Respiratory insufficiency is a complication of molar pregnancy that could result from embolization of tumor tissue to the pulmonary vessels, or cardiovascular complications of thyroid storm, preeclampsia, anemia, and massive fluid replacement.[4] Pulmonary compromise is generally observed in patients with excessive uterine size and high hCG levels. The typical presentation of these

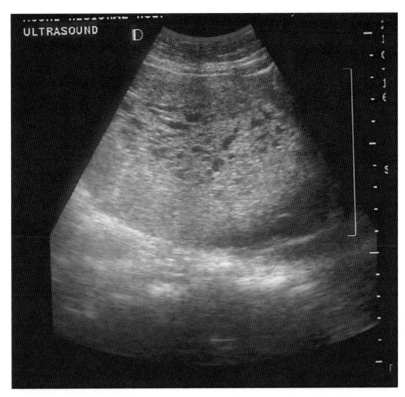

Figure 14.1 Ultrasound of complete mole. Uterus with mixed echogenic "snowstorm" pattern of solid/cystic components reflecting the multiple edematous villi.

patients is development of acute respiratory decompensation either on the operating table or in the recovery room after molar evacuation. Chest radiography may show bilateral pulmonary infiltrates, and auscultation of the chest usually reveals diffuse rales. Arterial blood gases may indicate respiratory acidosis and hypoxia. With appropriate cardiovascular and respiratory support, the signs and symptoms of respiratory distress usually resolve within 72 hours. However, it is important to recognize that some patients may require mechanical ventilation to provide adequate oxygenation.[10]

Gestational trophoblastic neoplasia

The prompt identification of malignant gestational trophoblastic neoplasia (GTN) is important because a delay in the diagnosis may increase the patient's risk and might adversely affect their response to treatment.[11] Malignant GTN is histologically classified into (1) invasive moles, (2) choriocarcinoma, and (3) placental-site trophoblastic disease (PSTT).

Diagnosis of gestational trophoblastic neoplasia

Gestational trophoblastic neoplasias can either be postmolar GTNs or malignant nonmolar GTNs. Approximately 50% to 70% of patients with postmolar GTN have persistent or invasive moles and 30% to 50% have postmolar gestational choriocarcinomas.[4] Gestational choriocarcinomas are derived from molar pregnancies in approximately half of all cases, while the remaining choriocarcinomas are derived from term pregnancies, spontaneous abortions, and ectopic pregnancies. Placental site trophoblastic tumors (PSTT) are a

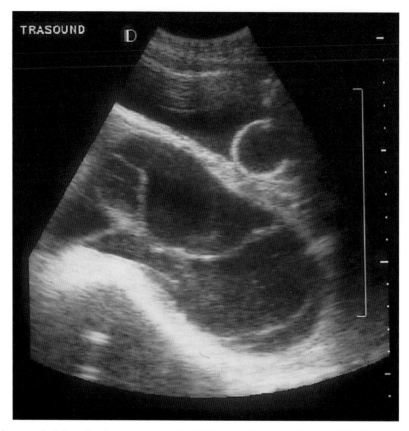

Figure 14.2 Ultrasound of theca lutein cyst associated with the complete mole illustrated in Figure 14.1. Note multiple thin septae.

rare form of GTN that can follow any pregnancy event.[11]

Patients diagnosed with GTN after molar evacuation are identified relatively early because the serial evaluation of post-evacuation hCG levels usually allows for intervention before the development of disseminated disease. The criteria for diagnosis of post-hydatidiform mole GTN according to FIGO 2000[12] are:

1 Four values or more of plateaued hCG ($\pm$ 10%) over at least 3 weeks: days 1, 7, 14, and 21.

2 A rise in hCG of 10% or greater for 3 values or more over at least 2 weeks: days 1, 7, and 14.

3 The histologic diagnosis of choriocarcinoma.

4 Persistence of hCG beyond 6 months after mole evacuation.

In contrast, patients with malignant GTN following nonmolar gestations often present with predominantly non-gynecologic symptoms and signs, which include hemoptysis, cerebral hemorrhage, gastrointestinal or urologic hemorrhage, or a clinical diagnosis of widely metastatic malignancy from an unknown primary site.[11] Most of these patients will have a history of irregular uterine bleeding, amenorrhea, or recent pregnancy event. However, the index pregnancy event may have occurred several years before presentation, or may have been a subclinical spontaneous abortion.[11]

The possibility of malignant GTN should be suspected in any woman of reproductive age who presents with metastatic disease from an unknown primary site or undiagnosed cerebral hemorrhage.[11] Under these circumstances, the diagnosis is facilitated by a high index of suspicion coupled with serum hCG testing and exclusion of a concurrent pregnancy, and most often without the need for tissue biopsy.

Staging of gestational trophoblastic neoplasia

Three staging systems have been used for patients with GTN: the revised 2000 FIGO staging system, the WHO prognostic index score, and the Clinical Classification System. The current standard for reporting results of treatment for GTN is the revised FIGO staging system, which incorporates both an anatomic staging system with a modification of the WHO prognostic index (Tables 14.2 and 14.3). The WHO scoring system was revised by FIGO, eliminating the determination of the patient and consort blood types. This modified scoring system consolidated the risk categories into low-risk and high-risk categories with scores of < 7 and ≥ 7, respectively. [11,13] According to FIGO, hydatidiform mole should be registered but not be staged as stage 0, because if hCG persists and the patient requires chemotherapy, restaging would be required. Patients with hydatidiform mole are placed on record but staging only applies to trophoblastic neoplasia. Cases that do not fulfill the criteria for any given stage should be listed separately as unstaged. It should be realized that most cases of stage I and II GTN are low-risk disease, while cases in stage III may be either low or high risk depending on their risk score. Virtually all patients with stage IV lesions have high-risk disease. Additionally, PSTT is not included in this staging (Table 14.2).

Patients with low-risk GTN are usually initially managed with single-agent methotrexate or dactinomycin regimens. Hysterectomy may be incorporated into treatment, but essentially all patients with low-risk disease can be cured, with the majority retaining child-bearing capacity, and only a few of these patients will require multiagent chemotherapy.[4]

In contrast, patients with high-risk GTN require multiagent chemotherapy and often require multimodality therapy directed against high-risk metastatic sites, or salvage treatment with surgery or

Table 14.2 FIGO anatomic staging of gestational trophoblastic neoplasia

Stage I	Disease confined to the uterus
Stage II	GTN extends outside of the uterus, but is limited to the genital structures (adnexa, vagina, broad ligament)
Stage III	GTN extends to the lungs, with or without known genital tract involvement
Stage IV	All other metastatic sites

From FIGO committee report. *Int J Gynecol Obstet.* 2002;77:285–287.

radiation later in their course of treatment. The most frequently used regimen is a combination of etoposide-methotrexate-dactinomycin alternating on a weekly basis with vincristine and cyclophosphamide (EMA/CO). These patients should be managed in a center with experience treating high-risk GTN, where cure rates of up to 86% among patients with high-risk disease have been reported.[4]

Clinical Scenario 1

A 23-year-old P0010 undergoes D&C for an ultrasound diagnosis of "missed SAB" at 9 weeks' gestation. Final pathology report indicates that this is a partial mole pregnancy.

What evaluation and follow-up are recommended?

When molar pregnancy is diagnosed after evacuation, a chest x-ray should be obtained to screen for metastatic lesions. Metastases complicate approximately 20% of complete moles compared to <5% in partial moles.[13]

Serial quantitative serum hCG determinations should be performed after molar evacuation using one of several commercially available assays capable of detecting β-hCG to baseline values (<5 international units/L). Ideally, serum hCG levels should be obtained within 48 hours of evacuation, every 1 to 2 weeks while elevated until 2 or 3 normal values are recorded, and then

Table 14.3 FIGO risk factor score for gestational trophoblastic neoplasia

Scores	0	1	2	4
Age	< 40	≥ 40	–	–
Antecedent pregnancy	Mole	Abortion	Term	–
Interval months from index pregnancy	< 4	4 – < 7	7 – < 13	≥ 13
Pretreatment serum hCG (IU/L)	$< 10^3$	$10^3 – < 10^4$	$10^4 – < 10^5$	$\geq 10^5$
Largest tumor size (including uterus)	–	3–5 cm	> 5 cm	–
Site of metastases	–	Spleen Kidney	GI tract	Liver Brain
Number of metastases	–	1–4	5–8	> 8
Previous failed chemotherapy	–	–	Single agent	≥ 2 drugs

From FIGO committee report. *Int J Gynecol Obstet.* 2002;77:285–287.

at 1 to 2-month intervals for an additional 6 to 12 months. While several studies have documented that the risk of developing postmolar GTN is low if a single normal hCG value is recorded after evacuation of complete and partial moles, all of these studies are limited by the large number of patients lost to follow-up.[4]

A pelvic examination should be performed often in order to recognize and diagnose early genital metastasis and any other signs that could indicate pelvic metastases of GTN.[4]

A reliable method of contraception is highly encouraged during the period of surveillance to avoid confusion between a new pregnancy and postmolar GTN. The intrauterine device should not be used due to a higher rate of uterine perforation when the hCG values are abnormal, in addition to a higher rate of expulsion or infection. Oral contraceptives have been shown to reduce the incidence of intercurrent pregnancies while not increasing the risk of postmolar GTN when compared with barrier contraception in a randomized trial conducted by the Gynecologic Oncology Group (GOG). Once the patient successfully achieves a period of 6 to 12 months of normal hCG levels, she may be encouraged to attempt another pregnancy.

Some authors recommend a period of surveillance to be tailored according to the patient's clinical course. For example, if the hCG value has fallen adequately within 8 weeks of evacuation, the follow-up might be safely reduced to 6 months because none of these patients has required chemotherapy.[1] On the other hand, among patients whose hCG values were elevated beyond 8 weeks post-evacuation, follow-up might continue for up to 2 years. Any elevation of hCG values during surveillance should be thoroughly investigated for the presence of persistent or metastatic gestational trophoblastic tumors, placental site trophoblastic disease, or a new pregnancy.

When a patient with previous mole or or history of treatment for GTN conceives, the new pregnancy should undergo an early ultrasound examination for evaluation of the placenta and fetus, because the risk for a second mole is 1% to 2%. Patients with a previous mole or GTN should have an hCG evaluation 6 to 10 weeks after completion of each subsequent pregnancy, because they are at risk for a disease recurrence.[1]

Clinical Scenario 2

A 43-year-old P3012 presents with uterine enlargement to 16 weeks' gestational size, bleeding and passing tissue from the cervix. Serum hCG is 250,000 IU/L. Ultrasound reveals a typical pattern for hydatidiform mole with bilateral theca lutein cysts (Fig. 14.2).

What is the preferred management for evaluation and evacuation of this patient?

A workup should be performed in preparation for molar evacuation if the clinical presentation was suggestive of molar pregnancy. Additionally, the patient should be carefully evaluated to identify the potential presence of medical complications including preeclampsia, electrolyte imbalance, hyperthyroidism, and anemia that might complicate surgical evacuation. A complete blood count, clotting function studies, renal and liver function tests, blood type and screen, pre-evacuation hCG level, and chest x-ray should be obtained before evacuation. A thyroid panel should be obtained if the uterus is enlarged >14 weeks' size or hCG elevated >50,000 U/L. The mole should be evacuated as soon as possible after stabilization of any medical complications.

The purpose of molar evacuation is the removal of all molar tissue from the uterus in a manner that decreases the chances of malignant sequelae. If the patient no longer desires to preserve fertility, a hysterectomy may be performed with aspiration of prominent theca lutein cysts at the time of surgery. Although this eliminates the risks of local invasion and reduces the risk of postmolar GTN, it does not prevent metastasis or eliminate the development of postmolar GTN.[1]

On the other hand, the majority of patients desire to preserve fertility, and the preferred method of evacuation is suction D&E.[4] Medical induction of labor with oxytocin or prostaglandin are not recommended for evacuation because they increase blood loss and increase the risk for malignant sequelae compared with suction D&E.[4] Additionally, patients most often require D&E to complete the evacuation of the mole after medical induction of labor.

Suction D&E for molar evacuation is usually performed under general anesthesia, but local or regional anesthesia may be used for a cooperative patient with a small uterus. Pre-evacuation insertion of cervical laminaria may facilitate cervical dilatation in a patient who is medically stable. After serial dilation of the cervix, the uterus is evacuated by introducing a suction cannula and allowing the uterus to involute while rotating the cannula, rather than sounding the uterus and performing sharp curettage. This reduces the chance of perforation and may be assisted with a bedside ultrasound. Intravenous oxytocin (20 U/L pitocin) is begun after the cervix is dilated. If there is failure or delay of uterine involution, bimanual uterine massage should be attempted in addition to the oxytocin infusion. The use of ergotamine in the form of methergine 0.2 mg every 2 to 4 hours is encouraged. Routine second and third evacuations were attempted in the past, but are discouraged because they do not decrease the risk of postmolar GTN[4] and may result in perforation or uterine synechiae. Anti-D immunoglobulin should be given to patients who are Rh negative because Rh D factor is expressed in the trophoblast.

What are potential complications during and following evacuation? How might they be prevented and managed?

Pulmonary complications are often observed around the time of molar evacuation among patients with uterine enlargement greater than 14 to 16 weeks gestational size.[4] Baseline arterial blood gases may be valuable in managing patients with uterine enlargement. Respiratory distress syndrome may be caused by trophoblastic embolization, high-output congestive heart failure caused by anemia, hyperthyroidism, preeclampsia, or iatrogenic fluid overload. In general, these complications should be treated aggressively with therapy directed by central hemodynamic monitoring and ventilator support as required. Patients with hyperthyroidism should undergo medical management prior to evacuation to prevent thyroid storm during anesthesia. Pregnancy-induced hypertension may require antihypertensive medications and magnesium therapy, but will rarely result in eclampsia. These medical complications usually regress promptly after evacuation of the mole and may not require specific therapy after evacuation.[4]

Theca lutein cysts (Fig. 14.2) are associated with hCG hyperstimulation of the ovaries.[9] The resolution of theca lutein cysts lags behind the drop in hCG values. They may take several months to resolve after molar evacuation but rarely require surgical intervention for rupture or torsion.

Blood loss during suction D&E is usually <500 mL, but patients with uterine enlargement >14 weeks size are at an increased risk for significant hemorrhage perioperatively. Often they present with anemia from previous bleeding, which places them at an increased risk of respiratory complications. These patients should have at least 2 U packed red blood cells available and a large-bore IV placed before beginning the evacuation. Pitocin and ergotamine should be used as previously discussed.

What are the chances a patient with a mole will ultimately have malignant GTN? Are there features that make some patients higher risk?

In the United States, approximately 20% of patients are treated for GTN after evacuation of a hydatidiform mole.[4] The following are recognized risk factors for developing postmolar GTN. It should be recognized that the risk of postmolar GTN is seven to ten times higher for complete moles than partial moles.

1 The size of the uterus at the time of diagnosis has been considered for many years to be significant with regard to malignant sequelae; 25% of patients with large-for-dates uteri developed GTN when compared to 11% in patients with small-for-dates.[4]

2 Theca lutein cysts (Fig. 14.2), irrespective of uterine size, are associated with subsequent GTN. In some series, patients with enlarged ovaries had a 49% chance of developing GTN.[1, 2]

3 Patients with signs of marked trophoblastic proliferation (elevated hCG >100,000 IU/mL, uterine size greater than gestational age, and theca lutein cysts > 6 cm) had an elevated risk

of local invasion and metastasis at 33% and 8.8%, respectively, when compared to 3.4% and 0.6% in those without these signs of marked trophoblastic growth.[1, 2]

4 The method of molar evacuation; 36% of those treated with hysterotomy developed GTN, compared to 19% and < 10% if D&E or hysterectomy were used, respectively.[4]

5 Patients who are more than 40 years of age have a higher chance of developing postmolar GTN. Tow and Xia and associates reported that 33% and 37% of women > 40 years old in their studies, respectively, developed GTN.[10, 14]

6 Previous molar gestation increases the chances of developing GTN. Parazzini and coworkers reported a threefold increased risk.[14]

7 The development of medical complications such as ARDS, preeclampsia, or hyperthyroidism also are associated with an increased risk of postmolar GTN.[4]

8 Other factors that have been reported to be associated with higher rates of postmolar GTN are the occurance of uterine subinvolution with bleeding after uterine evacuation, the degree of trophoblastic hyperplasia, nuclear atypia, fibrin deposition, hemorrhage, and necrosis on histologic examination.[4]

Despite these recognized risk factors, several studies have reported that "high-risk" moles accounted for only 35% of the patients who developed postmolar GTN after molar evacuation.

In patients with high-risk clinical features, is there a way to prevent malignant sequelae?

Chemoprophylaxis after complete molar evacuation is controversial. The debate concerns the strategy of exposing all patients to toxic chemotherapy when only approximately 20% of patients will develop GTN, and these patients can be identified promptly using serial hCG monitoring.[14] In two randomized studies,[4] prophylactic chemotherapy with brief methotrexate or dactinomycin regimens reduced the incidence of postmolar GTN in women with high-risk moles from 47.4% to 14.3% ($p < 0.05$) and 50% to 13.8% ($p < 0.05$), respectively.

One study found that the disease was diagnosed later and needed more chemotherapy courses to achieve remission in the treated cohort.[4] Although prophylactic chemotherapy reduced the incidence of persistent trophoblastic disease in high-risk patients, it likely increased tumor resistance and morbidity.

Also, there are anecdotal cases of fatalities caused by prophylactic chemotherapy, and it does not completely eliminate the need for post-evacuation follow-up. Because of the low morbidity and mortality achieved by monitoring patients with serial hCG determinations and instituting chemotherapy only in patients with a diagnosis of postmolar GTN, routine application of prophylactic chemotherapy is not recommended.[4] It may be useful in the management of the rare high-risk complete molar pregnancy when follow-up is unavailable or unreliable.

Three weeks after evacuation with D&E, the patient had an initial decline in hCG to 10,300 IU/L, but on the 4th week she has a rise of hCG to 12,500 IU/L with intermittent vaginal bleeding.

What are the criteria for the diagnosis of postmolar GTN? How should this patient be managed?

Those diagnosed with GTN after molar evacuation are recognized relatively early in the course of disease because of the serial evaluation of post-evacuation hCG levels and prompt identification of trophoblastic proliferation causing progressive elevation of hCG. The criteria for diagnosis of post-hydatidiform mole trophoblastic neoplasia as defined by FIGO consensus committee in 2000[12] are:

1 Four values or more of plateaued hCG (± 10%) over at least 3 weeks: days 1, 7, 14, and 21.
2 A rise of hCG of 10% or greater for 3 values or more over at least 2 weeks: days 1, 7, and 14.
3 The histologic diagnosis of choriocarcinoma.
4 Persistence of hCG beyond 6 months after mole evacuation.

A pretreatment evaluation of a patient with GTN should include:

1 A thorough history and physical examination that should include a detailed gynecologic examination to exclude vaginal or pelvic metastasis. A systematic examination of possible sites of metastasis, including a detailed neurological, examination is recommended.
2 A complete blood count, blood type and screening, and clotting function studies, in addition to liver and renal function tests.
3 An hCG quantitative test.
4 An evaluation of clinical risk factors to further direct chemotherapy.
5 Radiographic evaluation should include chest x-ray or CT scan, brain MRI or CT scans, and abdominopelvic CT or MRI scan.

High-risk sites of metastases rarely occur without symptoms from the metastases or pulmonary metastases (Fig. 14.3), but up to 40% of patients treated for postmolar GTN with negative chest x-rays have small pulmonary lesions detected on chest CT scan.[4] Therefore, complete radiographic evaluation is recommended in most cases of GTN before initiating treatment.

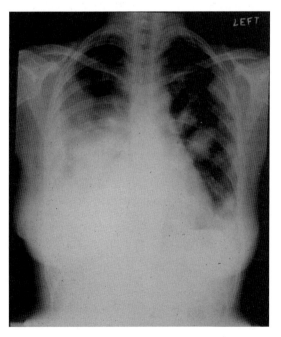

Figure 14.3 Multiple pulmonary metastases of GTN with large right pleural effusion.

Should this patient have a repeat D&C?

The role of a repeat D&C in the event of an hCG rise or plateau after molar evacuation is yet to be determined. In several studies, repeat curettage was reported to induce remission or influence treatment in less than 20% of patients and was complicated by uterine perforation in 4.8% to 8% of patients.[13, 15] In contrast, Pezeshki and associates[16, 17] reported that 368 (68%) of 544 patients entered spontaneous remission after repeat evacuation of a mole for rising hCG values, with no patient requiring hysterectomy for perforation. Patients with persistent histologic evidence of gestational trophoblastic disease and those with hCG levels above 1500 IU/L were significantly less likely to respond to the second curettage.[16, 17] A randomized clinical trial is obviously needed.

After establishing a diagnosis of GTN and staging, what are the management options?

A variety of chemotherapy agents have been used for non-metastatic and low-risk metastatic GTN and have achieved similar primary remission rates.[13] Essentially, all patients in these two categories can be cured, usually without the need for hysterectomy.[7] Most centers treat low-risk patients with methotrexate or with actinomycin D (Dactinomycin); various dosing schedules have been used and are beyond the scope of this book. Single-agent chemotherapy is preferred for patients who wish to retain their fertility.

Recently, the results of a prospective randomized trial comparing methotrexate and dactinomycin were reported.[18] This trial was conducted by the Gynecologic Oncology Group, comparing weekly methotrexate (30 mg/m^2 IM) with bi-weekly dactinomycin (1.25 mg/m^2 IV) as initial treatment for patients with low-risk GTN. Among responding patients, a median of 8 weekly cycles was required in the methotrexate arm and 4 bi-weekly cycles in the dactinomycin arm. Among eligible patients, complete responses were observed in 53% of patients in the methotrexate group and 69% in the dactinomycin group

($p = 0.015$). Both regimens were well tolerated.[18] Chemotherapy is continued until hCG values have achieved normal levels, and an additional course is administered after the first normal hCG value has been recorded. Hematologic indices, and renal and liver function tests, must be monitored, but significant toxicity during single-agent therapy is infrequent. Most gynecologic oncologists will use one agent at a time in order to expose the patient's tumor to the fewest chemotherapeutic agents.[4]

In contrast, patients with high-risk GTN require aggressive multiagent chemotherapy and often multimodality treatment for high-risk sites of metastases. The EMA/CO regimen is most frequently used as primary chemotherapy,[4] but management of high-risk GTN is beyond the scope of this book. These patients should be managed in centers with experience in treating these extremely complex patients.

If hCG values have not fallen by at least 10% over a cycle of therapy, treatment should be changed to an alternative single-agent regimen unless there are new high-risk metastases. If there is failure of alternative single-agent chemotherapy, the patient should be treated with multiagent chemotherapy. Hysterectomy should be considered for refractory disease that is confined to the uterus. Patients with non-metastatic disease are less likely to require second-line therapy than patients with low-risk metastatic disease.[4] There is no literature on performing a repeat suction curettage for patients who appear to be failing single-agent chemotherapy. Overall, 85% to 95% of patients in these categories can be cured without needing multiagent chemotherapy or hysterectomy. The overall cure rate for patients with low-risk disease approaches 100%, with recurrence rates less than 5%.[4]

When should a hysterectomy be considered in the management of a patient with GTN?

In the group of patients with low-risk disease, early hysterectomy will shorten the duration and amount of chemotherapy required to produce remission, but hysterectomy should not be used in lieu of chemotherapy.[4] Hysterectomy may be performed during the first cycle of chemotherapy. However, further chemotherapy and hCG monitoring should be employed similar to patients managed exclusively with chemotherapy.

What is the recommended monitoring following apparent remission? What is the risk of recurrence?

Following hCG remission, serial determinations of hCG levels at 2-week intervals for the first 3 months of remission and then at 1-month intervals is recommended until monitoring has completed 1 year of normal hCG levels. The risk of recurrence after 1 year of remission is less than 1%,[13] but late recurrences have been observed. Approximately 80% of recurrences are diagnosed within the first year after treatment and 95% by 18 months.[13] The risk for subsequent recurrence after a second remission is 50%, indicating the need for even closer long-term surveillance in patients successfully treated for recurrent GTN.

Clinical Scenario 3

A 32-year-old P0010 has been successfully treated for postmolar GTN and after 12 months of normal hCG values wishes to pursue childbearing.

What are her risks of having another molar pregnancy? If she does become pregnant, what should be the clinical management?

Pregnancy should be deferred for at least 1 year to prevent disruption of hCG surveillance. A reliable form of hormonal contraception during the first year of remission should be used.

There does not appear to be an increase in the risk of congenital malformations or other complications related to pregnancy after chemotherapy for GTN.[4] Because of the increased risk for repeat molar gestation (1–2%), these patients warrant early ultrasound to confirm fetal viability and placental appearance, chest x-ray to rule out occult metastases, histologic evaluation of the placenta at delivery to exclude choriocarcinoma, and follow-up serum hCG 6 to 8 weeks after delivery to rule out recurrent malignant GTN. Unlike the risk for repeat molar gestation, a second gestational choriocarcinoma following successful treatment of choriocarcinoma arising from a normal pregnancy has not been reported.

What are chronic toxicities after chemotherapy for GTN?

Most patients return to normal activity within a few months of treatment and most side effects are reversible.[1] Patients treated with multiagent regimens may develop secondary tumors such as acute myeloid leukemia (most likely related to etoposide), colon cancer, or melanoma. Fertility was also found to be adversely affected in patients treated for high-risk disease with multiagent chemotherapy or after the age of 35 years. Additionally, chemotherapy causes an earlier onset of menopause by approximately 1 year after methotrexate/folinic acid and by 3 years for EMA/CO.[1] Because this disease affects an integral part of a woman's being, depression can be severe and adequate support from multiple levels is necessary.

Clinical Scenario 4

A 27-year-old nulligravida presents with slightly irregular menses. Serum hCG is 80 IU/L. Ultrasound reveals a 2-cm simple cyst involving the right ovary and normal endometrial stripe. Repeat hCG values at 48 and 96 hours are 77 and 94 IU/L. A simple ovarian cyst is observed at laparoscopy with normal fallopian tubes, and secretory endometrium is obtained at D&C.

How should this patient be evaluated?

The measurement of apparent but spurious human chorionic gonadotropin (hCG) has been reported in the literature over the last 3 decades, and has recently been referred to as "phantom hCG." Such false-positive results have led to some women being mistakenly diagnosed with GTD and subsequently being subjected to a variety of diagnostic procedures, chemotherapy, hysterectomy, and other surgical procedures before it is recognized that the assay is giving spurious results, thus potentially leading to unwanted side effects such as infertility and induction of secondary malignancies. It is relatively rare, but immunoassay interference is still an important problem that can result in misdiagnosis and medical-legal or malpractice issues.[21]

Phantom hCG is caused by a substance in serum that interferes with the hCG immunoassay. Causes of false-positive hCG measurements have been summarized into four areas: (1) measurement of pituitary hCG-like substance; (2) production of free hCG alpha-subunit; (3) interference by non-hCG substances, including hLH or hLH alpha-subunit, both species-specific and heterophilic anti-animal immunoglobulin antibodies, rheumatoid factor, anti-hCG antibodies, and nonspecific serum factors; and (4) assay issues such as carryover by positive displacement pipettes and contaminants that affect label detection (radioactive iodine or fluorophores).[21]

Characteristics of false-positive hCG measurements include the following:

1 Low-level positive result (generally < 1,000 mIU/mL and usually < 150 mIU/mL).

2 Positive serum but negative urine assays; serial dilutions of serum that are not parallel to the hCG standard and yield higher or lower levels of hCG when multiplied by dilution factor.

3 Positive hCG results that are not consistent with clinical or surgical findings.

4 No substantial changes in in serial blood levels, even after therapeutic procedures.

5 Negative results using a different type of quantitative hCG assay.

When there are discordant hCG results or phantom hCG is suspected, the following steps are recommended[22]:

1 Measure urinary hCG—heterophilic antibodies are not excreted in the urine.

2 Re-measure the hCG concentration using a different method—some assays are affected less by heterophilic antibodies, or errors in performance may not be repeated.

3 Look for parallelism to the hCG standard in serial dilutions of the serum—lack of an expected drop in the hCG value during serial dilutions indicates nonspecific interference with the assay.

4 Add normal mouse serum or other animal serum to specimen prior to the assay—this strips antimurine antibodies from the specimen.

5 Test for anti-hCG antibodies.

6 Measure serial hCG concentrations over several days or weeks—random fluctuations in hCG levels are typical of false-positive assays.

The U.S. hCG Reference Service is a consulting service with a specialized clinical laboratory aiding physicians in the interpretation of conflicting or misrepresentative hCG results and can provide assistance in management of these patients. It is affiliated with the University of New Mexico. Access can be through the following web address: http://www.hcglab.com/.

Clinical Scenario 5

A 27-year-old Caucasian multigravida presents for routine antenatal ultrasound examination at 12 weeks' gestation. This reveals a placental tumor suspicious for hydatidiform mole and an hCG value of 278,666. The fetus, on the other hand, has no visible sonographic anomalies.

How should this patient be counseled?

Twin gestation comprising a normal fetus and hydatidiform mole is a rare entity and is described in the literature through small case series and case reports. Thus limited information is present to guide the appropriate management of such patients. It occurs in 1 of 22,000 to 100,00 pregnancies; both complete and partial moles with coexisting fetuses have been reported.[23, 24] Most of these are diagnosed by ultrasound examination during the antepartum period as a complex cystic placental component distinct from the feto-placental unit, but in a few cases the diagnosis was at the time of placental examination after delivery. A detailed antepartum sonographic examination is necessary to rule out other possible causes of placental pathology such as retroplacental hematoma, fibroids, or other placental abnormalities in addition to a detailed fetal ultrasound examination to exclude any anomalies. If molar pregnancy is still suspected and the pregnancy desired, fetal karyotyping to document normal fetal karyotype, chest x-ray to exclude metastases, and serial hCG levels may be of value in counseling the patient.

There is a higher rate of medical complications of pregnancy in addition to more frequent development of postmolar GTNs with a higher rate of metastatic lesions or requirement for multiagent chemotherapy when such pregnancies are compared to singleton hydatidiform moles.[13, 25] Matsui et al[13, 25] concluded from their national collaborative study that because the risk of malignancy is unchanged with advancement of gestational age, continued pregnancy may be allowed in patients with hydatidiform mole with twin fetus provided that severe maternal complications are controlled, and fetal karyotype and development are normal. Such patients should be counseled extensively prior to any treatment plan.

Viable infants delivered of such pregnancies have not been found to have any congenital malformations[4, 10]; on the other hand, there have been cases of documented choriocarcinoma of infants delivered to these mothers.[26–30] Because the disease can manifest up to 6 months after delivery, monitoring of hCG levels following delivery is recommended in these infants.[1]

References

1. Seckl MJ, Newlands ES. Management of gestational trophoblastic disease. In: Gershenson DM, McGuire WP, Gore M, eds. *Gynecologic Cancer: Controversies in Management.* Philadelphia: Elsevier; 2004:555–573.

2. Burger RA, Creasman WT. Gestational trophoblastic neoplasia. In: DiSaia PJ, Creasman WT, eds. *Clinical Gynecologic Oncology.* 6th ed. St. Louis: Mosby; 2002:185–210.

3. Ostor A. "God's first cancer and man's first cure": milestones in gestational trophoblastic disease. *Anat Pathol.* 1996;1:165–178.

4. Soper JT. Gestational trophoblastic disease. *Obstet Gynecol.* 2006;108:176–187.

5. Shih IM, Kurman RJ. Ki-67 labeling index in the differential diagnosis of exaggerated placental site, placental site trophoblastic tumor, and choriocarcinoma: a double immunohistochemical staining technique using Ki-67 and Mel-CAM antibodies. *Hum Pathol.* 1998;29:27–33.

6. Crum CP. The female genital tract. In: Kumar V, Abbas AK, Fausto N, eds. *Pathologic Basis of Disease.* 7th ed. Philadelphia: Elsevier Saunders; 2005:1059–1117.

7. Kohorn EI. Molar pregnancy: presentation and diagnosis. *Clin Obstet Gynecol.* 1984;27:181–191.

8. Kohorn EI. Hydatidiform mole and gestational trophoblastic disease in Southern Connecticut. *Obstet Gynecol.* 1982;59:78–84.

9. Osathanondh R, Berkowitz RS, de Cholnoky C, Smith BS, Goldstein DP, Tyson JE. Hormonal measurements in patients with theca lutein cysts and gestational trophoblastic disease. *J Reprod Med.* 1986;31:179–183.

10. Berkowitz RS, Goldstein DP. Gestational trophoblastic disease. In: Hoskins WJ, Perez CA, Young RC, eds. *Principals and Practice of Gynecologic Oncology.* 4th ed. Philadelphia: Lippincott Williams & Wilkins; 2005:1055–1076.

11. Soper JT. Staging and evaluation of gestational trophoblastic disease. *Clin Obstet Gynecol.* 2003;46:570–578.

12. Ngan HY, Bender H, Benedet JL, Jones H, Montruccoli GC, Pecorelli S. Gestational trophoblastic neoplasia, FIGO 2000 staging and classification. *Int J Gynaecol Obstet.* 2003;83(suppl):175–177.

13. ACOG practice bulletin 53. Diagnosis and treatment of gestational trophoblastic disease. *Obstet Gynecol.* 2004;103:1365–1377.

14. Parazzini F, Mangili G, Belloni C, La Vecchia C, Liati P, Marabini R. The problem of identification of prognostic factors for persistent trophoblastic disease. *Gynecol Oncol.* 1988;30:57–62.

15. van Trommel NE, Massuger LF, Verheijen RH, Sweep FC, Thomas CM. The curative effect of a second

curettage in persistent trophoblastic disease: a retrospective cohort survey. *Gynecol Oncol.* 2005;99:6–13.

16. Pezeshki M, Hancock BW, Silcocks P, *et al.* The role of repeat uterine evacuation in the management of persistent gestational trophoblastic disease. *Gynecol Oncol.* 2004;95:423–429.

17. Goldstein DP, Garner EI, Feltmate CM, Berkowitz RS. The role of repeat uterine evacuation in the management of persistent gestational trophoblastic disease. *Gynecol Oncol.* 2004;95:421–422.

18. Osborne R, Filiaci V, Schink JC, *et al.* A randomized phase III trial comparing weekly parenteral methotrexate and "pulsed" dactinomycin as primary management for low-risk gestational trophoblastic neoplasia: a Gynecologic Oncology Group study. *Gynecol Oncol.* 2008;108:S2–S3.

19. Lurain JR, Singh DK, Schink JC. Role of surgery in the management of high-risk gestational trophoblastic neoplasia. *J Reprod Med.* 2006;51:773–736.

20. Lurain JR. Treatment of gestational trophoblastic tumors. *Curr Treat Options Oncol.* 2002;3:113–124.

21. Tsai HJ. Phantom HCG and clinical management. *Taiwan J Obstet Gynecol.* 2006;45:92–94.

22. Braunstein GD. False-positive serum human chorionic gonadotropin results: causes, characteristics, and recognition. Am J Obstet Gynecol. l 2002;187:217–224.

23. Bruchim I, Kidron D, Amiel A, Altaras M, Fejgin MD. Complete hydatidiform mole and a coexistent viable fetus: report of two cases and review of the literature. *Gynecol Oncol.* 2000;77:197–202.

24. Steller MA, Genest DR, Bernstein MR, Lage JM, Goldstein DP, Berkowitz RS. Clinical features of multiple conception with partial or complete molar pregnancy and coexisting fetuses. *J Reprod Med.* 1994;39:147–154.

25. Fishman DA, Padilla LA, Keh P, Cohen L, Frederiksen M, Lurain JR. Management of twin pregnancies consisting of a complete hydatidiform mole and normal fetus. *Obstet Gynecol.* 1998;91:546–550.

26. Feldman K. Choriocarcinoma with neonatal anemia. *N Engl J Med.* 1977;296:880.

27. Heath JA, Tiedemann K. Successful management of neonatal choriocarcinoma. *Med Pediatr Oncol.* 2001;36:497–499.

28. Kelly DL, Jr., Kushner J, McLean WT. Neonatal intracranial choriocarcinoma. Case report. *J Neurosurg.* 1971;35:465–471.

29. Kim SN, Chi JG, Kim YW, *et al.* Neonatal choriocarcinoma of liver. *Pediatr Pathol.* 1993;13:723–730.

30. Parks DG. Maternal and neonatal death from advanced choriocarcinoma due to a delay in diagnosis: a case report. *J Reprod Med.* 2007;52:228–230.

Index